Fundus Autofluorescence

EDITED BY

Noemi Lois, MD, PhD, FRCS(Ed)

Ophthalmology Department
Grampian University Hospitals-NHS Trust, Foresterhill
Aberdeen, Scotland, United Kingdom

John V. Forrester, FMedSci, FRSE, FIBiol

Department of Ophthalmology
Institute of Medical Sciences, Foresterhill
University of Aberdeen
Aberdeen, Scotland, United Kingdom

Wolters Kluwer | Lippincott Williams & Wilkins
Health

Philadelphia • Baltimore • New York • London
Buenos Aires • Hong Kong • Sydney • Tokyo

Acquisitions Editor: Jonathan W. Pine, Jr.
Product Manager: Julia Seto
Senior Manufacturing Manager: Benjamin Rivera
Marketing Manager: Lisa Parry
Design Coordinator: Teresa Mallon
Production Service: Maryland Composition/ASI

© 2009 by LIPPINCOTT WILLIAMS & WILKINS, a WOLTERS KLUWER business
530 Walnut Street
Philadelphia, PA 19106 USA
LWW.com

Printed in the People's Republic of China

Library of Congress Cataloging-in-Publication Data

Fundus autofluorescence / [edited by] Noemi Lois, John V. Forrester.—1st ed.
   p. ; cm.
   Includes bibliographical references and index.
   ISBN 978-1-58255-799-1
 1. Fundus oculi. 2. Fluorescence angiography. 3. Lipofuscins. 4. Fluorescence. I. Lois, Noemi.
II. Forrester, John V.
   [DNLM: 1. Fluorescence. 2. Fundus Oculi. 3. Lipofuscin—physiology. 4. Ophthalmoscopy—
methods. 5. Retinal Diseases—diagnosis. WW 270 F9895 2010]
   RE545.F86 2010
   617.7′4—dc22
                                  2009003110

Care has been taken to confirm the accuracy of the information presented and to describe generally accepted practices. However, the authors, editors, and publisher are not responsible for errors or omissions or for any consequences from application of the information in this book and make no warranty, expressed or implied, with respect to the currency, completeness, or accuracy of the contents of the publication. Application of the information in a particular situation remains the professional responsibility of the practitioner.

The authors, editors, and publisher have exerted every effort to ensure that drug selection and dosage set forth in this text are in accordance with current recommendations and practice at the time of publication. However, in view of ongoing research, changes in government regulations, and the constant flow of information relating to drug therapy and drug reactions, the reader is urged to check the package insert for each drug for any change in indications and dosage and for added warnings and precautions. This is particularly important when the recommended agent is a new or infrequently employed drug.

Some drugs and medical devices presented in the publication have Food and Drug Administration (FDA) clearance for limited use in restricted research settings. It is the responsibility of the health care provider to ascertain the FDA status of each drug or device planned for use in their clinical practice.

To purchase additional copies of this book, call our customer service department at **(800) 638-3030** or fax orders to **(301) 223-2320**. International customers should call **(301) 223-2300**.

Visit Lippincott Williams & Wilkins on the Internet: at LWW.com. Lippincott Williams & Wilkins customer service representatives are available from 8:30 am to 6 pm, EST.

10 9 8 7 6 5 4 3 2 1

*To my wonderful and very supportive
husband, Augusto, and to our
children, Emilia and Yago, a blessing
from heaven.
—Noemi Lois*

*To my mother, Maire Frances Terese,
for all she has done for me.
—John V. Forrester*

CONTENTS

Ehab Abdelkader, MSc, FRCS
Ophthalmology Department
Grampian University Hospitals-NHS Trust
Aberdeen, Scotland, United Kingdom

Isabelle Audo, MD, PhD
Institute of Ophthalmology
London, United Kingdom
Laboratoire de Physiopathologie Cellulaire et
Moléculaire de la Rétine,
Institut de la Vision
Département de Génétique
Université Pierre et Marie Curie
Centre d'Investigation Clinique
CHNO des Quinze-Vingts
Paris, France

Caren Bellmann, MD
Institut Curie
Service d'Ophtalmologie
Paris, France

Almut Bindewald-Wittich, MD
Department of Ophthalmology
University of Bonn
Bonn, Germany

Alan C. Bird, MD
Emeritus Professor of Ophthalmology
Department of Genetics
Institute of Ophthalmology
University College of London

Ferdinando Bottoni, MD
University Eye Clinic
Luigi Sacco Hospital
University of Milan
Milan, Italy

Michael E. Boulton, PhD
Anatomy and Cell Biology
University of Florida College of Medicine
Gainesville, Florida

François Delori, PhD
Schepens Eye Research Institute
Harvard Medical School
Boston, Massachusetts

Susan. M. Downes, MD, FRCOphth
Consultant Ophthalmic Surgeon
Honorary Clinical Senior Lecturer, Oxford University
Oxford Eye Hospital
John Radcliffe Hospital
Oxford, United Kingdom

Robert P. Finger, MD
Department of Ophthalmology
University of Bonn
Bonn, Germany

Fred W. Fitzke, PhD
Visual Science
Institute of Ophthalmology
University College London
London, United Kingdom

Monika Fleckenstein, MD
Department of Ophthalmology
University of Bonn
Bonn, Germany

Carsten Framme, PD Dr. med., FEBO, MHM®
University Eye Hospital Regensburg
Regensburg, Germany

Frank G. Holz, MD
Professor of Ophthalmology
University of Bonn
Bonn, Germany

Phil Hykin, FRCS, FRCOpth
Moorfields Eye Hospital
London, United Kingdom

Simone Kellner, MD
AugenZentrum, Siegburg
RetinaScience, Bonn
Bonn, Germany

Ulrich Kellner, MD
AugenZentrum, Siegburg
RetinaScience, Bonn
Bonn, Germany

Lucia Kuffová, MD, PhD
Clinical Research Fellow
Department of Immunity and Inflammation
Division of Applied Medicine
University of Aberdeen
Aberdeen, Scotland, United Kingdom

Daniel Lavinsky, MD
Vision Institute
Department of Ophthalmology
Paulista School of Medicine
Federal University of Sao Paulo
São Paulo, Brazil

Rubens Belfort Mattos Jr., MD, PhD
Vision Institute
Department of Ophthalmology
Paulista School of Medicine
Federal University of São Paulo
São Paulo, Brazil

Rubens Belfort Mattos Neto, MD
Vision Institute
Department of Ophthalmology
Paulista School of Medicine
Federal University of São Paulo
São Paulo, Brazil

Vikki McBain, PhD
Ophthalmology Department
Grampian University Hospitals-NHS Trust
Aberdeen, Scotland, United Kingdom

Michel Michaelides, BSc, MB, BS, MRCOphth, MD
Medical Retina Fellow
Institute of Ophthalmology
University College London
Clinical Research Fellow
Moorfields Eye Hospital
London, United Kingdom

Eduardo V. Navajas, MD
Vision Institute
Department of Ophthalmology
Paulista School of Medicine
Federal University of São Paulo
São Paulo, Brazil

David A. Pearce, PhD
University of Rochester
School of Medicine & Dentistry
Center for Neuronal Development & Disease
Department of Biochemistry and Biophysics
Department of Neurology
Rochester, New York

Markus Preising, Dipl.-Biol.
Department of Ophthalmology
Laboratory of Molecular Ophthalmology
Justus Liebig University
Universitaetsklinikum Giessen and Marburg GmbH
Giessen Campus
Giessen, Germany

Pamela Rath, MD
Retina Vitreous Consultants
Pittsburgh, Pennsylvania

Agnes B. Renner, MD
Department of Ophthalmology
University of Regensburg
Regensburg, Germany

Anthony G Robson, PhD
Moorfields Eye Hospital
London, United Kingdom
Institute of Ophthalmology
London, United Kingdom

Steffen Schmitz-Valckenberg, MD
Visual Science, Institute of Ophthalmology
University College London
London, England
Department of Ophthalmology
University of Bonn
Bonn, Germany

Hendrik P.N. Scholl, MD, MA
Department of Ophthalmology
University of Bonn
Bonn, Germany

Dietrich Schweitzer, Dr.-Jng. habil
Experimental Ophthalmology
Department of Ophthalmology
University of Jena
Jena, Germany

Sabrina S. Seehafer, PhD
Graduate
Center for Neural Development & Disease
University of Rochester
Rochester, New York

R. Theodore Smith, MD, PhD
Associate Professor of Ophthalmology and Biomedical
Engineering
Columbia University
New York, New York

Stephen H. Tsang, MD, PhD
Department of Ophthalmology
Edward S. Harkness Eye Institute
Bernard & Shirlee Brown Glaucoma Laboratory
Department of Pathology & Cell Biology
College of Physicians and Surgeons
Columbia University
New York, New York

Irena Tsui, MD
Department of Ophthalmology
Edward S. Harkness Eye Institute
Columbia University
New York, New York

Andrea von Rückmann, PD Dr med
Zentrum für Augenheilkunde und Plastische
Lidchirurgie
Zürich, Switzerland

Bettina Wabbels, MD
Department of Ophthalmology
University of Bonn
Bonn, Germany

Andrew R. Webster, FRCOpth
Moorfields Eye Hospital
London, United Kingdom
Institute of Ophthalmology
London, United Kingdom

Heping Xu, MD, PhD
Department of Ophthalmology
School of Medicine
Institute of Medical Sciences, Foresterhill
University of Aberdeen
Aberdeen, Scotland, United Kingdom

The field of retinal imaging is evolving fast. After decades of rule by fundus angiography, several valuable new, non-invasive modalities of fundus imaging have appeared, including optical coherence tomography, fundus autofluorescence, and adaptive optics retinography. Each of these techniques reveals various characteristics of the retinal tissue, whereas retinal angiography shows only the vascular component of the retina and choroid and any abnormal dye leakage and pooling.

The emergence of these new imaging modalities was made possible not only by technological progress but also by the increasing interest shown by clinicians in the neuronal and epithelial impairment of the retina that occurs in macular diseases. In this respect the study of lipofuscin and macular pigments, using various wavelengths, is becoming increasingly important in inherited macular dystrophies and age-related macular degeneration, because it provides information not only on morphological changes in the macula but also, indirectly, on retinal cell metabolism.

Noemi Lois, who has been studying autofluorescence for a long time, and John Forrester, whose role in digital retinal imaging, retinal physiology, and immunology is well known, deserve praise for their achievement in gathering the best specialists in retinal autofluorescence in a book covering all aspects of the study of autofluorescence that today appear to be useful for the clinical diagnosis and management of retinal diseases. Fundus autofluorescence is the perfect complement to color, red-free, and blue-reflectance fundus photography, as well as optical coherence tomography, because in many cases the combination of these non-invasive fundus imaging modalities can replace fluorescein or indocyanine green angiography.

This book will facilitate understanding of the scientific bases and principles of the interpretation of fundus autofluorescence. It has also the merit of comparing the place of fundus autofluorescence to that of other fundus imaging techniques, and in this respect is essential reading for the retinal specialist or indeed for any ophthalmologist who has to treat retinal diseases.

Alain Gaudric, MD
Professor and Chairman, Department of Ophthalmology
Lariboisière Hospital
University of Paris
Paris, France

T he field of retina has been revolutionized in recent years with the advent of new imaging modalities that allow clinicians to perform a better and more detailed evaluation of their patients. Among these, fundus autofluorescence is increasingly used and has proven to be a very helpful tool assisting the clinician in the diagnosis of many retinal disorders. It has been used also to determine appropriate treatment options and to evaluate outcomes following these therapies in selected cases. Fundus autofluorescence provides different and complementary information to that gathered by other imaging modalities such as fluorescein angiography and optical coherence tomography and it has been a pleasant surprise to those in the field how much information can be gleaned from this conceptually simple modality. Indeed there is much more to discover.

We conceived this book with the goal of providing the reader with a detailed up-to-date resume of current knowledge on fundus autofluorescence, including (i) basic aspects of the synthesis and degradation of lipofuscin, the main fluorophore in the retina generating the fundus autofluorescence signal; (ii) information on techniques available to image and quantify fundus autofluorescence and their basis; (iii) the anatomo-pathologic correlations of autofluorescence findings established in animal models; (iv) the normal distribution of autofluorescence across the fundus; and (v) that associated with disease. The value of fundus autofluorescence as a diagnostic and prognostic tool is underlined in each of the clinical chapters, covering a variety of retinal diseases in which knowledge of the distribution of autofluorescence has been gathered since this imaging technique became available. The value of fundus autofluorescence in the evaluation of patients with posterior segment disorders is discussed in each chapter in the context of other available imaging techniques, such as fluorescein and indocyanine green angiography and optical coherence tomography. Furthermore, fundus autofluorescence findings are reviewed in light of their value for understanding the pathogenesis of the conditions imaged. Lastly, individual clinical chapters provide a comprehensive update on all aspects of each condition discussed.

Although this book has been written for ophthalmologists with special interest in retina, we believe it will also be of interest and value to other readers such as general ophthalmologists, ophthalmologists in training, basic researchers in the field of retina, and ophthalmic photographers and optometrists with special interest in imaging techniques, particularly as autofluorescence imaging as a diagnostic tool becomes more widespread.

It is our hope that this book will help clinicians to understand and interpret autofluorescence images of the retina and to recognize the different autofluorescence patterns observed in the retinal diseases discussed, helping subsequently, with the diagnosis and management of patients with retinal diseases.

Noemi Lois and John V. Forrester

ACKNOWLEDGMENTS

We are very grateful to all authors who have contributed chapters to this book for sharing their knowledge and expertise on the subjects discussed, and for having so generously given their time and effort toward the completion of this project. We thank Mr. Jonathan W. Pine Jr., Senior Executive Editor, Lippincott Williams & Wilkins, for his support and advice throughout the publication process of this book, and Ms. Molly M. Ward for her expert assistance.

Basic Science

CHAPTER 1

Sabrina S. Seehafer
David A. Pearce

Lipofuscin: The "Wear and Tear" Pigment

Many substances fluoresce spontaneously (autofluoresce, i.e., emit light of a particular wavelength) when illuminated by light of a different wavelength. Pathologists are well used to observing autofluorescence (AF) in certain cells, such as macrophages, when viewing specimens with a cobalt blue light filter in the microscope. More recently, ophthalmologists have become accustomed to visualizing AF in images of the fundus. This book reviews the basic science and clinical knowledge regarding fundus AF in the human eye, a phenomenon that was first noted when fluorescein angiographic imaging of the eye was introduced and has become more clearly evident with the development of scanning laser ophthalmoscopy. AF is thought to be due to lipofuscin present in cells of the retina, especially retinal pigment epithelial cells. This first chapter serves as an introduction to the biochemistry and mechanisms behind the accumulation of lipofuscin and other autofluorescent storage material in tissues, with a particular focus on the central nervous system (CNS).

Lipofuscin, commonly referred as the "wear and tear" pigment, is an autofluorescent storage material that accumulates as a result of cell senescence. Lipofuscin has also been termed lipopigment (LP), autofluorescent storage material, yellow-brown material, and aging pigment. Although all cells accumulate lipofuscin, it is seen in the highest quantity in tissues or cells that are postmitotic, such as neurons, retina, and muscle. However, aging is not the only phenomenon associated with accumulation of autofluorescent storage material. Autofluorescent LPs have also been shown to accumulate as a result of pathological conditions, in which case the autofluorescent storage material is known as ceroid. Such conditions include the pediatric neurodegenerative disorders called neuronal ceroid lipofuscinoses (NCLs). This distinction between ceroid (AF material that accumulates in disease) and lipofuscin (AF material that accumulates as a result of aging), however, is not generally used in ophthalmology. Both ceroid and lipofuscin have been shown to primarily accumulate in the lysosome; however, they have also been shown to accumulate in vesicles, in the cytoplasm, and in the perikaryon of neurons. Table 1.1 lists different disease states and aging pathologies reported to involve an accumulation of lipofuscin/ceroid. The mechanisms and biochemistry of lipofuscin will be primarily discussed in the context of LP accumulation in all tissue types; in the case of ceroid, the focus will be on the CNS.

All types of autofluorescent LPs were originally described as autofluorescent material in postmortem tissue. All autofluorescent storage materials are not identical. The LPs are often defined based on their fluorescent spectral properties, i.e., the wavelength of light use to excite the intrinsic fluorophore (excitation) and the light emitted as a result of this initial excitation (emission). Lipofuscin has a yellow-brown appearance and a wide range of spectral properties, with excitation wavelengths of 320–460 nm and emission wavelengths of 460–630 nm (1). A detailed

TABLE 1.1	Occurrences of LPs (Lipofuscin/Ceroid)
Aging	Best disease
Age-related macular degeneration	Stargardt disease
Neuronal ceroid lipofuscinoses	Maternal inherited diabetes and deafness
Mucolipodosis IV	Choroideremia
MPS III Sanfilippo disease	Osteopetrosis with neuronal storage disease
Alzheimer disease	Adult-onset glycogen storage disease type 2
Retinitis pigmentosa	Macular ABCA4 disease
Cone and cone-rod dystrophy	Wilson disease
X-linked retinoschisis	Crohn disease
Leber congenital amaurosis	Choroidal tumors
Pattern dystrophy	

description of the spectral characteristics of retinal lipofuscin can be found in Chapter 2. The most marked signal for the autofluorescent storage material is seen under far-ultraviolet excitation. Ceroid from NCLs has excitation and emission wavelengths similar to those of lipofuscin, with an excitation maximum of 460 nm and an emission maximum of 539 nm (2). The range of excitation and emission wavelengths for both lipofuscin and ceroid reflects the different methods of measurement used, different types of tissue studied, and different corrections for spectrum. It is important to use age-matched controls in studies of LP biology to distinguish between the accumulation of lipofuscin (the result of aging) and LPs (the result of different diseases).

Other properties examined in characterizing LPs are histochemical staining techniques, such as differential dyes, lectin binding, and ultrastructure analysis. Tissue sections for both NCLs and aging brains have been shown to stain with periodic acid Schiff, a carbohydrate stain, and Sudan black, a lipid stain (3–5). Lectin histochemistry has been shown to distinguish between ceroid in NCLs and lipofuscin in the aging brain, with both LPs binding concanavalin A, but only ceroid in NCL brain tissue binding to agglutinin (6).

Electron microscopy (EM) has also been carried out on LPs to determine their ultrastructure. It has been shown by EM that lipofuscin-loaded tissue has granular osmophilic deposits (GRODs) that appear as very densely packed vesicles with dark granules filling the entire vesicle (3,5). For ceroid from NCLs, EM has shown GRODS identical to lipofuscin (5). However, two unique ultrastructures are also found only in the ceroid: fingerprint and curvilinear profiles. Curvilinear profiles are vesicles that have an amorphous arrangement of lamellar structures forming C- or S-shaped forms. Fingerprint profiles also have lamellar structures in the vesicles; however, the arrangement is in swirling circles, similar to the skin on a fingertip, and has a more dense arrangement of the lamellar structures.

Although considerable work has been done to characterize lipofuscin/ceroid at the microscopic level, the basic components of lipofuscin and its pathological counterpart remain to be determined. Various studies have shown that lipofuscin is composed of 19% to 51% lipids and 30% to 58% proteins (reviewed in Ref. 7). Further examination of lipofuscin has shown that the lipid component consists of triglycerides, cholesterol, phospholipids, and free fatty acids. The protein component is a heterogeneous mixture of proteins, with only one identified component: amyloid β-precursor protein (AβPP) (8). The carbohydrate component of lipofuscin is also a heterogeneous mixture (9). Iron, copper, aluminum, zinc, calcium, and magnesium account for approximately 2% of the lipofuscin components (10). Retinal specific lipofuscin has been shown to have a very particular composition (11,12) (see Chapter 2). One study of lipofuscin isolated from retinal pigment epithelium (RPE) demonstrated that the components were highly damaged by peroxidation and glucoxidation (13). These components were specifically damaged at lysine and cysteine adducts, such as malondialdehyde (MDAs) and 4-hydroxynonenal (HNE). Moreover, the same study identified advanced glycation end products (AGEs). This and other studies suggest that the components of lipofuscin are highly modified by oxidative stress.

For ceroid in the NCLs, except for the infantile variant, it has been shown that the primary protein component (50%) is the subunit c of mitochondrial ATPase. In the infantile variant of NCL, the primary component is composed of sphingolipid activating proteins (saposins/SAPs) A and D (14–18). In other NCL variants, ceroid contains SAPs A and D, but not to the extent of subunit c accumulation. Other identified components include AβPP, dolichol pyrophosphate-linked oligosaccharides, lipid-linked oligosaccharides, and metals (primarily iron) (16,19–21). Although all LP components vary in terms of the types of autofluorescent storage material and tissue, they all appear to be composed of undegraded or partially degraded proteins.

To date, very little is known about the fluorescent components (fluorophores) in most LPs that generate the spectral properties of the autofluorescent storage material. Some have hypothesized that the fluorophore is a single compound. However, the fluorescent signal may also be generated after interactions between several different nonfluorescent molecules. It has also been hypothesized that the fluorescence comes from lipid oxidation; however, some favor the hypothesis that modifications to the stored proteins result in the fluorescence. It is certain that the ranges of spectral properties reported for autofluorescent material make identification of a single fluorophore challenging. Isolation of lipofuscin/ceroid has also proven problematic, with spectral properties decreasing or attenuating during the isolation process. In vitro studies have shown that reactions between carbonyls and amino compounds that produce Schiff bases such as 1,4 dihydropyridine and 2-hydroxy-1,2-dihydropyrrol-3-ones demonstrate natural lipofuscin-like spectral properties (reviewed in Ref. 22). In retinal lipofuscin, it has been shown that the major blue absorbing fluorophore is pyridinium bisretinoid (A2E) (23,24) (see Chapter 2). Ceroid is similar to lipofuscin outside of the retina and currently has no identified fluorophore. Furthermore, it cannot be excluded that each type of ceroid or lipofuscin might have a specific fluorophore, or multiple fluorophores with overlapping spectral properties that result in the overall autofluorescent signal. Numerous studies have examined the biochemical properties of LPs (Table 1.2), but the larger question is, Why does this autofluorescent storage material accumulate?

MECHANISMS OF LIPOFUSCIN ACCUMULATION

Three different mechanisms have been proposed for accumulation of lipofuscin/ceroid: lysosomal dysfunction, autophagy, and cellular stress. The accumulation of LP at the lysosome implies an underlying lysosomal dysfunction that results in a buildup of lipofuscin/ceroid. Autophagy, the major degradation/recycling pathway, could be altered, leading to LP/ceroid deposition. Cellular stresses in the form of oxidative stress or starvation could have an impact on the cell physiology and result in lipofuscin/ceroid accumulation.

TABLE 1.2	Biochemical Properties of LPs	
	Lipofuscin	**Ceroid**
Location	Primarily lysosome	Primarily lysosome
Spectral properties (nm)		
Excitation	320–460	320–460
Emission	460–630	460–630
Storage components		
Proteins	heterogeneous mix AβPP	subunit C mitochondria ATPase saposins A & D, AβPP
Lipids	triglycerides, cholesterol phospholipids, free fatty acids	phosphorylated dolichols, phospholipids neutral lipids
Carbohydrates	heterogeneous mix	dolichol-linked oligosaccharides
Metals	Fe, Cu, Al, Zn, Mn, Ca	predominantly Fe
Staining characteristics		
Sudan black B	Yes	Yes
Periodic Schiff base	Yes	Yes
Lectin	concanavalin A	concanavalin A, agglutinin
Ultrastructures	GRODS	GRODs, fingerprint, curvilinear

Lysosomal Dysfunction As a Cause for Lipofuscin Accumulation

A large percentage of lipofuscin/ceroid has been shown to accumulate in a specific organelle, the lysosome. There are two possible fundamental mechanisms that could result in accumulation of LP in the lysosomes: substrate accumulation due to mutation/dysfunction in enzymes, or an imbalance in lysosomal homeostasis resulting in an altered lysosomal environment changing multiple enzyme activities/functions. In the case of the NCLs, three variant diseases are caused by mutations in lysosomal enzymes: congenital, infantile, and late infantile NCL. These diseases are caused by mutations in the lysosomal enzymes cathepsin D, palmitoyl protein thioesterase 1, and tripeptyl protease, respectively (reviewed in Ref. 25). However, not all of the autofluorescent storage material can be accounted for by such specific enzymatic defects. Undefined ways to affect lysosomal enzymes, such as alterations in lysosomal homeostasis, are also likely. Other NCLs have defects in proteins that have not yet been assigned a definitive function. Juvenile NCL (JNCL) has a defect in the CLN3 protein, which resides in the lysosomal/late endosomal membrane (reviewed in Ref. 26). In fibroblasts from patients with JNCL, a decrease in lysosomal pH was observed. Most recently, the pH of lysosomes was shown to be regulated by a membrane channel protein (TRP-ML1). Defects in this protein lead to lysosomal accumulation of lipid deposits (27), so there may be a general mechanism at fault in the accumulation of lysosomal material related to the intralysosomal milieu. This shift in intralysosomal conditions may not be optimal for enzymatic activity. Suboptimal lysosomal enzyme activity could potentially underlie the accumulation of lipofuscin/ceroid (28). In support of this are studies demonstrating that administration of leupeptin, a general lysosome inhibitor, or chloroquine, an amine that raises lysosomal pH to an alkaline environment, in rats resulted in accumulation of lipofuscin-like autofluorescent storage material in brain tissue and hepatocytes (29–32) (see also Chapter 4).

Studies on the aging process have shown that as lipofuscin accumulates, lysosomal cysteine proteinases undergo a decrease in enzymatic activity (33,34). Other laboratories have shown an increased activity of lysosomal enzymes such as β-galactosidase and cathepsin B and D (35–37). In any case, there is enough evidence to suggest that changes occurring at the lysosomal level could be a possible cause of LP accumulation.

Autophagy

Autophagy is the process of transporting macromolecules and organelles to the lysosome for degradation. During this process, macromolecules and organelles are engulfed in double-membrane vesicles that are trafficked to the lysosome for the breakdown of proteins and organelles as basic precursors for recycling in the cell. Three forms of autophagy have been described in the mammalian cell (22,38–40). The first is macroautophagy, which is the process of engulfing large organelles such as mitochondria and/or large portions of the cytosol into a double-membrane vesicle called the autophagosome, followed by trafficking to the lysosome for degradation. This is the most widely studied form of autophagy. In contrast, microautophagy describes a mechanism in which small organelles or proteins are brought into the lysosome for degradation by invagination of the lysosome membrane. In the third form of autophagy, a chaperone complex aids in identifying cytosolic proteins for degradation by the lysosome (chaperone-mediated autophagy [CMA]). For a protein to enter the CMA pathway, it must be targeted by a KFERQ sequence (41). There is a degree of interplay between each type of autophagy, such that when there are defects in CMA, macroautophagy will compensate for those defects (42).

It has been shown in numerous studies that as cells age, all forms of autophagy slow down (43–47). Thus, as the rate of autophagy decreases, there may be increased formation of lipofuscin. To determine whether alterations in autophagy can result in lipofuscin accumulation, Stroikin et al. (48) treated dividing fibroblasts with 3-methyladenine (3-MA), which inhibits the first step of autophagy. In this process, called sequestration, the material is engulfed in double-membrane vesicles to form the autophagosome. Their study showed an accumulation of lipofuscin-like material in the fibroblasts as a result of the 3-MA treatment. Autophagy has been shown to be upregulated in all cells when cells are starved to the point where they break down all nonessential or slightly damaged proteins into amino acids for cell survival (49). In another study (50), fibroblasts that were exposed to prolonged hyperoxia and nutrient starvation and had accumulation of lipofuscin showed decreased survival compared to cells without lipofuscin. It was hypothesized that lipofuscin in the lysosome blocks the efficient breakdown of material to allow for further survival. However, there is as yet no consensus as to whether all lysosomal enzymes have attenuated activity in aging cells. What seems to be clear is that lysosomes loaded with lipofuscin are not able to degrade proteins, organelles, and macromolecules for recycling as efficiently. This could result in the further accumulation of lipofuscin.

Experimental models are available in which there appears to be an accumulation of lipofuscin/ceroid. In the Cathepsin D−/− mouse model for congenital NCL, there is a buildup of vesicles in the brain that are autofluorescent, contain subunit c of mitochondrial ATPase, and are positive for the autophagosome marker, LC3 (51). This study suggests that the ceroid is accumulating in autophagosome, and this accumulation of ceroid outside the lysosome itself is indicative of an increase in autophagy most likely caused by autophagic stress. A mouse model for juvenile NCL, Cln3$^{\Delta ex7-8}$ mouse, has also shown defects in autophagy. Brains from

Cln3$^{\Delta ex7-8}$ mice were shown to have an increase in LC3-positive vesicles, specifically LC3-II, suggesting an upregulation in autophagy but possible delays in autophagic vesicle maturation (52). Additional work carried out on cerebellar precursor cells from this mouse showed that upon stimulation of autophagy, the normal overlap between the lysosomal and autophagosome vesicles was decreased compared to wild-type mice. Taken together, these results illustrate a dysregulation of autophagy in JNCL.

Each field of research has supported alterations in autophagy as a cellular event that can occur both in disease and in the aging process. Studies using inhibitors specific for autophagy have shown that autophagy is a possible mechanism for lipofuscin/ceroid accumulation. However, alterations in autophagy, which are linked to the lysosome and other key organelles such as mitochondria, could be a result of a primary insult to the lysosome, protein trafficking, mitochondria function, or autophagy itself. The interplay between each organelle and the overall cellular environment may be synergistic in the formation of autofluorescent storage material.

Cellular Stress

Alterations in cell physiology could also contribute to or be a possible mechanism underlying lipofuscin/ceroid accumulation. Certain types of stress can cause cells to alter their intracellular microenvironment, for instance, via reactive oxygen species (ROS).

The major organelle responsible for the production of ROS (45) is the mitochondria (reviewed in Refs. 53–55). ROS are formed by the normal functioning of the electron transport chain (ECT) during ATP generation. Mitochondrial and cytosolic enzymes, including catalase, glutathione peroxidase, and superoxide dismutase (SOD), help rid the cell of harmful free radicals. However, this system is not perfect, and some ROS escape the mitochondria with the potential to oxidize proteins, lipids and other macromolecules. In a normal functioning cell, oxidized or damaged proteins are transported to the lysosome for degradation. Senescent mitochondria, also known as giant mitochondria, have been shown to swell, lose their cristae and, occasionally, the inner membrane, resulting in little or no ATP production (56–58). All of these characteristics of aging mitochondria would lead to the release of increasing amounts of free radicals. In younger cells, as mitochondria age, they are targeted by autophagy and degradation at the lysosome. Once the mitochondria reach the lysosome, they are degraded. As mitochondria are broken down, H_2O_2 is released into the lysosomal compartment. The lysosome itself is the perfect environment for Fenton chemistry to take place to propagate the free radical damage due to the available iron and cysteine pools, and the acidic pH. Lysosomes are responsible for recycling ferritin for the cell's continued use of the iron (59). Fenton chemistry refers to the reaction in which ferrous iron converts the less reactive free radical of H_2O_2 into the most reactive oxidative species of OH·. This basic conversion allows for an increasing amplification of oxidative damage because of an increase in the array of reactive reactions resulting from the increase in reactivity.

LP has components such as oxidized lipids and proteins; this, along with other experiments showing increased oxidative stress and slow degradation of mitochondria, is known as the mitochondrial-lysosomal axis theory of aging (7). This theory supports the hypothesis that oxidative damage may lead to the accumulation of autofluorescent storage material. However, it has yet to be determined whether this oxidation occurs inside the lysosome itself or elsewhere in the cell, as ROS are membrane-permeable and can diffuse throughout the cell. With slowing autophagy, there could be a buildup of giant mitochondria in the cytosol leading to an increased ROS in the cytosol, as well as the hydroxyl radical emanating from the lysosome from the reactions discussed above. This increase in ROS could lead to damage to nucleic acids, intracellular proteins, extracellular proteins, organelles, lipids, and membranes. Additionally, if the ROS interacts with reactive metabolites, such as nitrogen species, this could lead to the formation of a further class of reactive species, namely, reactive nitrogen species (RNS) or peroxynitirites, which would further propagate damage across the cell. Regardless of whether the ROS or RNS arise in the lysosome or in the cytosol, the effect would be across the whole cell.

In the case of ceroid in NCLs, it has been shown that subunit c of mitochondrial ATPase is the most prevalent protein stored. A study in the English Setter model of NCL showed partial uncoupling between electron transport and ATP production in liver mitochondria (60). In NCL fibroblasts, mitochondria were shown to have damaged fatty acid oxidation (61). Recently, our laboratory showed that in the brain of the JNCL knockout mouse model, progressive oxidative damage occurs throughout the CNS (62). That study demonstrated an increased amount of protein oxidation, a decrease in glutathione, and an increase in one form of SOD in the CNS. A similar study examining two other variants of NCLs found that the protein and gene expressions of SOD were also upregulated (63). Therefore, ceroid accumulation in NCLs may be the result of oxidative damage.

Cell starvation alters a cell's ability to use nonessential processes. Under such harsh stress, cells will induce autophagy of nonessential proteins and organelles in the lysosome, with the subsequent breakdown of these macromolecules into small basic precursors that can then be used by the cell to maintain its life. This additional stress could propagate lipofuscin/ceroid formation in a cell with already present autophagy defects or oxidative stress. Specifically, during starvation the buffering enzymes to reduce ROS exposure are down-regulated, whereas more macromolecules are being transported to the very reactive oxidative environment of the lysosome, as discussed above. Additionally, deficiencies in various nutrients, such as vitamin E, have been shown to cause accumulation of lipofuscin and ceroid (64). This accumulation of LP is hypothesized to occur due to the loss of the antioxidant property normally provided by vitamin E. All of these types of stress may play a role in the same oxidative pathway that leads to lipofuscin/ceroid accumulation.

CONCLUDING REMARKS ON LIPOPIGMENT ACCUMULATION

Overall, there is evidence to support all three basic mechanisms of LP accumulation in both aging and NCLs. Figure 1.1 summarizes each mechanism of lipofuscin/ceroid accumulation. The lysosome plays a role in the deposition of LP in each of these basic mechanisms. The mitochondria are also affected in all. It is possible that in some cases lipofuscin/ceroid accumulation occurs mainly due to a defect in a single pathway; however, it is likely that in most instances this accumulation results from deficiencies or subtle alterations in all three pathways. The varying contributions of these pathways may result in differences in the makeup of the autofluorescent storage material, challenging the characterization of this material.

Implications of Lipofuscin/Ceroid in the Central Nervous System

Does lipofuscin accumulation result in cell death, or is the LP internalized into the lysosomes as a protective mechanism to help avoid apoptosis? Lipofuscin accumula-

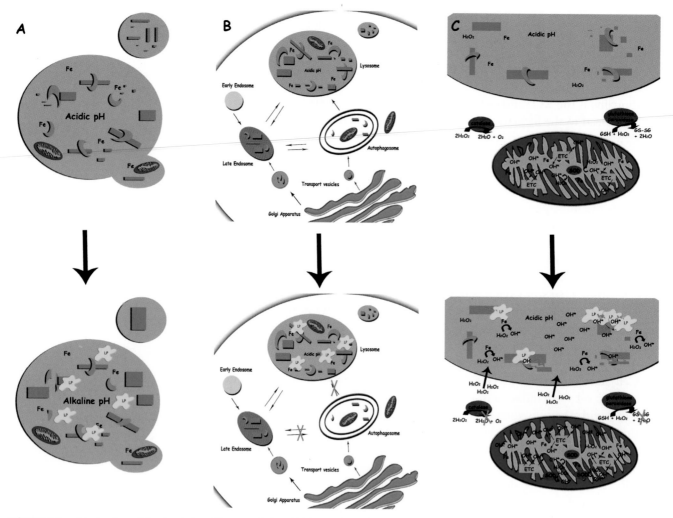

FIGURE 1.1. Mechanism of lipofuscin/ceroid accumulation. **(A)** Lysosomal dysfunction. The top panel illustrates a normally functioning lysosome with vesicles delivering organelles, such as mitochondria, and proteins/macromolecules for degradation. The lysosomal enzymes (blue half circles) are properly degrading the material and maintaining an acidic pH. This organelle is also transporting the basic precursors that have already broken down to other locations in the cell to be recycled back into proteins. However, in aging or NCLs, there are alterations to the lysosome, as seen in the bottom part of the panel. Lysosomal pH is raised to a more alkaline environment and/or lysosomal enzymes are not properly functioning. This results in the accumulation of LPs in the lysosome because the lysosome is incapable of transporting them out of the lysosome. **(B)** Autophagy defects. During the process of autophagy in a normal cell, an autophagosome surrounds the mitochondria and protein/macromolecules and transports them to the lysosome for degradation by direct fusion to the lysosome or fusion to the late endosome (top panel). Transport vesicles move lysosomal enzymes to the late endosome for maturation into a lysosome or additionally to the autophagosome itself. In aging cells or in cells with LP pathologies, the trafficking of these vesicles slows. Although there may not be a permanent block, if transport is delayed, proteins and organelles targeted for degradation can become trapped in an environment that is not conducive to degradation, and alterations to the components may then occur. Proteins/organelles may undergo modifications before they finally reach the lysosome, rendering them nondegradable. Additionally, the lysosomal enzymes involved in the trafficking would also experience delays in trafficking, which would affect the cell. There could be a shortage of enzymes in lysosomes, or the enzymes could be held in environments that lead to their modification, both resulting in lowered enzymatic activity. Any slowing down or blocking of autophagy can result in accumulation of LP. **(C)** Cellular stress (oxidation). The mitochondria are the power plant of all mammalians. The ETC (shown in orange) produces ATP, but as a result of this process, harmful ROS (44) such as OH· and H_2O_2 form. However, the cell has enzymes to control the effects of ROS. In the mitochondria, the enzyme SOD converts OH· to H_2O_2, a membrane-permeable form of ROS that goes across the mitochondrial membranes. Once it reaches the cytosol, another set of enzymes detoxify H_2O_2. Catalase and glutathione peroxidase convert $2H_2O_2$ into 2 H_2O. This system is not perfect, and some ROS reach other organelles; however, the effect is minimal. Top panel: As cells age, they start to accumulate mitochondria that are less functional and have an increased production of ROS. This could be a result of slowed trafficking for degradation or of degradation itself. The end result is that the enzymes (purple) are not able to keep up with the increased concentration of ROS. With more H_2O_2 in the cellular environment, the lysosome is an attractive location for accumulation because as a result of the high quantity of iron (Fe), the lysosome can use Fenton chemistry to convert H_2O_2 to OH·, a more reactive ROS. Oxidation alters lysosomal enzymes, proteins, lipids, and organelles, resulting in slowed degradation because of the crosslinks and modifications (pink zigzags) and possible lowered enzymatic activity resulting in the accumulation of LP (a substrate for oxidative damage), propagating the cycle. Large gray ovals: lysosomes; green squares and rectangles: proteins/macromolecules; blue half circles: lysosomal enzymes.

tion has been implicated in the pathology of neurodegenerative disease and in aging, particularly in association with neuronal loss and increasing reactivity and number of glial cells (64). Storage of neuronal lipofuscin has also been associated with increased oxidative stress and decreased antioxidant defense (reviewed in Refs. 7 and 66). It has also been shown that neuronal lipofuscin destroys neuron structure and is correlated with the development of cytoskeletal defects (67–69). Overall, it has been assumed that lipofuscin in the brain is detrimental, impacting neuronal and glial homeostasis, which affects the brain physiology (reviewed in Refs. 65 and 70). For the NCLs, ceroid, although clearly a hallmark of disease, has not been demonstrated to be the primary disease defect. Accumulated ceroid, while damaging cells, may occur as the consequence of a yet-to-be-determined initial disease insult. It has not been determined whether neurons are trying to remove lipofuscin/ceroid as a harmful component. It has also not been demonstrated that LP accumulation arises from the need to rid the cell of certain components. However, it has been shown that LP triggers apoptotic cascades to initiate cell death (reviewed in Refs. 71–73).

Continued research needs to pursue the different mechanisms that underlie accumulation of lipofuscin/ceroid. Depending on the tissue type and autofluorescent storage material pathology involved, different mechanisms may be the culprits in the complex biology of this accumulation.

REFERENCES

1. Dowson JH. The evaluation of autofluorescence emission spectra derived from neuronal lipopigment. J Microsc 1982;128(Pt 3):261–270.
2. Dowson JH, Armstrong D, Koppang N, et al. Autofluorescence emission spectra of neuronal lipopigment in animal and human ceroidoses (ceroid-lipofuscinoses). Acta Neuropathol (Berl) 1982;58:152–156.
3. Elleder MA. Histochemical and ultrastructural study of stored material in neuronal ceroid lipofuscinosis. Virchows Arch B Cell Pathol 1978;28:167–178.
4. Elleder M. Deposition of lipopigment—a new feature of human splenic sinus endothelium (SSE). Ultrastructural and histochemical study. Virchows Arch A Pathol Anat Histopathol 1990;416:423–428.
5. Elleder M. Primary extracellular ceroid type lipopigment. A histochemical and ultrastructural study. Histochem J 1991;23:247–258.
6. Wisniewski KE, Maslinska D. Lectin histochemistry in brains with juvenile form of neuronal ceroid-lipofuscinosis (Batten disease). Acta Neuropathol (Berl) 1990;80:274–279.
7. Brunk UT, Terman A. The mitochondrial-lysosomal axis theory of aging: accumulation of damaged mitochondria as a result of imperfect autophagocytosis. Eur J Biochem 2002;269:1996–2002.
8. Bancher C, Grundke-Iqbal I, Iqbal K, et al. Immunoreactivity of neuronal lipofuscin with monoclonal antibodies to the amyloid beta-protein. Neurobiol Aging 1989;10:125–132.
9. Brunk UT, Terman A. Lipofuscin: mechanisms of age-related accumulation and influence on cell function. Free Radic Biol Med 2002;33:611–619.
10. Jolly RD. Batten disease (ceroid-lipofuscinosis): the enigma of subunit c of mitochondrial ATP synthase accumulation. Neurochem Res 1995;20:1301–1304.
11. Katz ML, Drea CM, Eldred GE, et al. Influence of early photoreceptor degeneration on lipofuscin in the retinal pigment epithelium. Exp Eye Res 1986;43:561–573.
12. Katz ML, Drea CM, Robison Jr WG. Relationship between dietary retinol and lipofuscin in the retinal pigment epithelium. Mech Ageing Dev 1986;35: 291–305.
13. Schutt F, Bergmann M, Holz FG, et al. Proteins modified by malondialdehyde, 4-hydroxynonenal, or advanced glycation end products in lipofuscin of human retinal pigment epithelium. Invest Ophthalmol Vis Sci 2003;44:3663–3668.
14. Palmer DN, Martinus RD, Cooper SM, et al. Ovine ceroid lipofuscinosis. The major lipopigment protein and the lipid-binding subunit of mitochondrial ATP synthase have the same NH2-terminal sequence. J Biol Chem 1989;264:5736–5740.
15. Palmer DN, Barns G, Husbands DR, et al. Ceroid lipofuscinosis in sheep. II. The major component of the lipopigment in liver, kidney, pancreas, and brain is low molecular weight protein. J Biol Chem 1986;261:1773–1777.
16. Palmer DN, Martinus RD, Barns G, et al. Ovine ceroid-lipofuscinosis. I: Lipopigment composition is indicative of a lysosomal proteinosis. Am J Med Genet Suppl 1988;5:141–158.
17. Palmer DN, Fearnley IM, Walker JE, et al. Mitochondrial ATP synthase subunit c storage in the ceroid-lipofuscinoses (Batten disease). Am J Med Genet 1992;42:561–567.

18. Tyynela J, Palmer DN, Baumann M, et al. Storage of saposins A and D in infantile neuronal ceroid-lipo-fuscinosis. FEBS Lett 1993;330:8–12.
19. Kitaguchi T, Wisniewski KE, Maslinski S, et al. Beta-protein immunoreactivity in brains of patients with neuronal ceroid lipofuscinosis: ultrastructural and biochemical demonstration. Neurosci Lett 1990;112:155–160.
20. Wisniewski, KE, Gordon-Krajcer W, Kida E. Abnormal processing of carboxy-terminal fragment of beta precursor protein (beta PP) in neuronal ceroid-lipofuscinosis (NCL) cases. J Inherit Metab Dis 1993;16: 312–316.
21. Wisniewski KE, Maslinska D, Kitaguchi T, et al. Topographic heterogeneity of amyloid B-protein epitopes in brains with various forms of neuronal ceroid lipofuscinoses suggesting defective processing of amyloid precursor protein. Acta Neuropathol (Berl) 1990;80:26–34.
22. Terman A, Brunk UT. Lipofuscin: mechanisms of formation and increase with age. APMIS 1998;106: 265–276.
23. Sakai N, Decatur J, Nakanishi K, et al. Ocular age pigment "A2-E": an unprecedented pyridinium bis-retinoid. J Am Chem Soc 1996;118:1559–1560.
24. Reinboth JJ, Gautschi K, Munz K, et al. Lipofuscin in the retina: quantitative assay for an unprecedented autofluorescent compound (pyridinium bis-retinoid, A2-E) of ocular age pigment. Exp Eye Res 1997;65:639–643.
25. Ramirez-Montealegre D, Rothberg PG, Pearce DA. Another disorder finds its gene. Brain 2006;129(Pt 6):1353–1356.
26. Phillips SN, Benedict JW, Weimer JM, et al. CLN3, the protein associated with Batten disease: structure, function and localization. J Neurosci Res 2005;79:573–583.
27. Miedel MT, Rbaibi Y, Guerriero CJ, et al. Membrane traffic and turnover in TRP-ML1-deficient cells: a revised model for mucolipidosis type IV pathogenesis. J Exp Med 2008;205:1477–1490.
28. Holopainen JM, Saarikoski J, Kinnunen PK, et al. Elevated lysosomal pH in neuronal ceroid lipofuscinoses (NCLs). Eur J Biochem 2001;268:5851–5856.
29. Ivy GO, Schottler F, Wenzel J, et al. Inhibitors of lysosomal enzymes: accumulation of lipofuscin-like dense bodies in the brain. Science 1984;226:985–987.
30. Ivy GO, Kanai S, Ohta M, et al. Lipofuscin-like substances accumulate rapidly in brain, retina and internal organs with cysteine protease inhibition. Adv Exp Med Biol 1989;266:31–45; discussion 45–47.
31. Ivy GO, Roopsingh R, Kanai S, et al. Leupeptin causes an accumulation of lipofuscin-like substances and other signs of aging in kidneys of young rats: further evidence for the protease inhibitor model of aging. Ann NY Acad Sci 1996;786:12–23.
32. Ivy GO, Kanai S, Ohta M, et al. Leupeptin causes an accumulation of lipofuscin-like substances in liver cells of young rats. Mech Ageing Dev 1991;57:213–231.
33. Amano T, Nakanishi H, Kondo T, et al. Age-related changes in cellular localization and enzymatic activities of cathepsins B, L and D in the rat trigeminal ganglion neuron. Mech Ageing Dev 1995;83:133–141.
34. Gracy RW, Chapman ML, Cini JK, et al. Molecular basis of the accumulation of abnormal proteins in progeria and aging fibroblasts. Basic Life Sci 1985;35:427–442.
35. Gerland LM, Peyrol S, Lallemand C, et al. Association of increased autophagic inclusions labeled for beta-galactosidase with fibroblastic aging. Exp Gerontol 2003;38:887–895.
36. Keppler D, Walter R, Perez C, et al. Increased expression of mature cathepsin B in aging rat liver. Cell Tissue Res 2000;302:181–188.
37. Nakanishi H, Tominaga K, Amano T, et al. Age-related changes in activities and localizations of cathepsins D, E, B, and L in the rat brain tissues. Exp Neurol 1994;126:119–128.
38. Sundelin S, Wihlmark U, Nilsson SE, et al. Lipofuscin accumulation in cultured retinal pigment epithelial cells reduces their phagocytic capacity. Curr Eye Res 1998;17:851–857.
39. Yin D, Brunk U. Autofluorescent ceroid/lipofuscin. Methods Mol Biol 1998;108:217–227.
40. Terman A, Brunk UT. Ceroid/lipofuscin formation in cultured human fibroblasts: the role of oxidative stress and lysosomal proteolysis. Mech Ageing Dev 1998;104:277–291.
41. Dice JF. Peptide sequences that target cytosolic proteins for lysosomal proteolysis. Trends Biochem Sci 1990;15:305–309.
42. Massey AC, Kaushik S, Sovak G, et al. Consequences of the selective blockage of chaperone-mediated autophagy. Proc Natl Acad Sci USA 2006;103:5805–5810.
43. Cuervo AM, Dice JF. Age-related decline in chaperone-mediated autophagy. J Biol Chem 2000;275: 31505–31513.
44. Dice JF. Altered degradation of proteins microinjected into senescent human fibroblasts. J Biol Chem 1982;257:14624–14627.
45. Bergamini E, Del Roso A, Fierabracci V, et al. A new method for the investigation of endocrine-regulated autophagy and protein degradation in rat liver. Exp Mol Pathol 1993;59:13–26.
46. Donati A, Cavallini G, Paradiso C, et al. Age-related changes in the autophagic proteolysis of rat isolated liver cells: effects of antiaging dietary restrictions. J Gerontol A Biol Sci Med Sci 2001;56:B375–B383.
47. Donati A, Cavallini G, Paradiso C, et al. Age-related changes in the regulation of autophagic proteolysis in rat isolated hepatocytes. J Gerontol A Biol Sci Med Sci 2001;56:B288–B293.
48. Stroikin Y, Dalen H, Loof S, et al. Inhibition of autophagy with 3-methyladenine results in impaired turnover of lysosomes and accumulation of lipofuscin-like material. Eur J Cell Biol 2004;83: 583–590.
49. Finn PF, Dice JF. Proteolytic and lipolytic responses to starvation. Nutrition 2006;22:830–844.

50. Terman A, Dalen H, Brunk UT. Ceroid/lipofuscin-loaded human fibroblasts show decreased survival time and diminished autophagocytosis during amino acid starvation. Exp Gerontol 1999;34:943–957.

51. Shacka JJ, Klocke BJ, Young C, et al. Cathepsin D deficiency induces persistent neurodegeneration in the absence of Bax-dependent apoptosis. J Neurosci 2007;27:2081–2090.

52. Cao Y, Espinola JA, Fossale E, et al. Autophagy is disrupted in a knock-in mouse model of juvenile neuronal ceroid lipofuscinosis. J Biol Chem 2006;281:20483–20493.

53. Balaban RS, Nemoto S, Finkel T. Mitochondria, oxidants, and aging. Cell 2005;120:483–495.

54. Lenaz G, Bovina C, D'Aurelio M, et al. Role of mitochondria in oxidative stress and aging. Ann NY Acad Sci 2002;959:199–213.

55. Richter C, Gogvadze V, Laffranchi R, et al. Oxidants in mitochondria: from physiology to diseases. Biochim Biophys Acta 1995;1271:67–74.

56. Beregi E, Regius O, Huttl T, et al. Age-related changes in the skeletal muscle cells. Z Gerontol 1988; 21:83–86.

57. Ermini M. Ageing changes in mammalian skeletal muscle: biochemical studies. Gerontology 1976;22: 301–316.

58. Terman A, Dalen H, Eaton JW, et al. Mitochondrial recycling and aging of cardiac myocytes: the role of autophagocytosis. Exp Gerontol 2003;38:863–876.

59. Radisky DC, Kaplan J. Iron in cytosolic ferritin can be recycled through lysosomal degradation in human fibroblasts. Biochem J 1998;336(Pt 1):201–205.

60. Siakotos AN, Blair PS, Savill JD, et al. Altered mitochondrial function in canine ceroid-lipofuscinosis. Neurochem Res 1998;23:983–989.

61. Dawson G, Kilkus J, Siakotos AN, et al. Mitochondrial abnormalities in CLN2 and CLN3 forms of Batten disease. Mol Chem Neuropathol 1996;29:227–235.

62. Benedict JW, Sommers CA, Pearce DA. Progressive oxidative damage in the central nervous system of a murine model for juvenile Batten disease. J Neurosci Res 2007;85:2882–2891.

63. Heine C, Tyynela J, Cooper JD, et al. Enhanced expression of manganese-dependent superoxide dismutase in human and sheep CLN6 tissues. Biochem J 2003;376(Pt 2):369–376.

64. Fattoretti P, Bertoni-Freddari C, Casoli T, et al. Morphometry of age pigment (lipofuscin) and of ceroid pigment deposits associated with vitamin E deficiency. Arch Gerontol Geriatr 2002;34:263–268.

65. Riga S, Riga D, Schneider F, et al. Processing, lysis, and elimination of brain lipopigments in rejuvenation therapies. Ann NY Acad Sci 2006;1067:383–387.

66. Terman A, Brunk UT. Aging as a catabolic malfunction. Int J Biochem Cell Biol 2004;36:2365–2375.

67. Fifkova E, Morales M. Aging and the neurocytoskeleton. Exp Gerontol 1992;27:125–136.

68. Vickers JC, Delacourte A, Morrison JH. Progressive transformation of the cytoskeleton associated with normal aging and Alzheimer's disease. Brain Res 1992;594:273–278.

69. Grune T, Jung T, Merker K, et al. Decreased proteolysis caused by protein aggregates, inclusion bodies, plaques, lipofuscin, ceroid, and 'aggresomes' during oxidative stress, aging, and disease. Int J Biochem Cell Biol 2004;36:2519–2530.

70. Riga D, Riga S, Halalau F, et al. Brain lipopigment accumulation in normal and pathological aging. Ann NY Acad Sci 2006;1067:158–163.

71. Kurz T, Terman A, Gustafsson B, et al. Lysosomes in iron metabolism, ageing and apoptosis. Histochem Cell Biol 2008;129:389–406.

72. Kurz T, Terman A, Gustafsson B, et al. Lysosomes and oxidative stress in aging and apoptosis. Biochim Biophys Acta 2008;1780:1291–1303.

73. Kurz T, Terman A, Brunk UT. Autophagy, ageing and apoptosis: the role of oxidative stress and lysosomal iron. Arch Biochem Biophys 2007;462:220–230.

Lipofuscin of the Retinal Pigment Epithelium

ipofuscin accumulation is strongly associated with retinal aging and the progression of age-related macular degeneration (AMD) (1). Such lipofuscin accumulation is typical of highly metabolic, postmitotic cells in a variety of aging mammalian tissues (e.g., liver, heart, brain, testes, and retina) that accumulate nondegradable lipid-protein aggregates within lysosomes (2–4). In the retinal pigment epithelium (RPE), lipofuscin can be derived from autophagy (degradation of spent intracellular organelles such as mitochondria, Golgi, and endoplasmic reticulum) (1,2,5) or the ingestion of photoreceptor outer segments (POS) (2,6). The failure of the RPE lysosomal system to completely degrade this material is probably the result of preoxidative modifications. The high level of lipofuscin in the RPE leads to cellular dysfunction, which in turn contributes to photoreceptor dysfunction and degeneration (1,4).

RETINAL PIGMENT EPITHELIUM LIPOFUSCIN

RPE lipofuscin granules accumulate in the central to basal portion of the cell as spherical membrane-bound granules of 1–2 μm diameter (Fig. 2.1) (7). In addition, in aged donors lipofuscin can be observed complexed with melanin-forming aggregates of heterogeneous composition and size, in which case they are termed melanolipofuscin. Ex vivo and in vivo analyses demonstrate an age-related increase in lipofuscin content, up until the age of about 70 years (6,8–10). Thereafter, lipofuscin levels plateau or even decline (9). The reason for this decline is not clear, but it may involve one or a combination of lipofuscin degradation routes, e.g., voiding into the extracellular space (as basal laminar deposits or precursor material to drusen) or association with melanosomes. Concomitant with the accumulation of lipofuscin granules are a decrease in melanosomes and an increase in melanolipfuscin granules (8). On the basis of early morphometric data, the accumulation of RPE lipofuscin was erroneously considered to be bimodal (6), but it is now apparent that such accumulation is linear—at least up until the later decades, when the effects of age-related pathology begin to have an impact (Fig. 2.2) (9). Lipofuscin demonstrates a regional distribution across the fundus (9–11) (see Chapter 3). The distribution of lipofuscin demonstrates a retinal topography similar to that of rod photoreceptors, suggesting that ingested POS are a major substrate for RPE lipofuscin (11). Alternatively, the highest density of photoreceptors will require the highest level of metabolic activity for the RPE, and thus mitochondrial turnover and autophagy will be much higher.

The cytoplasmic volume occupied by lipofuscin increases significantly with age (Fig. 2.1). Feeney-Burns and colleagues demonstrated that 8% of the cytoplasmic volume of the central RPE is occupied by lipofuscin granules by 40 years of age, and this increases to 19% by 80 years of age (8). It is likely that this would affect metabolic function, intracellular compartmentalization of organelles, and lysosomal activity,

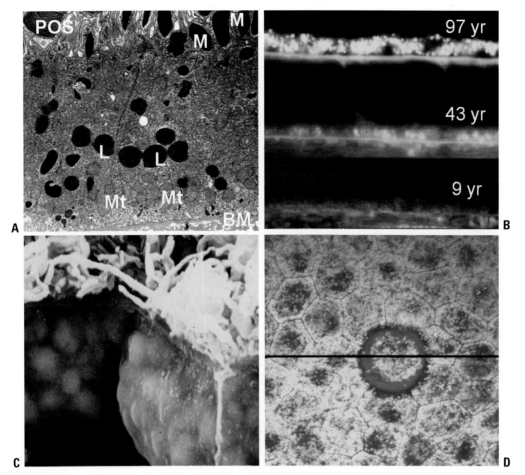

FIGURE 2.1.   Micrographs showing the accumulation of lipofuscin in human RPE cells. **(A)** Transmission electron micrograph of human RPE from a 52-year-old donor (reproduced courtesy of John Marshall, St. Thomas's Hospital, London). Note, photoreceptor outer segment (POS); melanosomes (M) located toward the apical portion of the cell; lipofuscin granules (L) in the central to basal region; a high density of basally located mitochondria (Mt); Bruch's membrane (BM). **(B)** Fluorescence microscopy of tissue sections from 9-, 43-, and 97-year-old donors showing an increase in fluorescent lipofuscin granules with increasing age. **(C)** A scanning electron micrograph showing RPE cells from an 85-year-old donor. The cells are so packed with lipofuscin granules that their outline can be seen pressing against the cell membrane. (Reproduced courtesy of John Marshall, St. Thomas's Hospital, London). **(D)** A confocal image of flat-mount human RPE showing the variable distribution of lipofuscin between individual cells. The annulus devoid of lipofuscin surrounds a druse. (Image provided by Boulton and Njoh.)

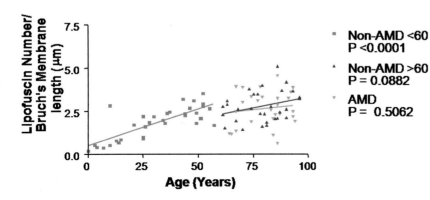

- **Non-AMD <60**
  P <0.0001

- **Non-AMD >60**
  P = 0.0882

- **AMD**
  P = 0.5062

FIGURE 2.2.   Graph showing the number of lipofuscin granules/μm of Bruch's membrane for non-AMD donors and donors with AMD as a function of age. Regression analysis showed a significant increase in RPE lipofuscin granules up to age 50 and a tendency to plateau between 60 and 100 years. (Data provided by Boulton and Njoh.)

reducing the functional capacity of the RPE with increasing age. In old age, the cytoplasmic volume occupied by the equatorial and peripheral RPE is considerably less than that in the central retina.

In addition to the regional distribution of lipofuscin across the fundus, there is considerable cell-to-cell heterogeneity in lipofuscin density in any particular region of the retina (Fig. 2.1) (12). It is evident that two adjacent cells (presumably with the same functional and metabolic load) can have high, intermediate, or minimal levels of lipofuscin. This would support the proposal by Burke and Hjelmeland (12) that mosaicism of the RPE is a natural result of normal mechanisms regulating gene expression during development and postnatal aging. This heterogeneity may help explain the highly focal nature of the lesions associated with pathologies such as AMD.

Among the different tissue lipofuscins, RPE lipofuscin has a number of unique properties that determine its photophysical properties and its potential for contributing to RPE dysfunction, as will be discussed in more detail below. First, RPE lipofuscin is derived at least in part from POS and thus contains significant quantities of retinoids (4,13), including the diretinal conjugate A2E (4). Second, RPE lipofuscin is a broadband absorber that is constantly exposed to visible light and is located in a high-oxygen environment, which makes it an ideal substrate for retinal photodamage (1).

LIPOFUSCIN GENESIS AND COMPOSITION

Although RPE lipofuscin is believed to result from the incomplete degradation of POS and autophagy of spent or damaged intracellular organelles, the relative contributions of these pathways remain unknown. It is thought that prior oxidative damage to these substrates renders them undegradable by the lysosomal system, the universal intracellular degradation machinery that contains over 40 hydrolytic enzymes. However, prior oxidation does not account for the fluorescent properties of lipofuscin, since Eldred and Katz (14,15) showed that the autofluorescent products of lipid peroxidation differ from those of lipofuscin. Although we have gained an understanding of the initial substrates involved in lipofuscin genesis, we still have a limited understanding of the composition of the mature lipofuscin granules. Probably the first attempt at analysis was made by Eldred and Katz (13), who used Folch's extraction to separate lipofuscin into three fractions: chloroform-soluble, methanol-soluble, and insoluble (Fig. 2.3A). Thin-layer chromotography analysis of the chloroform fraction revealed 10 discrete fluorophores: two green-emitting, which comigrated with retinol and retinyl palmitate; three emitting yellow/green; and one golden-yellow and four orange-red fluorophores, the most prominent of which was subsequently identified as A2E (Fig. 2.3) (16). Further studies by other researchers identified the fluorophores as retinoid derivatives (4,17). This was followed by many studies on the role of A2E, the only readily synthetic component of lipofuscin, and demonstrations of its phototoxic and lysosomotrophic properties. However, the content of the bulk (>70%) of lipofuscin material, which is located at the insoluble interface on Folch's extraction, has largely been ignored (18).

It has long been considered that lipofuscin consists of cross-linked oxidatively modified lipids, proteins, and sugars, with the protein content ranging from 10% to 70% of the lipofuscin granule. The first proteome for RPE lipofuscin was reported by Schutt and colleagues (19) in 2002. They identified over 65 abundant cellular proteins, including cytoskeleton proteins, proteins of transduction, enzymes of metabolism, proteins of the mitochondrial respiratory chain, ion channel proteins, and chaperones, which supported the origin of lipofuscin as a combination of photoreceptor phagocytosis and autophagy. Furthermore, analysis of the samples revealed that many of

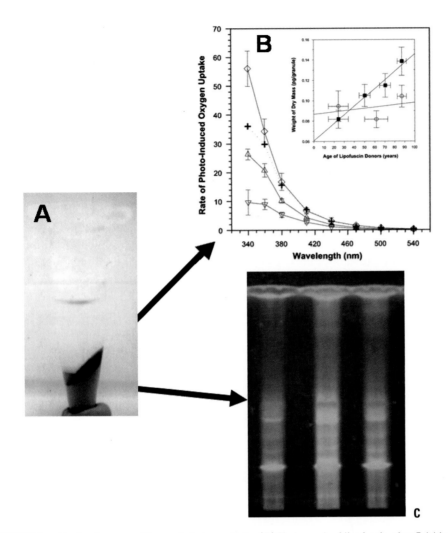

FIGURE 2.3. Lipofuscin composition and photoreactivity. **(A)** Photograph of lipofuscin after Folch's extraction. The top layer is the methanol/water phase, the bottom layer is the chloroform-soluble phase, and insoluble material is located at the interface. **(B)** Comparison of the action spectra of initial rates of photo-induced oxygen uptake in suspensions of DMPC liposomes containing both the chloroform-soluble (△) and insoluble (▽) interfacial material plus a combination ("reconstituted lipofuscin", ◇). The arithmetic addition (+) is shown of the rates measured separately for the chloroform-soluble and chloroform-insoluble fractions. The inset shows the change in content of dry mass of the chloroform-soluble (○) and chloroform-insoluble (■) material extracted from lipofuscin granules as a function of donor age. Horizontal bars: SD of the donors of the pooled samples; vertical bars: SD of the dry mass measurements (reproduced courtesy of Investigative Ophthalmology and Visual Science from Ref. 18). **(C)** Comparison of the thin-layer chromatography profile of the chloroform-soluble fraction of pooled lipofuscin granules from donors of different ages: 1) 50–59 years; 2) 60–69 years; 3) 70–79 years. The fractions show a number of different fluorophores when excited by UV irradiation.

these proteins were damaged by the aberrant covalent modifications of MDA, 4-HNE and AGEs (20). In a subsequent proteome analysis of RPE lipofuscin, Warburton et al. (21) identified 41 cellular proteins; surprisingly, only 11% these proteins had been identified in the proteomic analysis of Schutt and colleagues (19). Although there are numerous explanations for this discrepancy, the likely problem lies in the purity of the starting material. Lipofuscin is generally isolated by repeated sucrose density gradient centrifugation (19,21,22); however, there is usually some residual contamination by cellular debris (22). While investigating this further, we demonstrated that highly purified debris-free RPE lipofuscin granules contain little or no protein, but do contain significant amounts of modified material, such as carboxyethylpyrrole adducts (23). In conclusion, although our understanding of the composition of lipofuscin in the RPE remains limited, it does appear that protein makes only a very small contribution, if any, and that oxidized and modified lipids from outer-segment and mitochondrial membranes may be major contributors.

Spectral Characteristics of RPE Lipofuscin

RPE lipofuscin granules exhibit a broad and wavelength-dependent absorption spectrum with a decrease in absorption toward increasing wavelengths (22). The excitation and emission spectra of lipofuscin granules are shown in Figure 2.4, and a summary of excitation and emission peaks is provided in Table 2.1. RPE lipofuscin granules typically exhibit four main regions of interest in the emission spectra when excited at 364 nm: the main peak located at 600–610 nm, a blue-green shoulder located at 470 nm, a green-yellow shoulder at 550 nm, and, in the case of lipofuscin from individuals over 50 years, a far red shoulder at 680 nm. Similar emission peaks are observed at 500, 610, and 680 nm when lipofuscin is excited at 476 nm, which is similar to the excitation employed by in vivo autofluorescence (AF) systems (≥488 nm) (24,25). Excitation spec-

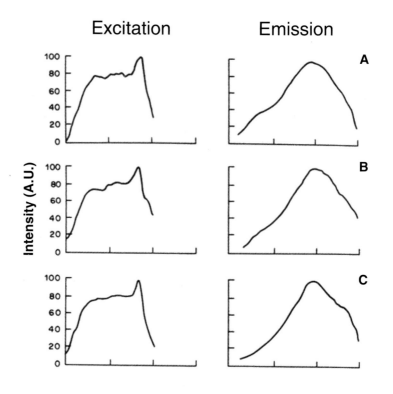

FIGURE 2.4.   Excitation and emission spectra of intact lipofuscin granules isolated from donors of different ages. Excitation spectra were monitored with emission performed at 570 nm and emission spectra were monitored with excitation performed at 364 nm. Lipofuscin granules were prepared from different age groups: **(A)** 5–29 years; **(B)** 30–49 years; **(C)** >50 years. Excitation and emission spectra are expressed in arbitrary units (A.U.). (Modified from Ref. 22.)

TABLE 2.1	Summary of the Main Fluorescence Peaks for Lipofuscin Granules From Different Age Groups Observed in Figure 2.4. Excitation spectra were monitored with emission performed at 570 nm, and emission spectra were monitored with excitation performed at 364 nm.

Sample age (yr)	Excitation (nm)	Emission (nm)	Total Peak Amplitude[a]
5–29	370, 405, 470	470, 550, 600	1.00
30–49	370, 405, 470	470, 550, 600	1.71
50–80	370, 470	570, 600, 680	1.95

[a]Normalized to the 5–29 yr group.

tra with emissions monitored at 610 nm or 570 nm show a main excitation peak at 470 nm, with two subsidiary peaks at 370 and 405 nm (22). Time-resolved fluorescence microscopy has identified four decay components in lipofuscin with decay times of approximately 0.21, 0.65, 1.75, and 6.6 ns (26). Wavelength-resolved decay analysis demonstrated that the three main fluorescing components of lipofuscin do not strongly interact and thus appear to be excited directly. The spectral characteristics of melano-lipofuscin are intermediate between those of lipofuscin and melanin.

The fluorescence properties of lipofuscin granules exhibit age-related changes. The fluorescence intensity of lipofuscin granules increases by up to 40% with increasing age (22). Whether this is due to increased deposition of material in the lipofuscin or a change in composition is unclear. It should also be emphasized that there is considerable heterogeneity in the fluorescence properties between individual lipofuscin granules, with variations in both emission maxima and spectral shape (27,28). Thus, lipofuscin spectra generally represent an average of all these spectral differences.

Aging, Lipofuscin, and the Potential for Chronic Light Damage

The spectral characteristics of lipofuscin together with its localization in a high-oxygen environment and diurnal exposure to visible light make it an ideal substrate for photochemical reactions. Our laboratory was the first to demonstrate that lipofuscin is able to photogenerate reactive oxygen species (ROS) when we demonstrated that exposure of isolated human RPE lipofuscin granules to light results in the generation of the superoxide anion (29). That study also showed that the photogeneration of ROS was dependent on both light intensity and wavelength, with the highest levels of superoxide anions being generated at higher visible light intensities and shorter (blue) wavelengths of visible light. Subsequent studies demonstrated that isolated human lipofuscin granules are able to photogenerate significant quantities of singlet oxygen, hydroxyl radical, hydrogen peroxide, and the longer-lived lipid hydroperoxides (30–32). There is evidence that the overall photoreactivity of lipofuscin increases with increasing age (18). It appears that this is due to an increase in one or more of the components in the chloroform-insoluble fraction obtained from lipofuscin granules (Fig. 2.3). Analyses of blue-light photoreactivity in isolated RPE cells from donors of different ages demonstrated a significant age-related increase in oxygen photo-uptake (an indicator of ROS formation), primarily due to the presence of lipofuscin within the cells (30). Not surprisingly, the lipofuscin-photogenerated ROS are capable of eliciting oxidative modification to lipids, proteins, and nucleic acids. Lipofuscin granules exposed to light induce oxidation of both intra- and extragranular lipids, and inactivate critical RPE enzymes, including the lysosomal and antioxidant enzymes (33). The impact of these photo-oxidative reactions on cell function was assessed in a cell culture system in which lipofuscin-containing RPE cultures were exposed to 2.8 mWcm^2 blue light (390–550 nm) or amber light (550–700 nm), or maintained in the dark (34,35). Exposure of lipofuscin-containing cells to blue light resulted in lipid peroxidation, formation of the aldehydes MDA and 4HNE, protein-carbonyl formation indicative of protein oxidation, nuclear but not mitochondrial DNA damage, loss of lysosomal integrity, cytoplasmic vacuolation, and membrane blebbing culminating in cell death within 48 hours (Fig. 2.5) (34,35). RPE dysfunction could be observed within 3 hours of exposure of lipofuscin-containing cells to blue light and was associated with DNA damage, a reduction in antioxidant status, and a decrease in lysosomal enzyme activity (34,36). Neither cells exposed to equivalent irradiant energy amber light nor cells maintained in the dark exhibited any oxidative changes or loss of cell function. The ability of lipofuscin to cause photo-oxidative damage to all components extrinsic to the lysosomal compartment indicates the importance of longer-lived and less reactive ROS, such as lipid peroxides, that have a greater chance to cause oxidative damage throughout the cell.

The most studied of the potential photosensitizers of RPE lipofuscin is A2E (4,32,37). Although A2E makes a major contribution to lipofuscin fluorescence by serving as an energy acceptor from other blue-light-absorbing molecules within lipofus-

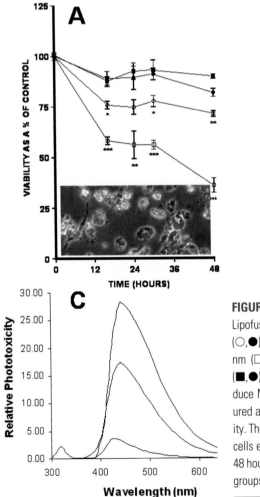

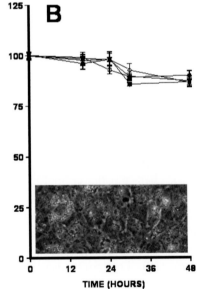

FIGURE 2.5. The photoreactivity of RPE lipofuscin. Lipofuscin-fed RPE cells (□,■) and cells lacking lipofuscin (○,●) were exposed to 2.8 m/WCm^2 light; **(A)** 390–550 nm (□,○); **(B)** 550–800 nm; or maintained in the dark (■,●) for up to 48 hour. The ability of the RPE cells to reduce MTT to a blue formazan product (absorbance measured at 590/630 nm) was used as a measure of cell viability. The insets show light micrographs of lipofuscin-fed RPE cells exposed to light **(A)** or maintained in the dark **(B)** for 48 hour. Phototoxicity action spectra for three different age groups **(C)** are shown. (Modified from Refs. 34 and 41.)

cin (38), it is itself only weakly photoreactive compared to the hydrophobic components of lipofuscin (31,39). Despite its weak photoreactivity, A2E can, at high concentrations, elicit blue-light-induced RPE cell dysfunction and cell death in cell culture. However, other A2E-related molecules, such as A2E epoxides, are also present in lipofuscin and these may be more photoreactive than A2E itself (4,40). Based on the spectral characteristics and photoreactivity of lipofuscin, there is strong evidence to suggest that lipofuscin may contribute to the pathogenesis of AMD (41) (see also Chapter 10). First, longitudinal studies of in vivo fluorescence have shown that areas of the retina with the highest lipofuscin levels are most susceptible to degeneration (24,42,43). Second, the chronology of RPE lipofuscin accumulation is coincident with the development of AMD (6). Third, since the RPE is composed of postmitotic cells, ROS damage will accumulate throughout life. Fortunately, the crystalline lens attenuates the shorter wavelengths of light reaching the retina, and this effect will be greater in older brunescent lenses. However, even when the age-related changes in the transmission characteristics of the ocular media are taken into account, the overall phototoxicity of lipofuscin increases substantially with age because the protective effects of lens senescence are partly offset by a substantial increase in the concentration of photoreactive lipofuscin granules in the retina (Fig. 2.5) (41). Although this phototoxicity increases steadily with age, the potential for photoinducible damage will be many times greater where there are focal "hot spots" of lipofuscin.

A2E and Lipofuscin

Eldred and Lasky (16) were the first to identify the major fluorophore in the chloroform-soluble extract of lipofuscin as A2E. The formation of A2E begins in the POS with condensation reactions between phosphatidylethanolamine (PE) and two molecules of all-trans-retinal (ATR) released from activated rhodopsin (4,17). The product of the initial Schiff-base reaction between a single ATR and PE is N-retinylidine-PE (NRPE). The biosynthetic pathway continues through a number of steps, including the addition of the second ATR to form the phosphatidyl-pyridinium bisretinoid that is the immediate precursor to A2E (4,44) and the fluorescent pigment that accumulates in POS. Although there is general agreement that A2-PE undergoes enzymatic cleavage to form A2E (17,45), it is unclear whether this cleavage occurs in the outer segment prior to ingestion or after uptake into secondary lysosomes (4,17). However, A2E ends up within the lysosomes containing lipofuscin granules and, because of its nondegradable qualities, its overall concentration in the RPE, not unexpectedly, increases in parallel with lipofuscin accumulation. It is also evident that A2E can undergo a variety of changes, including photoisomerization and oxidation, to produce a variety of A2E derivatives (4).

Although A2E has been shown to be present in lipofuscin, and exposure of RPE cell cultures to chemically synthesized A2E in solution can cause cell dysfunction and death, the actual importance of A2E to the overall composition and cytotoxicity of lipofuscin has never really been proven and a number of contradictions can be found in the literature (45). First, the absorption properties of A2E account for only a small proportion of the visible light absorbed by lipofuscin (45). Second, it is unclear to what extent A2E contributes to the fluorescence spectrum of lipofuscin, since intracellular A2E has a maximum emission at 560–575 nm and lipofuscin granules have maximum emissions at 600–610 nm (9). Third, low concentrations of A2E protect against UV-induced DNA damage in RPE cells in vitro (46). Fourth, A2E is not the major photosensitizer responsible for the generation of ROS by mature lipofuscin granules (34). Fifth, the bioavailability of A2E in the RPE remains difficult to determine, and to date there is no evidence that A2E or its derivatives can be released from lipofuscin granules once it has been sequestered.

Notwithstanding these observations, it is known that synthetic A2E applied directly to RPE cells in culture is phototoxic when exposed to blue light; it can cause oxidation of cellular constituents through the photogeneration of singlet oxygen (40); it upregulates the expression of angiogenic factors such as VEGF (47); it is lysosomotrophic and able to destabilize lysosomal membranes, resulting in reduced lysosomal enzyme activity (48); and it can reduce mitochondrial capacity, leading to apoptosis (37). In addition, photo-oxidation products of A2E can lead to complement activation (49). Thus it is clear that A2E has the potential to cause RPE cell damage, but whether in vivo this occurs pre- or postincorporation into lipofuscin granules remains to be shown.

Association Between Lipofuscin and Retinal Degeneration

Elevated lipofuscin levels, as demonstrated by fundus AF imaging, are associated with a variety of retinal degenerations (24,43,50,51) (see "Fundus Autofluorescence in the Diseased Eye" section). Although all of these conditions demonstrate increased AF and elevated numbers of lipofuscin granules within the RPE, the composition of the granules may well vary significantly. Furthermore, it is difficult to determine whether lipofuscin is a cause or consequence of these conditions. However, in the case of AMD, there is considerable circumstantial evidence linking lipofuscin with the etiology of the disease. First, lipofuscin can be observed in early drusen, and these may serve as an immunogenic stimulus for the localized activation of dendritic cells and deposition of inflammatory factors (52). Confocal microscopy demonstrates two lipofuscin profiles in the overlying RPE. One presents as a ring of hypofluorescence surrounding drusen, and the other presents as a central area with decreased lipofuscin (Njoh and Boulton, unpublished results). Furthermore, subretinal exocytosis of lipofuscin granules appears to be a feature of eyes >60 years of age and results in degradation of these granules in the extracellular sub-RPE space (Hageman, Boulton, and Njoh, unpublished results). Second, the highest density of lipofuscin is located in the central retina, where the density of rod outer segments is at its highest and where there is a preferential loss of rod cells in AMD (53). Third, the accumulation of lipofuscin is reported to be greater in whites than in blacks (54,55), and AMD is more prevalent among whites than among black persons (56). Fourth, chronic phototoxicity, lysosomotrophic damage, and occupation of cytoplasmic volume in RPE cells by lipofuscin and its constituent A2E throughout life will contribute to RPE dysfunction and put added stress on a highly metabolically active cell type (1,4). Fifth, longitudinal in vivo monitoring of fundus AF has demonstrated that the presence of focal increased AF is a risk factor for progression of AMD (57) (Fig. 2.6). Furthermore, zones of RPE exhibiting increased fundus AF signal are prone to atrophy (24,43,58), and these areas exhibit a variable loss of retinal sensitivity that suggests an association between RPE dysfunction and excessive accumulation of lipofuscin (59). Sixth, synthetic A2E when photoactivated can induce the expression of angiogenic factors in RPE cells (47). Seventh, photo-oxidation products of A2E can activate complement, and this may contribute to the chronic inflammation associated with AMD (49). Eighth, lipofuscin levels have been observed to be elevated in rodent models for AMD (60–62). Furthermore, in Stargardt disease there is an abnormality in the *abcr* gene that leads to a buildup of the lipofuscin fluorophore A2E (see also Chapter 11G) (63). The predisposition for excessive lipofuscin accumulation in retinal degenerations such as AMD and, in particular, its elevation during the early stages of disease progression suggest that lipofuscin makes a significant contribution to the pathogenesis of AMD rather than simply being a consequence of the disease.

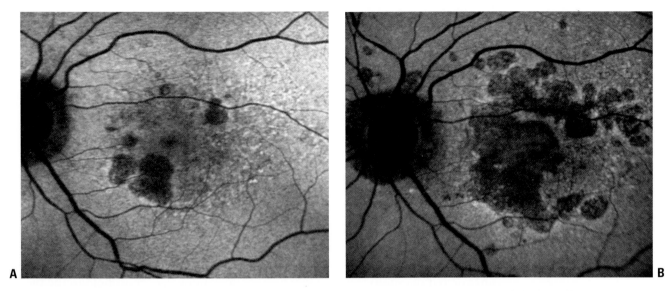

FIGURE 2.6.   (A) Fundus AF image of a 74-year-old patient with visual acuity 20/40 taken in 2005 with a Heidelberg HRA II scanning laser ophthalmoscope. Several areas of RPE atrophy are noted, with a few small areas of increased AF at the borders of the larger lesions. At this time the AF in the fovea was regular and the patient was told that progression of his condition was imminent. **(B)** Two years later the patient was reexamined and visual acuity had decreased to 20/200; AF taken with the same instrument showed extensive geographic atrophy, including the foveal area. (Image and caption provided by Dr. Erik Van Kuijk, Ophthalmology and Visual Sciences, University of Texas Medical Branch, Galveston, Texas.)

Reducing the Impact of Lipofuscin on Aging and Retinal Degeneration

If, as the evidence above suggests, lipofuscin is cytotoxic and contributes to the pathogenesis of retinal degenerations such as AMD and Stargardt disease, then a strategy to remove or prevent further formation of lipofuscin would be efficacious. There are a number of paradigms to support this: (a) lipofuscin can be voided into sub-RPE space, where it appears to be degraded; (b) lipofuscin deposition can be decreased with appropriate modification of the lysosomal compartment (64); and (c) knockout or modification of the RPE specific protein RPE65, a critical component of the retinoid cycle, prevents accumulation of the retinoid component of lipofuscin (65,66). The most popular approach to date is to inhibit A2E formation by reducing retinoid turnover in the visual cycle (see also Chapters 10C and 11G).

A2E deposition is an endpoint that can be easily measured both in vitro in cultured RPE cells and in vivo using the *abcr−/−* mouse model for Stargardt disease (67). Isotretinoin (Accutane) and the small-molecule isoprenoid RPE65 antagonists reduce the formation and accumulation of A2E and other retinoid pigments in *abcr−/−* mice (68). An alternative approach is to reduce A2E accumulation by reducing serum vitamin A using N-(4-hydroxyphenyl)retinamide (69). Although all of these approaches are promising, they have two major limitations: (a) targeting the retinoid cycle is likely to affect visual functions, and there is clear evidence that many of these agents slow dark adaptation and/or reduce impaired electroretinogram (ERG) responses (67,70); and (b) although A2E fluorophores are reduced, there has been little morphometric analysis to confirm a significant reduction in the lipofuscin granules within the RPE. Fenretinide, currently in clinical trial (see also Chapter 10C), is the most recently developed agent aimed at reducing the retinoid cycle, but evidence suggests that this may actually promote choroidal neovascularization (CNV) in compromised eyes (71).

Alternative approaches that are aimed primarily at attacking the nonretinoid composition of lipofuscin include reducing the accumulation of lipofuscin by either a) preventing the formation of intralysosomal ROS, which crosslink intralysosomal material using iron chelators (64), or b) preventing the formation of cross-linking adducts in lipofuscin by increasing levels of intralysosomal glutathione-s-transferase and facilitating the degradation of lipofuscin substrates. There is no doubt that the next decade will see the development of a variety of therapeutic approaches for preventing or removing lipofuscin accumulation.

LIPOFUSCIN—THE UNANSWERED QUESTIONS

In the last two decades there has been a major emphasis on RPE lipofuscin research, and studies have provided invaluable information on the composition, photobiological properties, and association of lipofuscin with retinal degenerations such as AMD and Stargardt disease. However, despite our increased knowledge, there are still many unanswered questions. First, to what extent does autophagy contribute to the biogenesis of RPE lipofuscin? Research would suggest that the mitochondria, which are abundant in RPE cells, are compromised in aging and AMD (72) and thus their turnover may be much greater. Second, if protein is only a minor component in lipofuscin, what are the nonretinoid constituents? Of interest, autofluorescent lipofuscin-like granules accumulate in long-term RPE cultures without exposure to POS or retinoids (73,74). These granules are highly photoreactive. Third, what is the importance of A2E within the lipofuscin granule? Is it inactive when sequestered into the lipofuscin granule, and can it be released? Fourth, what are the fluorophores in lipofuscin? Clearly A2E is one, but there must be many more since A2E does not account for a large part of the excitation or emission spectra of lipofuscin granules either in vivo or in vitro. Fifth, is lipofuscin immunogenic and does its release into the sub-RPE space lead to a localized inflammatory response? Sixth, what is melanolipofuscin? Given the heterogeneous composition of these granules, they cannot be simply derived from the fusion of melanosomes and lipofuscin granules as suggested in some textbooks. Seventh, can we degrade existing lipofuscin or prevent its accumulation by pharmacological intervention? Finally, is lipofuscin a cause or a consequence of retinal degenerations? It is hoped that research over the next decade will clarify these issues and both improve our understanding of retinal pathogenesis and identify effective pharmacological treatments for diseases in which lipofuscin is prevalent.

REFERENCES

1. Boulton M, Rozanowska M, Rozanowski B, et al. The photoreactivity of ocular lipofuscin. Photochem Photobiol Sci 2004;3:759–764.
2. Sohal RS. Age Pigments. Amsterdam: Elsevier/North-Holland Biomedical Press, 1981.
3. Seehafer S, Pearce P. You say lipofuscin, we say ceroid. Defining autofluorescent storage material. Neurobiol Aging 2006;27:576–588.
4. Sparrow JR, Boulton ME. RPE lipofuscin and its role in retinal pathology. Exp Eye Res 2005;80:595–606.
5. Terman A, Gustafsson B, Brunk UT. Autophagy, organelles and ageing. J Pathol 2007;211:134–143.
6. Boulton M. Ageing of the retinal pigment epithelium. In: Osborne N, Chader G, eds. Progress in Retinal Research. Oxford: Pergamon Press, 1991:125–151.
7. Feeney L. Lipofuscin and melanin of human retinal pigment epithelium. Fluorescence, enzyme cytochemical, and ultrastructural studies. Invest Ophthalmol Vis Sci 1978;17:583–600.
8. Feeney-Burns L, Hilderbrand ES, Eldridge S. Aging human RPE: morphometric analysis of macular, equatorial, and peripheral cells. Invest Ophthalmol Vis Sci 1984;25:195–200.
9. Delori FC, Goger DG, Dorey CK. Age-related accumulation and spatial distribution of lipofuscin in RPE of normal subjects. Invest Ophthalmol Vis Sci 2001;42:1855–1866.
10. Wing GL, Blanchard GC, Weiter JJ. The topography and age relationship of lipofuscin concentration in the retinal pigment epithelium. Invest Ophthalmol Vis Sci 1978;17:601–607.

11. Marshall J. The ageing retina: physiology or pathology? Eye 1987;1:282–295.
12. Burke JM, Hjelmeland LM. Mosaicism of the retinal pigment epithelium: seeing the small picture. Mol Interv 2005;5:241–249.
13. Eldred GE, Katz ML. Fluorophores of the human retinal pigment epithelium: separation and spectral characterization. Exp Eye Res 1988;47:71–86.
14. Eldred GE, Katz ML. The autofluorescent products of lipid peroxidation may not be lipofuscin-like. Free Radic Biol Med 1989;7:157–163.
15. Eldred GE, Katz ML. The lipid peroxidation theory of lipofuscinogenesis cannot yet be confirmed. Free Radic Biol Med 1991;10:445–447.
16. Eldred GE, Lasky MR. Retinal age pigments generated by self-assembling lysosomotropic detergents. Nature 1993;361:724–726.
17. Lamb LE, Simon JD. A2E: a component of ocular lipofuscin. Photochem Photobiol 2004;79:127–136.
18. Rozanowska M, Pawlak A, Rozanowski B, et al. Age-related changes in the photoreactivity of retinal lipofuscin granules: role of chloroform-insoluble components. Invest Ophthalmol Vis Sci 2004;45:1052–1060.
19. Schutt F, Ueberle B, Schnolzer M, et al. Proteome analysis of lipofuscin in human retinal pigment epithelial cells. FEBS Lett 2002;528:217–221.
20. Schutt F, Bergmann M, Holz FG, et al. Proteins modified by malondialdehyde, 4-hydroxynonenal, or advanced glycation end products in lipofuscin of human retinal pigment epithelium. Invest Ophthalmol Vis Sci 2003;44:3663–3668.
21. Warburton S, Southwick K, Hardman RM, et al. Examining the proteins of functional retinal lipofuscin using proteomic analysis as a guide for understanding its origin. Mol Vis 2005;11:1122–1134.
22. Boulton M, Docchio F, Dayhaw-Barker P, et al. Age-related changes in the morphology, absorption and fluorescence of melanosomes and lipofuscin granules of the retinal pigment epithelium. Vision Res 1990;30:1291–1303.
23. Ng KP, Gugiu B, Renganathan K, et al. Retinal pigment epithelium lipofuscin proteomics. Mol Cell Proteomics 2008;7:1397–1405.
24. Holz FG, Bindewald-Wittich A, Fleckenstein M, et al. Progression of geographic atrophy and impact of fundus autofluorescence patterns in age-related macular degeneration. Am J Ophthalmol 2007;143:463–472.
25. von Ruckmann A, Fitzke FW, Gregor ZJ. Fundus autofluorescence in patients with macular holes imaged with a laser scanning ophthalmoscope. Br J Ophthalmol 1998;82:346–351.
26. Docchio F, Boulton M, Cubeddu R, et al. Age-related changes in the fluorescence of melanin and lipofuscin granules of the retinal pigment epithelium: a time-resolved fluorescence spectroscopy study. Photochem Photobiol 1991;54:247–253.
27. Clancy KMR, Krogmeier JR, Pawlak A, et al. Atomic force microscopy and near-field scanning optical microscopy measurements of single human retinal lipofuscin granules. J Phys Chem B 2000;104:12098–12101.
28. Haralampus-Grynaviski NM, et al. Probing the spatial dependence of the emission spectrum of single human retinal lipofuscin granules using near-field scanning optical microscopy. Photochem Photobiol 2001;74:364–368.
29. Boulton M, Lamb LE, Simon JD, et al. Lipofuscin is a photoinducible free radical generator. J Photochem Photobiol B 1993;19:201–204.
30. Rozanowska M, Jarvis-Evans J, Korytowski W, et al. Blue light-induced reactivity of retinal age pigment. In vitro generation of oxygen-reactive species. J Biol Chem 1995;270:18825–18830.
31. Rozanowska M, Wessels J, Boulton M, et al. Blue light-induced singlet oxygen generation by retinal lipofuscin in non-polar media. Free Radic Biol Med 1998;24:1107–1112.
32. Sparrow JR, Nakanishi K, Parish CA. The lipofuscin fluorophore A2E mediates blue light-induced damage to retinal pigmented epithelial cells. Invest Ophthalmol Vis Sci 2000;41:1981–1989.
33. Wassell J, Davies S, Bardsley W, et al. The photoreactivity of the retinal age pigment lipofuscin. J Biol Chem 1999;274:23828–23832.
34. Davies S, Elliott MH, Floor E, et al. Photocytotoxicity of lipofuscin in human retinal pigment epithelial cells. Free Radic Biol Med 2001;31:256–265.
35. Godley BF, Shamsi FA, Liang FQ, et al. Blue light induces mitochondrial DNA damage and free radical production in epithelial cells. J Biol Chem 2005;280:21061–21066.
36. Shamsi FA, Boulton M. Inhibition of RPE lysosomal and antioxidant activity by the age pigment lipofuscin. Invest Ophthalmol Vis Sci 2001;42:3041–3046.
37. Sparrow JR, Cai B. Blue light-induced apoptosis of A2E-containing RPE: involvement of caspase-3 and protection by Bcl-2. Invest Ophthalmol Vis Sci 2001;42:1356–1362.
38. Haralampus-Grynaviski NM, Lamb LE, Clancy CM, et al. Spectroscopic and morphological studies of human retinal lipofuscin granules. Proc Natl Acad Sci USA 2003;100:3179–3184.
39. Gaillard ER, Atherton SJ, Eldred G, et al. Photophysical studies on human retinal lipofuscin. Photochem Photobiol 1995;61:448–453.
40. Ben-Shabat S, Itagaki Y, Jockusch S, et al. Formation of a nonaoxirane from A2E, a lipofuscin fluorophore related to macular degeneration, and evidence of singlet oxygen involvement. Angew Chem Int Ed Engl 2002;41:814–817.
41. Margrain TH, Boulton M, Marshall J, et al. Do blue light filters confer protection against age-related macular degeneration? Prog Retin Eye Res 2004;23:523–531.
42. Bindewald A, Bird AC, Dandekar SS, et al. Classification of fundus autofluorescence patterns in early age-related macular disease. Invest Ophthalmol Vis Sci 2005;46:3309–3314.

43. Lois N, Owens SL, Coco R, et al. Fundus autofluorescence in patients with age-related macular degeneration and high risk of visual loss. Am J Ophthalmol 2002;133:341–349.

44. Parish CA, Hashimoto M, Nakanishi K, et al. Isolation and one-step preparation of A2E and iso-A2E, fluorophores from human retinal pigment epithelium. Proc Natl Acad Sci USA 1998;95:14609–14613.

45. Rozanowska M, Sarna T. Light-induced damage to the retina: role of rhodopsin chromophore revisited. Photochem Photobiol 2005;81:1305–1330.

46. Roberts JE, Kukielczak BM, Hu DN, et al. The role of A2E in prevention or enhancement of light damage in human retinal pigment epithelial cells. Photochem Photobiol 2002;75:184–190.

47. Zhou J, Cai B, Jang YP, et al. Mechanisms for the induction of HNE- MDA- and AGE-adducts, RAGE and VEGF in retinal pigment epithelial cells. Exp Eye Res 2005;80:567–580.

48. Holz FG, Schütt F, Kopitz J, et al. Inhibition of lysosomal degradative functions in RPE cells by a retinoid component of lipofuscin. Invest Ophthalmol Vis Sci 1999;40:737–743.

49. Zhou, J, Jang YP, Kim SR, et al. Complement activation by photooxidation products of A2E, a lipofuscin constituent of the retinal pigment epithelium. Proc Natl Acad Sci USA 2006;103:16182–16187.

50. von Ruckmann A, Fitzke FW, Bird AC. Distribution of pigment epithelium autofluorescence in retinal disease state recorded in vivo and its change over time. Graefes Arch Clin Exp Ophthalmol 1999;237:1–9.

51. von Ruckmann A, Fitzke FW, Bird AC. In vivo fundus autofluorescence in macular dystrophies. Arch Ophthalmol 1997;115:609–615.

52. Hageman GS, Mullins RF. Molecular composition of drusen as related to substructural phenotype. Mol Vis 1999;5:28.

53. Curcio CA, Medeiros NE, Millican CL. Photoreceptor loss in age-related macular degeneration. Invest Ophthalmol Vis Sci 1996;37:1236–1249.

54. Weiter JJ, Delori FC, Wing GL, et al. Retinal pigment epithelial lipofuscin and melanin and choroidal melanin in human eyes. Invest Ophthalmol Vis Sci 1986;27:145–152.

55. Dorey CK, Wu G, Ebenstein D, et al. Cell loss in the aging retina. Relationship to lipofuscin accumulation and macular degeneration. Invest Ophthalmol Vis Sci 1989;30:1691–1699.

56. Friedman DS, O'Colmain BJ, Muñoz B, et al. Prevalence of age-related macular degeneration in the United States. Arch Ophthalmol 2004;122:564–572.

57. Solbach U, Keilhauer C, Knabben H, et al. Imaging of retinal autofluorescence in patients with age-related macular degeneration. Retina 1997;17:385–389.

58. Holz FG, Bellman C, Staudt S, et al. Fundus autofluorescence and development of geographic atrophy in age-related macular degeneration. Invest Ophthalmol Vis Sci 2001;42:1051–1056.

59. Schmitz-Valckenberg S, Bültmann S, Dreyhaupt J, et al. Fundus autofluorescence and fundus perimetry in the junctional zone of geographic atrophy in patients with age-related macular degeneration. Invest Ophthalmol Vis Sci 2004;45:4470–4476.

60. Ambati J, Anand A, Fernandez S, et al. An animal model of age-related macular degeneration in senescent Ccl-2- or Ccr-2-deficient mice. Nat Med 2003;9:1390–1397.

61. Malek G, Johnson LV, Mace BE, et al. Apolipoprotein E allele-dependent pathogenesis: a model for age-related retinal degeneration. Proc Natl Acad Sci USA 2005;102:11900–11905.

62. Justilien V, Pang JJ, Renganathan K, et al. SOD2 knockdown mouse model of early AMD. Invest Ophthalmol Vis Sci 2007;48:4407–4420.

63. Mata NL, Weng J, Travis GH. Biosynthesis of a major lipofuscin fluorophore in mice and humans with ABCR-mediated retinal and macular degeneration. Proc Natl Acad Sci USA 2000;97:7154–7159.

64. Kurz T. Can lipofuscin accumulation be prevented? Rejuvenation Res 2008;11:441–443.

65. Katz ML, Redmond TM. Effect of Rpe65 knockout on accumulation of lipofuscin fluorophores in the retinal pigment epithelium. Invest Ophthalmol Vis Sci 2001;42:3023–3030.

66. Kim SR, Fishkin N, Kong J, et al. Rpe65 Leu450Met variant is associated with reduced levels of the retinal pigment epithelium lipofuscin fluorophores A2E and iso-A2E. Proc Natl Acad Sci USA 2004;101:11668–11672.

67. Radu RA, Mata NL, Nusinowitz S, et al. Treatment with isotretinoin inhibits lipofuscin accumulation in a mouse model of recessive Stargardt's macular degeneration. Proc Natl Acad Sci USA 2003;100:4742–4747.

68. Maiti P, Kong J, Kim SR, et al. Small molecule RPE65 antagonists limit the visual cycle and prevent lipofuscin formation. Biochemistry 2006;45:852–860.

69. Radu RA, Han Y, Bui TV, et al. Reductions in serum vitamin A arrest accumulation of toxic retinal fluorophores: a potential therapy for treatment of lipofuscin-based retinal diseases. Invest Ophthalmol Vis Sci 2005;46:4393–4401.

70. Travis GH, Golczak M, Moise AR, et al. Diseases caused by defects in the visual cycle: retinoids as potential therapeutic agents. Annu Rev Pharmacol Toxicol 2007;47:469–512.

71. Sreekumar PG, Zhou J, Sohn J, et al. N-(4-hydroxyphenyl) retinamide augments laser-induced choroidal neovascularization in mice. Invest Ophthalmol Vis Sci 2008;49:1210–1220.

72. Xu H, Zhong X, Lin H, et al. Endogenous ROS production increases and mitochondrial redox function decreases in the RPE as a function of age and stage of AMD. Invest Ophthalmol Vis Sci 2008;49:ARVO E-abstract.

73. Wassell J, Ellis S, Burke J, et al. Fluorescence properties of autofluorescent granules generated by cultured human RPE cells. Invest Ophthalmol Vis Sci 1998;39:1487–1492.

74. Burke JM, Skumatz CM. Autofluorescent inclusions in long-term postconfluent cultures of retinal pigment epithelium. Invest Ophthalmol Vis Sci 1998;39:1478–1486.

Lipofuscin: The Origin of the Autofluorescence Signal

The retinal pigment epithelium (RPE) digests the tips of the outer segment of the photoreceptors, which are phagocytosed on a daily basis. The digestion process of these materials, which contain polysaturated fatty acids and byproducts of the visual cycle, is overall very efficient, but a tiny fraction is chemically incompatible for degradation and accumulates in lysosomes of the RPE. This undigested fraction is called lipofuscin (LF). Above the age of 70, as much as 20% to 33% of the free cytoplasmic space of the RPE cell may be occupied by LF granules and melano-lipofuscin granules, a compound product of LF and melanin (1).

LF is a pigment that exhibits a characteristic autofluorescence (AF) when excited in ultraviolet (UV) or blue light. Fluorescence microscopy of the RPE using UV or blue excitation light reveals distinctly bright orange-red or golden-yellow granules. This fluorescence also makes it possible to visualize and measure LF noninvasively, since the absorption spectrum of LF is monotonic (2) without any distinct spectral signature, and it would be very challenging to measure it by fundus reflectometry.

SPECTROFLUOROMETRY AND IMAGING OF FUNDUS AUTOFLUORESCENCE

Fundus AF was initially demonstrated in vivo by vitreous fluorophotometry, which revealed in preinjection scans a distinct "retinal" peak whose magnitude increased with age, as would be expected from LF fluorescence (3,4). These observations led to the development of a fundus spectrofluorometer (5,6) designed to measure the excitation and emission spectra of the AF from small retinal areas (2 degrees diameter) of the fundus and to allow absolute measurements of the fluorescence. The device incorporated an image-intensifier-diode-array as detector, beam separation in the pupil, and confocal detection to minimize the contribution of AF from the crystalline lens. This device was used initially to demonstrate that fundus AF essentially exhibits the characteristics of RPE LF (7).

Fundus AF is about 2 orders of magnitude less intense than the background fluorescence of a sodium fluorescein angiogram at the brightest part of the dye transit. As a result, AF imaging systems with high sensitivity and/or image averaging capabilities (8) are required to record the fundus AF with acceptable signal/noise ratios and safe retinal exposures. Confocal scanning laser ophthalmoscopy (SLO) (9) optimally addressed these requirements, and the first clinical AF imaging system was introduced at Moorfields in London with an excitation wavelength of 488 nm (10,11). Subsequent developments using confocal SLO systems, nonconfocal cameras, and different excitation wavelengths have further broadened the field of AF imaging (12–16).

RETINAL DISTRIBUTION OF AUTOFLUORESCENCE

AF images of the fundus show a central dark area caused by the light absorption by both RPE melanin and macular pigment that strongly absorbs wavelengths shorter than 540 nm (17). The AF signal is believed to originate posterior to the photoreceptors because it is affected by absorption by the visual pigments when the latter are not fully bleached. Indeed, the parafoveal difference spectrum, log (dark-adapted AF) − log (light-adapted AF), clearly reveals the spectrum of rhodopsin (7,18). Similarly, the AF is believed to originate anterior to the choriocapillaris because its emission spectrum does not reveal absorption bands of oxyhemoglobin (in contrast, the reflectance spectrum of the fundus shows these absorption bands at 540 and 575 nm) (19). These observations are consistent with the notion that the bulk of the AF emanates from the RPE. Clinical interpretations of AF images reinforce this conclusion. The AF emission spectrum in a full-thickness macular hole is similar in magnitude and shape to that measured at about 7 degrees eccentricity because the neurosensory retinal tissues are absent in the hole and the RPE is roughly intact (7,10). Conversely, RPE atrophy causes the AF emission spectrum from geographic atrophy in age-related macular degeneration (AMD) to be significantly reduced and distorted (20).

SPECTRAL PROPERTIES OF FUNDUS AUTOFLUORESCENCE

The emission spectra of fundus AF are broad (Fig. 3.1) and maximal in the 600–640 nm region of the spectrum, shifting slightly toward longer wavelengths with increasing excitation wavelength (21). This "red shift" occurs for excitations at the long wavelength end of the absorption spectrum for some fluorophores in viscous or polar environments (22). The red shift in large part explains the variability of emission spectra maxima reported in the literature; with excitation wavelengths ranging from 364 nm (lamp used in microscopy) to 580 nm (16), the emission peak will vary between 590 and 660 nm.

The excitation spectra have maxima between 490 and 530 nm. In contrast to the spectra measured 7 degrees temporal to the fovea, the foveal spectra are attenuated and distorted. This is due in part to the lower amount of LF in the foveal area (23), and to the absorption of the excitation light by macular pigment. The difference spectrum, log(foveal AF) − log(parafoveal AF), has the shape of the absorption spectrum of macular pigment (Fig. 3.1, inset), and this serves as the basis for the two-wavelength AF method to measure macular pigment (24). Note that the difference spectrum still decreases with increasing wavelength at 550–570 nm (arrow), where macular pigment does not absorb substantially. This is because of the absorption by RPE melanin, which decreases with wavelength and is larger at the fovea than at the parafovea (RPE melanin is located on the apical side of the RPE cell) (23,25).

INFLUENCE OF CRYSTALLINE LENS ABSORPTION

Excitation and emission spectra of fundus AF are affected by absorption and scattering in the lens and the other ocular media. For example, an excitation at 488 nm is attenuated, on average, by factors of 2.2 and 3.3 for ages 20 and 70 years, respectively (26). The AF emission is also attenuated, but to a lesser extent, because it occurs at longer

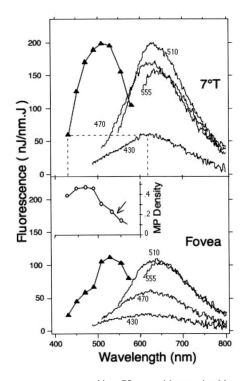

FIGURE 3.1. Fluorescence spectra measured in a 52-year-old normal subject at 7 degrees temporal to the fovea (7 degrees T) and at the fovea (sampling area: 2 degrees in diameter) (21). Continuous lines: emission spectra (excitation wavelength as indicated); line with filled triangle: excitation spectrum for emission at 620 nm. The excitation spectrum is not measured, but is constructed from the fluorescence at 620 nm and plotted against the excitation wavelength (*dotted line*). The foveal spectra are lower than at 7 degrees temporal, particularly for excitation wavelengths shorter than 490 nm, where absorption of the excitation light by macular pigment is revealed. *Inset*: Difference spectrum, [log(foveal AF) — log(parafoveal AF)], converted to macular pigment density using the absorption coefficients of the macular pigment.

wavelengths (factors of 1.4 and 1.5, respectively, when averaged over emissions from 500 to 700 nm). If absolute AF levels are needed, then corrections to account for the excitation and emission losses are required. These losses can be estimated for each subject by psychophysical (27) or reflectometric (28,29) methods. Alternatively, algorithms that predict the average light loss at a given wavelength and age can be used in population studies (26,30). Corrections obtained with such algorithms (26) result in a marked increase in AF. The corrected excitation spectrum is shifted toward shorter wavelengths (where lens absorption is highest), but the shape of the emission spectrum does not change substantially (Fig. 3.2, top, spectra A and B).

AGE AND FUNDUS AUTOFLUORESCENCE

Fundus AF has been shown to increase significantly with age (4,7,11,21,31), confirming data obtained in ex vivo studies (32,33). The rate and time course of this increase varies among different studies, probably as a result of differences in population selection, techniques, correction method for media absorption, and other factors (31). The increase of fundus AF with age for a population of normal subjects (Fig. 3.3) shows a large but constant variability (the coefficient of variation per decade of age is about

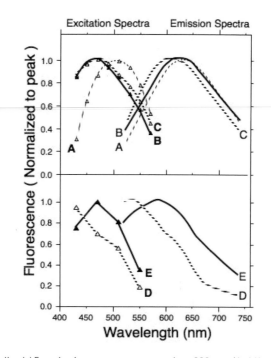

FIGURE 3.2. Normalized LF excitation spectra measured at 620 nm (*boldface letters*) and emission spectra for 470 nm excitation (*lightface letters*). The pairs of spectra are: **(A)** spectra from the 52-year-old subject of Fig. 3.1 (7 degrees T) not corrected for ocular media absorption; **(B)** the same as A but corrected for media absorption (the AF at 620 nm was 4.2 times larger than for A); **(C)** ex vivo spectra measured in the RPE of a donor eye (age: 83 years); **(D)** spectra measured on a large druse in a 70-year-old ARM patient; and **(E)** spectra measured in the same patient in an area devoid of visible drusen. Spectra B, D, and E were corrected for media absorption using the algorithm of van de Kraats and van Norren (26).

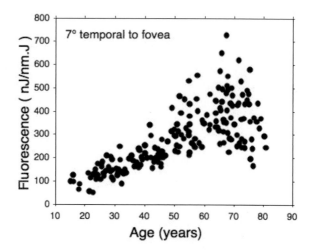

FIGURE 3.3. Age-related changes in fundus AF for subjects with normal retinal status (21). The excitation wavelength was 550 nm and the fluorescence was measured in the 610–630 nm spectral range. The data were corrected to account for absorption by the ocular media.

25% and 28%). Foveal AF increases similarly with age; however, the ratio of the AF at the fovea to that at 7 degrees temporal to the fovea does not vary with age.

We observed a decrease in AF in subjects above the age of 70, contrary to other studies that demonstrated a continuous increase in AF above age 70, albeit with a decreasing rate of increase (11,32,33). The decrease in AF at ages higher than 70 years could result, in part, from an undercorrection by our media optical density estimates, or from changes in AF efficiency (2,34).

RETINAL PIGMENT EPITHELIUM FLUOROPHORES

Emission spectra measured in vivo are consistent with those obtained in ex vivo measurements on donor RPE (Fig. 3.2) (7,35) and individual LF granules (2). The emission spectra in vivo correspond with that of the most efficient fluorophore (fluorophore VIII) of the several identified by Eldred and Katz (36) from chloroform/methanol extracts of human RPE. Fluorophore VIII was later identified as a bisretinoid, called A2E (37,38), and is the most extensively studied LF component (39,40). The photophysical and harmful properties of A2E were recently expertly reviewed by Sparrow (41).

The excitation spectrum in vivo corresponds well with ex vivo measured excitation spectra from donor RPE (Fig. 3.2, spectra B and C) (7,35). However, the in vivo excitation spectra correspond only roughly with those obtained from LF granules (2) and are substantially broader than the absorption and excitation spectra for A2E in solution (42). The latter are maximal at 440 nm and their spectral width is about half that of the in vivo excitation spectra. This implies that A2E is only one of the LF fluorophores responsible for fundus AF. Other byproducts of the visual cycle, such as the ATR-dimer (43), could account for the observed differences.

RPE melanin, particularly in its oxidized form (44), also exhibits fundus AF when excited in the near infrared (45). Because the absorption spectrum of melanin is very broad, it is possible that RPE melanin contributes to the AF measured with short-wavelength excitations. The contribution of the AF of RPE melanin to the total AF for short-wavelength excitations is still not known; it was estimated to be 3% to 10% from the absorption spectrum of melanin (46), and 5% to 25% from ex vivo experiments on LF and melanin granules (2,47). Melanolipofuscin is increasingly present in the aging RPE cell, and it is likely that it contributes the AF signal. Docchio et al. (47) showed that melanolipofuscin has a fluorescence efficiency intermediate between those of melanin and LF, and that its emission spectrum was blue-shifted compared to that of RPE LF.

AUTOFLUORESCENCE OF BRUCH'S MEMBRANE DEPOSITS

Evidence of a substantial secondary contribution to the fundus AF signal comes from changes in the shape of the emission spectra observed with age and disease. Indeed, the three emission spectra in Fig. 3.2 (spectra B, E, and D) are increasingly shifted toward shorter wavelengths as age and the expected amount of Bruch's membrane deposits (BMD, or drusen) at the measurement site increase. This blue shift is best characterized by the wavelength of maximum emission or the ratio (emission at 560 nm / emission at 660 nm) (Fig. 3.4). At 7 degrees temporal to the fovea, the emission peak wavelength decreases and the ratio increases with age, indicating that the blue shift is

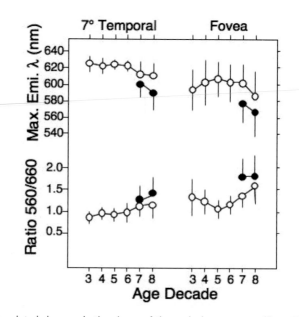

FIGURE 3.4.   Age-related changes in the shape of the emission spectrum (Exc.: 470 nm) as characterized by the maximum wavelength (*top*) and the ratio of the AF at 560 nm to that at 660 nm (*bottom*). Open circles: normal subjects; filled circles: patients with ARM. The spectra were corrected to account for absorption of the ocular media. A decrease in the peak wavelength and an increase in the ratio results in the "blue shift" of the emission spectra.

more substantial in older subjects. Furthermore, the blue shift is also more pronounced for spectra measured in age-related maculopathy (ARM) patients (Fig. 3.4).

Although an increase in the amount of melanolipofuscin could contribute to this shift (see above), the magnitude of the changes and the additional blue shift at the site of drusen suggest that BMD are responsible for the shift. This confirms ex vivo measurements (48) indicating that the emission from Bruch's membrane and BMD is similarly blue-shifted compared to the emission spectrum of LF. Spectral analyses predicted the BMD emission spectrum to be somewhat narrower than the LF emission and to have a maximum around 540 nm (49). Spectral deconvolution of spectra from ARM patients showed that the AF (Exc.: 488 nm) from BMD contributed on average 20% (range 5%–45%) of the total AF detected between 500 and 700 nm. This AF could play a role in the varying appearance of drusen in AF images in ARM patients.

The unique AF of drusen is also demonstrated by ratio imaging using pairs of AF images obtained with different excitation and emission bands, as shown in Fig. 3.5. One image (Fig. 3.5A) was obtained using bands similar to those used in routine AF imaging (Exc.: 470 nm), whereas the other (Fig. 3.5B) was obtained with excitation at 550 nm. The ratio image (Fig. 3.5D) thus reflects the difference in the local excitation spectra for both the macular pigment and the drusen. The latter are seen in the ratio image as uniform areas corresponding to their location in the monochromatic image (Fig. 3.5C). Differences in the excitation spectra of drusen and their neighboring area are thought to be responsible for this effect.

OTHER SECONDARY FLUOROPHORES

The blue shift at the fovea in the youngest subjects (Fig. 3.4; decades 3 and 4 compared with decade 5) must be related to other secondary fluorophores. The AF from

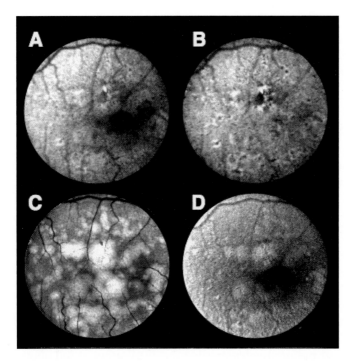

FIGURE 3.5.   LF images **(A,B)** and a 550-nm monochromatic image **(C)** from a 65-year-old ARM patient. **(A)** Obtained with excitation at 470 nm and a detection >510 nm, and **(B)** obtained with an excitation at 550 nm and a detection >600 nm. **(D)** The ratio (after alignment) of **A** to **B**. All images were recorded with a nonconfocal camera (15). Note that the attenuation by the macular pigment seen in **A** is not seen in **B**, allowing examination of the foveal RPE.

LF at the fovea in young subjects is very low. Therefore, secondary fluorophores emitting in the 500–540 nm spectral range may become relatively more important. This fluorescence is believed to originate anterior to the macular pigment and could be from the macular pigment itself (50), from flavins in the inner retina, from collagen (51) and hyaluronic acid (52) in the vitreous, and/or from lens LF reflected by the fundus.

AF from microglia in the inner retina of normal mice has been observed by AF imaging in some (53) but not all (54,55) studies. When seen (53), the AF emission of microglia appears to have LF-like characteristics (see also Chapter 4), although determination of the excitation spectrum would be required for comparison with RPE LF. However, AF of microglia has not been observed in normal human eyes by AF imaging. If the density and AF characteristics of microglia in normal human and mice were similar, then their observation in mice but not in humans might be explained by a lower AF emanating from the mice RPE than from the human RPE, causing their contrast to be high enough to be observed. This could result from a lower amount of RPE LF in mice and from a higher density of RPE melanin (larger attenuation of the AF of RPE LF in AF images).

Finally, AF contributions from the choroid and sclera have been estimated in AMD patients (69–81 years old) with geographic atrophy to be 6% to 15% of the total fundus AF for dark- and light-pigmented subjects, respectively (45). This suggests that choroidal melanin absorption modulates the AF from other choroidal fluorophores. The contribution of choroidal AF to total fundus AF will be less in younger subjects because of the higher concentrations and absorption by melanin in the RPE and choroid (23,25,56). Emission spectra measured in geographic atrophy give little information about the origin of the weak AF, because of distortion by blood absorption and noise in the spectral data. Endogenous fluorophores in the choroid may include stromal elastin and collagen, porphyrins, melanocytic melanofuscin, and macrophages (containing blue-emitting LF) (51,57,58).

TOPOGRAPHICAL DISTRIBUTION

Ex vivo studies have shown that the amount of RPE LF is low at the fovea, increases gradually to a maximum about 10 degrees from the fovea, and then decreases toward the periphery (23). Topographical distribution of fundus AF, measured with an excitation at 550 nm (and thus not affected by macular pigment absorption), confirms these findings; the AF is maximal at an eccentricity of 7 to 13 degrees, where the AF is about 1.7 times higher than at the fovea (31,59). The central minimum is caused principally by LF in the RPE, since the higher concentration of RPE melanin at the fovea has been estimated to be only 1.15 higher than at the parafovea (31). Fundus AF is not symmetrically distributed around the fovea (Fig. 3.6); the AF is maximal at about 12 degrees temporally and superiorly, lower inferiorly and nasally where it is maximal at about 7–8 degrees from the fovea.

The AF distribution roughly matches the distribution of rod photoreceptors (60), which is not surprising given that LF derives from precursors within phagocytosed photoreceptor outer segments. However, the distribution does not reflect the narrow distribution of cones at the fovea (60). The rate of LF formation from cones may be slower, as suggested by the observation in rhesus monkeys that the number of foveal cone-derived-phagosomes in the RPE was only one-third that of extrafoveal rod-derived-phagosomes (61). Other effects, such as high absorption by RPE melanin at the fovea, cone/rod differences in the fractional content of indigestible materials in the phagosomes, and spatially dependent protection by the macular pigment could also play a role in reducing foveal LF formation.

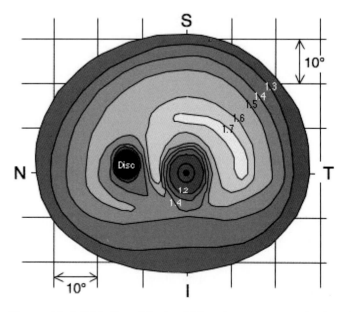

FIGURE 3.6. Topographical distribution of fundus AF based on measurements along the horizontal (nasal–temporal: N-T) and vertical (superior–inferior: S-I) meridians (data from about 40 subjects) (31). The AF is expressed relative to that at the fovea.

SUMMARY

The fundus LF signal derives principally from RPE LF, as evidenced by its spatial distribution, its spectral characteristics, and its relation to age. This signal is affected by absorption by the ocular media, macular pigment, retinal blood vessels and capillaries, and RPE melanin. Secondary sources of LF in humans are BMD and vitreous fluorescence. The AF of drusen may provide specific information about the type or content of drusen.

A case can be made for using excitation wavelengths longer than the 488 nm currently used in most fundus AF imaging systems. Indeed, there would be less ocular media absorption and scattering, and errors associated with correction for media absorption would be decreased. Macular pigment absorption would be reduced, if not eliminated, allowing for clear visualization of the foveal RPE (Fig. 3.5B). One would also expect an overall increase in the signal intensity and signal/noise ratio. Finally, longer wavelengths are less susceptible to photochemical damage to the retina.

REFERENCES

1. Feeney-Burns L, Hilderbrand ES, Eldridge S. Aging human RPE: morphometric analysis of macular, equatorial, and peripheral cells. Invest Ophthalmol Vis Sci 1984;25:195–200.
2. Boulton MD, Docchio F, Dayhaw-Barker P, et al. Age-related changes in the morphology, absorption and fluorescence of melanosomes and lipofuscin granules of the retinal pigment epithelium. Vision Res 1990;30:1291–1303.
3. Delori FC, Bursell S-E, Yoshida A, et al. Vitreous fluorophotometry in diabetics: study of artifactual contributions. Graefe's Arch Clin Exp Ophthalmol 1985;222:215–218.
4. Kitagawa K, Nishida S, Ogura Y. In vivo quantification of autofluorescence in human retinal pigment epithelium. Ophthalmologica 1989;199:116–121.
5. Delori FC. Spectrophotometer for noninvasive measurement of intrinsic fluorescence and reflectance of the ocular fundus. Appl Optics 1994;33:7439–7452.
6. Delori FC. Fluorophotometer for noninvasive measurement of RPE lipofuscin. Noninvasive assessment of the visual system. OSA Technical Digest 1992;1:164–167.
7. Delori FC, Dorey CK, Staurenghi G, et al. In vivo fluorescence of the ocular fundus exhibits retinal pigment epithelium lipofuscin characteristics. Invest Ophthalmol Vis Sci 1995;36:718–729.
8. Wade AR, Fitzke FW. A fast, robust pattern recognition system for low light level image registration and its application to retinal imaging. Opt Express 1998;3:190–197.
9. Webb RH, Hughes GW, Delori FC. Confocal scanning laser ophthalmoscope. Appl Opt 1987;26:1492–1449.
10. von Rückmann A, Fitzke FW, Bird AC. Distribution of fundus autofluorescence with a scanning laser ophthalmoscope. Br J Ophthalmol 1995;119:543–562.
11. von Rückmann A, Fitzke FW, Bird AC. Fundus autofluorescence in age-related macular disease imaged with a laser scanning ophthalmoscope. Invest Ophthalmol Vis Sci 1997;38:478–486.
12. Solbach U, Keilhauer C, Knabben H, et al. Imaging of retinal autofluorescence in patients with age-related macular degeneration. Retina 1997;17:385–389.
13. Holz FG, Bellmann C, Margaritidis M, et al. Patterns of increased in vivo fundus autofluorescence in the junctional zone of geographic atrophy of the retinal pigment epithelium associated with age-related macular degeneration. Graefes Arch Clin Exp Ophthalmol 1999;237:145–152.
14. Gray DC, Merigan W, Wolfing JI, et al. In vivo fluorescence imaging of primate retinal ganglion cells and retinal pigment epithelial cells. Opt Express 2006;14:7144–7158.
15. Delori FC, Fleckner MR, Goger DG, et al. Autofluorescence distribution associated with drusen in age-related macular degeneration. Invest Ophthalmol Vis Sci 2000;41:496–504.
16. Spaide RF. Fundus autofluorescence and age-related macular degeneration. Ophthalmology 2003;110:392–399.
17. Bone RA, Landrum JT, Cains A. Optical density spectra of the macular pigment in vivo and in vitro. Vision Res 1992;32:105–110.
18. Prieto PM, McLellan JS, Burns SA. Investigating the light absorption in a single pass through the photoreceptor layer by means of the lipofuscin fluorescence. Vision Res 2005;45:1957–1965.
19. Delori FC, Pflibsen KP. Spectral reflectance of the human ocular fundus. Appl Opt 1989;28:1061–1077.
20. Arend OA, Weiter JJ, Goger DG, et al. In-vivo fundus-fluoreszenz-messungen bei patienten mit alterabhangiger makulardegeneration. Ophthalmologie 1995;92:647–653.
21. Delori FC, Keilhauer C, Staurenghi G, et al. Origin of fundus autofluorescence. In: Holz FG, Schmitz-Valkenberg S, Spaide RF, Bird AC, eds. Atlas of Fundus Autofluorescence Imaging. Berlin, Heidelberg, New York: Springer, 2007:17–29.

22. Lakowicz JR, Keating-Nakamoto S. Red-edge excitation of fluorescence and dynamic properties of proteins and membranes. Biochemistry 1984;23:3013–3021.

23. Weiter JJ, Delori FC, Wing G, et al. Retinal pigment epithelial lipofuscin and melanin and choroidal melanin in human eyes. Invest Ophthalmol Vis Sci 1986;27:145–152.

24. Delori FC, Goger DG, Hammond BR, et al. Macular pigment density measured by autofluorescence spectrometry: comparison with reflectometry and heterochromatic flicker photometry. J Opt Soc Am A Opt Image Sci Vis 2001;18:1212–1230.

25. Feeney-Burns L, Berman ER, Rothman H. Lipofuscin of human retinal pigment epithelium. Am J Ophthalmol 1980;90:783–791.

26. van de Kraats J, van Norren D. Optical density of the aging human ocular media in the visible and the UV. J Opt Soc Am A Ophthalmol Image Sci Vis 2007;24:1842–1857.

27. Savage GL, Johnson CA, Howard DL. A comparison of noninvasive objective and subjective measurements of the optical density of human ocular media. Optom Vis Sci 2001;78:386–395.

28. Delori FC, Burns SA. Fundus reflectance and the measurement of crystalline lens density. J Opt Soc Am A 1996;13:215–226.

29. Berendschot TT, Broekmans WM, Klopping-Ketelaars IA, et al. Lens aging in relation to nutritional determinants and possible risk factors for age-related cataract. Arch Ophthalmol 2002;120:1732–1737.

30. Pokorny J, Smith VC, Lutze M. Aging of the human lens. Appl Opt 1987;26:1437–1440.

31. Delori FC, Goger DG, Dorey CK. Age-related accumulation and spatial distribution of lipofuscin in RPE of normal subjects. Invest Ophthalmol Vis Sci 2001;42:1855–1866.

32. Wing GL, Blanchard GC, Weiter JJ. The topography and age relationship of lipofuscin concentration in the retinal pigment epithelium. Invest Ophthalmol Vis Sci 1978;17:601–607.

33. Okubo A, Rosa Jr RH, Bunce CV, et al. The relationships of age changes in retinal pigment epithelium and Bruch's membrane. Invest Ophthalmol Vis Sci 1999;40:443–449.

34. Sparrow JR, Zhou J, Ben-Shabat S, et al. Involvement of oxidative mechanisms in blue-light-induced damage to A2E-laden RPE. Invest Ophthalmol Vis Sci 2002;43:1222–1227.

35. Delori FC, Goger DG, Sparrow JR. Spectral characteristics of lipofuscin autofluorescence in RPE cells of donor eyes. Invest Ophthalmol Vis Sci 2003;44:1715.

36. Eldred GE, Katz ML. Fluorophores of the human retinal pigment epithelium: separation and spectral characterization. Exp Eye Res 1988;47:71–86.

37. Eldred GE, Laskey MR. Retinal age pigments generated by self-absorbing lysomotropic detergents. Nature 1993;361:724–726.

38. Sakai N, Decatur J, Nakanishi K, et al. Ocular age pigment "A2-E": an unprecedented pyridinium bis-retinoid. J Am Chem Soc 1996;118:1559–1560.

39. Sparrow JR, Cai B, Fishkin N, et al. A2E, a fluorophore of RPE lipofuscin: can it cause RPE degeneration? Adv Exp Med Biol 2003;533:205–211.

40. Sparrow JR, Fishkin N, Zhou J, et al. A2E, a byproduct of the visual cycle. Vision Res 2003;43: 2983–2990.

41. Sparrow JR. Lipofuscin of the retinal pigment epithelium. In: Holz FG, Schmitz-Valkenberg S, Spaide RF, Bird AC, eds. Atlas of Fundus Autofluorescence Imaging. Berlin, Heidelberg, New York: Springer, 2007:3–16.

42. Sparrow JR, Nakanishi K, Parish CA. The lipofuscin fluorophore A2E mediates blue light-induced damage to retinal pigmented epithelial cells. Invest Ophthalmol Vis Sci 2000;41:1981–1989.

43. Fishkin NE, Sparrow JR, Allikmets R, et al. Isolation and characterization of a retinal pigment epithelial cell fluorophore: an all-trans-retinal dimer conjugate. Proc Natl Acad Sci USA 2005;102:7091–7096.

44. Kayatz P, Thumann G, Luther TT, et al. Oxidation causes melanin fluorescence. Invest Ophthalmol Vis Sci 2001;42:241–246.

45. Keilhauer CN, Delori FC. Near-infrared autofluorescence imaging of the fundus: visualization of ocular melanin. Invest Ophthalmol Vis Sci 2006;47:3556–3564.

46. Jacques SL, McAuliffe DJ. The melanosome: threshold temperature for explosive vaporization and internal absorption coefficient during pulsed laser irradiation. Photochem Photobiol 1991;53:769–775.

47. Docchio F, Boulton M, Cubeddu R, et al. Age-related changes in the fluorescence of melanin and lipofuscin granules of the retinal pigment epithelium: a time-resolved fluorescence spectroscopy study. J Photochem Photobiol 1991;54:247–253.

48. Marmorstein AD, Marmorstein LY, Sakaguchi H, et al. Spectral profiling of autofluorescence associated with lipofuscin, Bruch's membrane, and sub-RPE deposits in normal and AMD eyes. Invest Ophthalmol Vis Sci 2002;43:2435–2441.

49. Delori FC. RPE lipofuscin in aging and age related macular degeneration. In: Piccolino FC, Coscas G, eds. Retinal Pigment Epithelium and Macular Diseases. Dordrecht, The Netherlands: Kluwer Academic Publishers, 1998:37–45.

50. Gellermann W, Ermakov IV, Ermakova MR, et al. In vivo resonant Raman measurement of macular carotenoid pigments in the young and the aging human retina. J Opt Soc Am A Opt Image Sci Vis 2002;19:1172–1186.

51. Monici M. Cell and tissue autofluorescence research and diagnostic applications. Biotechnol Annu Rev 2005;11:227–256.

52. Ueno N, Chakrabarti B. Liquefaction of human vitreous in model aphakic eyes by 300-nm UV photolysis: monitoring liquefaction by fluorescence. Curr Eye Res 1990;9:487–492.

53. Xu H, Chen M, Manivannan A, et al. Age-related accumulation of lipofuscin in perivascular and sub-retinal microglia in experimental mice. Aging Cell 2008;7:58–68.
54. Paques M, Simonutti M, Roux MJ, et al. High resolution fundus imaging by confocal scanning laser oph-thalmoscopy in the mouse. Vision Res 2006;46:1336–1345.
55. Coffey PJ, Gias C, McDermott CJ, et al. Complement factor H deficiency in aged mice causes retinal ab-normalities and visual dysfunction. Proc Natl Acad Sci USA 2007;104:16651–16656.
56. Schmidt SY, Peisch RD. Melanin concentration in normal human retinal pigment epithelium; Regional variation and age-related reduction. Invest Ophthalmol Vis Sci 1986;27:1063–1067.
57. Forrester JV, McMenamin PG, Holthouse I, et al. Localization and characterization of major histocom-patibility complex class II-positive cells in the posterior segment of the eye: implications for induction of autoimmune uveoretinitis. Invest Ophthalmol Vis Sci 1994;35:64–77.
58. McMenamin PG. The distribution of immune cells in the uveal tract of the normal eye. Eye (London, England) 1997;11:183–193.
59. Delori FC, Goger DG, Keilhauer CN, et al. Bimodal spatial distribution of macular pigment: evidence of a gender relationship. J Opt Soc Am A Opt Image Sci Vis 2006;23:521–538.
60. Curcio CA, Sloan KR, Kalina RE, et al. Human photoreceptor topography. J Comp Neural 1990;292:497–523.
61. Anderson DH, Fisher SK, Erickson PA, et al. Rod and cone disc shedding in the rhesus monkey retina: a quantitative study. Exp Eye Res 1980;30:559–574.

Lipofuscin and Autofluorescence in Experimental Animal Models

Fundus autofluorescence (AF) imaging is increasingly being used in ophthalmic practice to aid in the diagnosis and monitoring of patients with a variety of retinal disorders. Thus, it is particularly important to understand the molecular and cellular sources of fundus AF. Only with such an understanding can doctors interpret and judge the significance of fundus AF changes in various pathological conditions. However, it is very difficult to obtain such information from human studies; in this context experimental animal studies may have great additional value. Improvements in in vivo fundus AF imaging techniques and the development of various animal models of disease enable us to carry out direct clinicopathological correlations as well as dissect the detailed mechanisms of lipofuscin formation.

THE VALUE OF EXPERIMENTAL ANIMAL MODELS

Experimental animal studies are valuable because they allow us to investigate the clinicopathological correlations of fundus AF and the pathological changes related to various AF patterns. Such information is critical for clinicians to correctly interpret AF images. Although a variety of animal models representing different types of human retinal diseases have been developed over the years, only a few AF clinicopathological studies have been published (1,2), including a study from the author's laboratory in normal aged mice. Another important use of experimental animal studies is to investigate the mechanisms of lipofuscin formation. Studies in this field have identified a few important factors involved in in vivo lipofuscin formation, including the RPE65 gene and vitamin A. In addition, animal studies are of great value for testing the effectiveness of various treatments, particularly those targeting the formation of lipofuscin.

IMAGING TECHNIQUES

In Vivo Imaging

Currently, confocal scanning laser ophthalmoscopy (cSLO) is the most widely used technique to image fundus AF in vivo. Because all commercial cSLOs are designed to image the human fundus, slight modifications, such as the use of special lenses, are needed to image rat or mouse retina. Various groups have used this system to image the rodent fundus. In the author's laboratory, a custom-built cSLO is used in experimental animal studies. To be able to image the mouse fundus, we use a +25D lens placed 1 cm in front of the mouse cornea to further focus the laser beam. In addition, a mouse hard contact lens is also used to prevent tear evaporation and keep the eyelids open. We are able to image a 43 × 32 degrees field of the mouse fundus (3). This in vivo imaging technique is noninvasive, and therefore changes in the fundus can be followed up at different stages of disease in the same animal.

Ex Vivo Imaging

As with human samples, lipofuscin in animal tissues can be extracted and examined in vitro by various techniques. Traditionally, tissue AF has been imaged in situ with the use of various fluorescence microscopes (4,5). Fluorescence microscopy is still a simple, straightforward, and useful technique to detect lipofuscin. Currently, however, more advanced and sophisticated technologies are used to quantify lipofuscin content and examine the detailed fluorescence emission spectra of lipofuscin. Bui and colleagues (6) used a fluorescence microplate reader (Tecan Safire II Fluorescence Microplate Reader, Tecan US, Research Triangle Park, NC) to examine the fluorescence emission spectra of RPE-choroid and retina explants. In their system, fresh samples were placed side up in a modified 384-well microplate. Emission spectra were measured following excitation at 420 nm using the top read mode (6). This technique allows one to measure the emission spectra as well as the relative fluorescent units of RPE-choroid and retina explants. In the author's laboratory, the lambda mode of a confocal scanning laser microscope (LSM510 META, Carl Zeiss) is used to image fluorescence emission spectra of mouse RPE-choroid and retina explants (1). This technique has several advantages: (i) samples can be excited with different lasers and the characteristics of the emission spectra excited by the different lasers can be studied; (ii) it detects the emission spectra of individual cells or regions but not the whole tissue, allowing comparisons of the emission spectra of different cells or different regions; and (iii) the fluorescent intensity of different tissues or different regions can be quantitatively recorded and analyzed. The lambda mode of the LSM510 META confocal microscope is designed to separate the fluorochromes with widely overlapping emission spectra or fluorochromes that are excited by the same laser. It is widely used to eliminate sample background AF. With the META scanning system, the emission fingerprints of each fluorochrome can be collected and a spectral database can be built (Fig. 4.1). It is therefore an ideal means of studying the fluorescence spectra

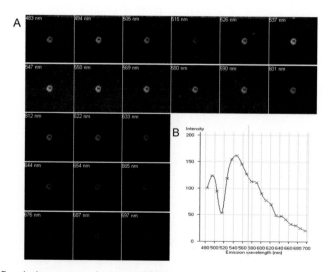

FIGURE 4.1.   AF emission spectra of a mouse RPE cell. The RPE flatmount was prepared from a 2-year-old C57BL/6 mouse and examined with the use of a LSM510 META confocal microscope (lambda model). The sample was excited with a 458 nm HeNe laser and the emission signals were collected from 460 to 697 nm. **(A)** Emission spectra database of the RPE cell. **(B)** AF intensity at different emission wavelengths extracted from the database in A.

of lipofuscin. With the META scanning mode, emission signals are detected by a polychromatic 32-channel detector, which allows the fast acquisition of lambda stacks. Samples can be excited with lasers at 448 nm, 477 nm, 488 nm, 514 nm, 543 nm, and 633 nm separately. For each excitation, the emission spectral range for lambda stack acquisition can be controlled as required, and the upper limit is 790 nm. For all lambda acquisitions, the pinhole needs to be set to 1 airy unit and the scanning speed set to 6. To be able to compare the emission fingerprints acquired from different cells/tissues, the configuration, including the detector gain, amplifier offset, and amplifier gain, should not be changed during the process of acquisition. An example of mouse RPE lipofuscin emission spectra excited by 458 nm is shown in Figure 4.1.

CLINICOPATHOLOGICAL CORRELATION OF FUNDUS AUTOFLUORESCENCE IN EXPERIMENTAL ANIMALS

Although various pathological studies in retinal/RPE lipofuscin have been carried out in postmortem human eyes over the past decade, direct clinicopathological correlation is lacking. To date, the clinicopathological correlation of fundus AF findings in the majority of retinal diseases is still largely unknown.

Fundus AF in Normal Mouse

To be able to understand fundus AF changes in various animal models of diseases of the posterior segment, the characteristics of fundus AF in healthy control animals need to be established. We have investigated the fundus AF in normal C57BL/6 mice of different ages. The overall fundus AF increased with age in normal C57BL/6 mice by cSLO (1). Increasingly strong AF signals were observed with age in the neuroretina and subretinal/RPE layer (Fig. 4.2A). Unlike fundus AF detected in normal human subjects, fundus AF appeared as discrete foci distributed throughout the retina (Fig. 4.2A). Most of the AF signals in the neuroretina were distributed around retinal vessels (1). Immunohistological studies of retinal or RPE-choroidal flatmounts indicated that most of the AF signals derived from Iba-1+ perivascular and subretinal microglia (Fig. 4.2B,C), and some derived from RPE cells (Fig. 4.3) (1).

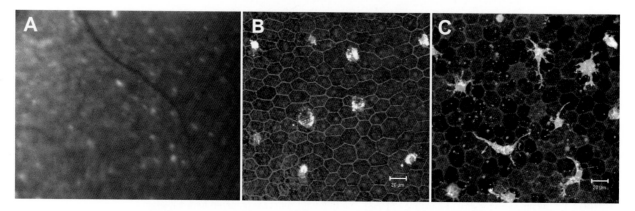

FIGURE 4.2. Fundus AF in a normal aged mouse. **(A)** Fundus AF in an 18-month-old C57BL/6 mouse. **(B)** Confocal microscopy of RPE flatmount of the same mouse reveals many autofluorescent cells located on the surface of the RPE cells. **(C)** The autofluorescent cells on the RPE cell surface stained positive for the microglia marker Iba-1.

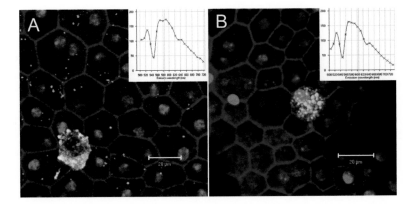

FIGURE 4.3. Lipofuscin in subretinal microglia and RPE cells. **(A)** Subretinal microglia with lipofuscin. *Inset*: Emission spectra of subretinal microglial lipofuscin excited with 488 nm. **(B)** RPE cell with lipofuscin. *Inset*: Emission spectra of RPE cell lipofuscin excited with 488 nm.

The number of subretinal microglia and the amount of intracellular lipofuscin increased with age (1). Transmission electron microscopy (TEM) revealed many lipufuscin granules in the cytoplasm of subretinal microglia (1). Emission spectra detected by the META scanning mode of the confocal microscope indicated that the spectra of the lipofuscin in subretinal microglia and the RPE cells were the same (Fig. 4.3), suggesting that they may have the same chemical components.

Fundus AF in Mouse Models of Disease

CCR2/CCL2 Knockout Mice

Mice deficient in either monocyte chemoattractant protein-1 (CCL2, also known as MCP-1) or its cognate C-C chemokine receptor-2 (CCR2) develop the cardinal fundus features observed in patients with age-related maculopathy (ARM) or age-related macular degeneration (AMD) (7). These include drusen, geographic atrophy, and choroidal neovascularization. Both strains of mice develop drusen-like changes at the age of 9 months. By 16 months, geographic atrophy can be observed. Choroidal neovascularization (CNV) can be detected in one-fourth of $CCL2^{-/-}$ and $CCR2^{-/-}$ mice at the age of 18 months. Such mice are therefore considered good models for ARM/AMD. Clinically, we observed drusen-like and geographic atrophy-like changes in our *CCR2* and *CCL2* knockout mice (purchased from the Jackson Laboratory), but no subretinal neovascularization. Fundus AF imaging using cSLO indicated many more autofluorescent foci present in CCL2- or CCR2-deficient mice compared to age-matched wild-type control mice (Fig. 4.4).

Ex vivo confocal imaging of retinal flatmounts from this animal model revealed many perivascular and subretinal Iba-1+ microglia with autofluorescent lipofuscin, similar to those seen in normal aged mice, but in significantly higher numbers.

CFH Knockout Mice

Genetic studies have revealed a strong association between a broad range of AMD phenotypes and variants in the gene encoding complement factor H (CFH). CFH is the major plasma protein that exclusively regulates the alternative pathway of complement activation. CFH protein has been detected in drusen, the pathogenic hallmark of AMD. CFH-deficient mice exhibit significantly reduced rod responses on electroretinography compared to age-matched controls (2). Fundus AF of these mice by

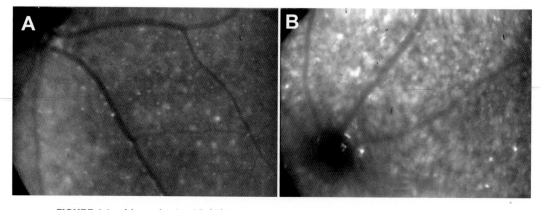

FIGURE 4.4. Mouse fundus AF. **(A)** Fundus AF of a 18-month-old C57BL/6 mouse. **(B)** Fundus AF of an 18-month-old CCL2 knockout mouse.

SLO revealed an increase in autofluorescent subretinal deposits, similar to those observed in CCR2- and CCL2-deficient mice. More recently, using ex vivo confocal microscopy of retinal and RPE/choroidal flatmounts, we showed that the majority of the autofluorescent signals were from subretinal microglia (Fig. 4.5).

Fundus Autofluorescence in Experimental Autoimmune Uveoretinitis

Clinical studies have shown altered AF in various chorioretinal inflammatory diseases (see Chapter 12). Inflammation may alter RPE and photoreceptor cell function and subsequently affect the production of autofluorescent molecules. Furthermore, inflammatory cells, in particular macrophages, may contain autofluorescent materials as a result of active phagocytosis of oxidized substances at the site of inflammation. It is therefore important to understand the correlation between AF patterns and pathological changes in chorioretinal inflammation.

We have carried out clinicopathological studies in a mouse model of experimental autoimmune uveoretinitis (EAU). EAU was induced by immunizing C57BL/6 mice

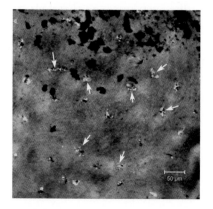

FIGURE 4.5. AF cells in the subretinal space. The retinal flatmount was prepared from a 12-month-old CFH knockout mouse and imaged by confocal microscope (LSM510 META). The image was taken from the photoreceptor side of the retinal flatmount. Many AF cells (*arrows*) are seen within the outer segment of the photoreceptor cells.

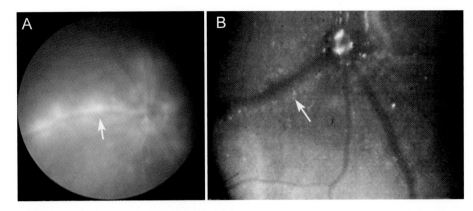

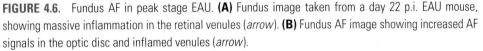

FIGURE 4.6.   Fundus AF in peak stage EAU. **(A)** Fundus image taken from a day 22 p.i. EAU mouse, showing massive inflammation in the retinal venules (*arrow*). **(B)** Fundus AF image showing increased AF signals in the optic disc and inflamed venules (*arrow*).

with human interphotoreceptor retinoid-binding protein (IRBP) peptide 1–20. In this EAU model, retinal inflammation starts at day 10–12 postimmunization (p.i.), peaks at day 20–25 p.i., and resolves at about day 30 (8). Fundus AF was imaged at disease initiation (day 12 p.i.), peak (day 25 p.i.), and resolution (day 35 p.i.) stages, respectively. At day 12 p.i., when inflammation was very mild and localized in the optic disc or venule fragments, fundus AF was largely normal; neither an increased nor a decreased AF signal was observed in inflamed retina areas compared to noninflamed ones. As inflammation progressed, increased AF signals began to appear in areas of inflammation at peak stage EAU. AF signals appeared as discrete small dots of increased AF surrounding inflamed vessels (Fig. 4.6).

At the late stages of inflammation (i.e., day 35 p.i., disease-resolution stage), a massive destruction of photoreceptor cells was observed. Highly increased AF signals were seen throughout the entire retina (Fig. 4.7).

Ex vivo confocal microscopy of retinal RPE-choroidal flatmounts revealed many autofluorescent cells at sites where inflammation was present, particularly in the area around the inflamed vessel segments. Immunofluorescent studies indicated that these autofluorescent cells were F4/80[+] macrophages.

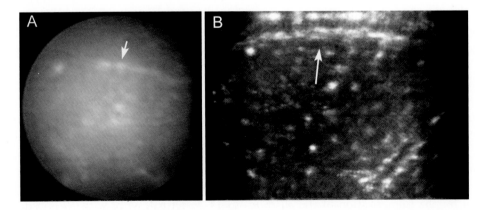

FIGURE 4.7.   Fundus AF in late-stage EAU. Images were taken from a day 35 p.i. EAU mouse. **(A)** Fundus image showing atrophic retina and inflamed venule segment (*arrow*). **(B)** Many small foci of increased AF distribute throughout the retina, with more in the perivascular area (*arrow*). The AF background is lower than that of the peak-stage EAU retina (Fig. 4.6).

EXPERIMENTAL ANIMAL STUDIES TO DISSECT THE MECHANISM OF LIPOFUSCIN FORMATION

Studies on the mechanism of lipofuscin formation in the eye have exclusively focused on RPE cells. It is believed that the formation of lipofuscin in RPE cells involves the visual cycle between RPE and photoreceptors and the reduced lysosomal function in RPE cells, in addition to other mechanisms (see also Chapter 2).

The visual cycle is a tightly regulated cycle in which retinoid (vitamin A) moves back and forth from RPE cells to photoreceptor outer segments through the interphotoreceptor matrix (IPM) and is strongly retained in this loop. Retinoid is released from the bloodstream to RPE cells. With light illumination, retinoid moves from the retina to RPE cells, and with dark adaptation the process is reversed. Substantial evidence indicates that vitamin A derivatives (retinoids) are required for RPE lipofuscin formation. In normal rat retinas, age-related lipofuscin accumulation occurs in RPE cells, and vitamin A deficiency has been shown to reduce RPE lipofuscin (9). In the Royal College of Surgeons (RCS) rat, a strain with an inherited retinal dystrophy, lipofuscin-like AF develops in the degenerating photoreceptor cells, and vitamin A deficiency substantially reduces the AF associated with degenerating photoreceptor cells. Furthermore a vitamin A-dependent fluorophore was isolated from these retinas with the use of thin-layer chromatography (TLC) (10). However, this fluorophore differs (in fluorescence intensity and mobility in TLC) from that of aged RPE cells of normal rats. It appears that the fluorophore generated in the photoreceptor cells must undergo chemical modification once it has been taken up by the RPE (10).

The requirement of vitamin A for lipofuscin formation is further supported by a study in which lipofuscin was induced in RPE cells by intravitreal injection of the lysosomal protease inhibitor leupeptin. Intravitreal injection of leupeptin caused rapid accumulation of inclusions with lipofuscin-like AF in the RPE of albino rats (11). However, in vitamin A-deprived animals, similar inclusions formed in response to leupeptin treatment, but they did not become AF (11). It appears likely that retinoids are directly incorporated into these inclusions. In another animal study, in which all-*trans* retinol was labeled with ^{3}H and injected into rats that were treated with an intravitreal injection of leupeptin, the radiolabel in the RPE was primarily associated with the leupeptin-induced inclusion bodies. Label was also present in the photoreceptor outer segments. The localization of vitamin A to the leupeptin-induced inclusions in the RPE strongly suggests that vitamin A is covalently bound to outer segment proteins that have been phagocytosed by the RPE but remain undegraded as a result of protease inhibition. Vitamin A is not likely to be bound through a Schiff base linkage, since retinal-Schiff base compounds do not exhibit lipofuscin-like fluorescence (12).

The importance of a normal visual cycle in the formation of lipofuscin is also supported by studies in *RPE65* knockout mice. *RPE65* is essential in the operation of the visual cycle and functions as a chaperone for all-*trans*-retinyl esters, the substrates for isomerization in the visual cycle. During the visual cycle, the visual pigment chromophore, 11-*cis*-retinal, is photoisomerized to the all-*trans* configuration and then enzymatically reisomerized to the 11-*cis* isomer. *RPE65* proteins are essential for the isomerization of the all-*trans*- to 11-*cis*-retinal. Mice with *RPE65* deficiency (i.e., *RPE65*$^{-/-}$ mice) accumulate almost no lipofuscin in RPE cells (4), and *RPE65*$^{+/-}$ mice also have significantly reduced accumulation of lipofuscin fluorophores in RPE cells. Further experiments in *RPE65* knockout mice with protease inhibitor (leupeptin) treatment showed that although lipofuscin-like inclusions were observed in both WT and RPE65 knockout mice, only the inclusions from WT RPE (and not $RPE65^{-/-}$ RPE) autofluoresce (13). These observations suggest that the formation of RPE lipofuscin fluorophores is almost completely dependent on a normal visual cycle.

In line with these experimental studies in mice, a lack of AF in patients with early-onset severe retinal rod-cone dystrophy has been observed (14). Early-onset severe rod-cone dystrophy is believed to be associated with *RPE65* mutations (15).

The fact that leupeptin treatment induces lipofuscin-like inclusions suggests that loss of lysosomal function is also responsible for the formation of lipofuscin. The inclusions are derived from photoreceptor outer segments, which are normally phagocytosed and degraded by the RPE. A normal lysosomal function is essential for the degradation of phagocytized materials. The tripeptide leu-gly-gly, which is similar to leupeptin except that it does not inhibit proteolysis, has no effect on RPE AF content. Likewise, netilmicin, a purported inhibitor of lysosomal phospholipases, does not increase AF in the RPE (11).

In summary, experimental studies on the formation of lipofuscin in RPE cells suggest that loss of lysosomal function is essential for the formation of lipofuscin inclusions, whereas a normal visual cycle is required for lipofuscin formation.

TESTING ANTILIPOFUSCIN COMPOUNDS IN ANIMAL MODELS

Increasing knowledge regarding the mechanism of lipofuscin formation will enable the development of antilipofuscin drugs, which could be of benefit in various retinal degenerative diseases. As summarized above, inhibiting visual cycle function with small molecules has been shown to be an effective approach to prevent lipofuscin formation. Various animal models have been used to test the effectiveness of compounds designed to inhibit lipofuscin formation (16). The effect of isotretinoin (Accutane), which has been shown to slow the synthesis of 11-*cis*-retinaldehyde and regeneration of rhodopsin, has been tested in $ABCA4^{-/-}$ knockout mice, a mouse model of Stargardt disease (see Chapter 11G). Fenretinide (N-[4-hydroxyphenyl]retinamide [HPR]) potently and reversibly reduces serum retinol. Administration of HPR to $ABCA4^{-/-}$ mice caused immediate, dose-dependent reductions in serum retinol and retinol binding protein (RBP). Chronic administration can produce commensurate reductions in visual cycle retinoids and arrest accumulation of A2E and lipofuscin AF in RPE cells. Physiologically, HPR treatment causes modest delays in dark adaptation. Chromophore regeneration kinetics, light sensitivity of photoreceptors, and phototransduction processes are normal. HRP could be a novel therapeutic approach with the potential to halt the accumulation of lipofuscin fluorophores in the eye (18). In this regard, a Phase II randomized, double-masked, placebo-controlled, multicenter study using fenretinide is currently under way (see also Chapter 10C).

Nonretinoid isoprenoid compounds have been shown to serve as antagonists of *RPE65*. These *RPE65* antagonists block regeneration of 11-*cis*-retinal, the chromophore of rhodopsin. Chronic treatment of a mouse model of Stargardt disease with *RPE65* antagonists abolished the formation of A2E. Thus, *RPE65* is also on the rate-limiting pathway of A2E formation. These nontoxic isoprenoid *RPE65* antagonists are candidates for treating forms of macular degeneration in which lipofuscin accumulation is an important risk factor. These antagonists will also be used to probe the molecular function of *RPE65* in vision (19).

SUMMARY

Although AF imaging has been used in the clinic for almost a decade, our understanding of fundus AF is still limited. Animal models are important tools for gaining insight into pathological changes and their correlation to observed fundus AF changes, and the mechanisms underlying the formation of lipofuscin. They are also valuable for developing effective drugs targeting lipofuscin formation with the goal of preventing retinal degeneration. Studies conducted so far on the mechanisms of lipofuscin formation have revealed many important molecules, and consequently new treatment approaches are being developed. The study of clinicopathological correlations of fundus AF has just begun. It has been demonstrated that other cells besides RPE cells may produce lipofuscin. Further work, in particular using different animal models of disease, is needed to understand the abnormalities in the distribution of fundus AF observed in different retinal diseases, as well as their significance. It should be remembered, however, that any observations made in animal models should subsequently be validated clinically in humans.

ACKNOWLEDGMENTS

The author thanks Dr. A. Manivannan (University of Aberdeen) for helping with the SLO imaging, and Professor J. Greenwood (Institute of Ophthalmology, London) for providing the *CFH* knockout mouse samples.

REFERENCES

1. Xu H, Chen M, Manivannan A, Lois N, et al. Age-dependent accumulation of lipofuscin in perivascular and subretinal microglia in experimental mice. Aging Cell 2008;7:58–68.
2. Coffey PJ, Gias C, McDermott CJ, et al. Complement factor H deficiency in aged mice causes retinal abnormalities and visual dysfunction. Proc Natl Acad Sci USA 2007;104:16651–16656.
3. Xu H, Manivannan A, Goatman KA, et al. Improved leukocyte tracking in mouse retinal and choroidal circulation. Exp Eye Res 2002;74:403–410.
4. Katz ML, Redmond TM. Effect of Rpe65 knockout on accumulation of lipofuscin fluorophores in the retinal pigment epithelium. Invest Ophthalmol Vis Sci 2001;42:3023–3030.
5. Marmorstein AD, Marmorstein LY, Sakaguchi H, et al. Spectral profiling of autofluorescence associated with lipofuscin, Bruch's membrane, and sub-RPE deposits in normal and AMD eyes. Invest Ophthalmol Vis Sci 2002;43:2435–2441.
6. Bui TV, Han Y, Radu RA, et al. Characterization of native retinal fluorophores involved in biosynthesis of A2E and lipofuscin-associated retinopathies. J Biol Chem 2006;281:18112–18119.
7. Ambati J, Anand A, Fernandez S, et al. An animal model of age-related macular degeneration in senescent Ccl-2- or Ccr-2-deficient mice. Nat Med 2003;9:1390–1397.
8. Broderick C, Hoek RM, Forrester JV, et al. Constitutive retinal CD200 expression regulates resident microglia and activation state of inflammatory cells during experimental autoimmune uveoretinitis. Am J Pathol 2002;161:1669–1677.
9. Robison Jr WG, Kuwabara T, Bieri JG. Deficiencies of vitamins E and A in the rat. Retinal damage and lipofuscin accumulation. Invest Ophthalmol Vis Sci 1980;19:1030–1037.
10. Katz ML, Eldred GE, Robison Jr WG. Lipofuscin autofluorescence: evidence for vitamin A involvement in the retina. Mech Ageing Dev 1987;39:81–90.
11. Katz ML, Shanker MJ. Development of lipofuscin-like fluorescence in the retinal pigment epithelium in response to protease inhibitor treatment. Mech Ageing Dev 1989;49:23–40.
12. Katz ML, Gao CL. Vitamin A incorporation into lipofuscin-like inclusions in the retinal pigment epithelium. Mech Ageing Dev 1995;84:29–38.
13. Katz ML, Wendt KD, Sanders DN. RPE65 gene mutation prevents development of autofluorescence in retinal pigment epithelial phagosomes. Mech Ageing Dev 2005;126:513–521.
14. Lorenz B, Wabbels B, Wegscheider E, et al. Lack of fundus autofluorescence to 488 nanometers from childhood on in patients with early-onset severe retinal dystrophy associated with mutations in RPE65. Ophthalmology 2004;111:1585–1594.

15. Lorenz B, Gyurus P, Preising M, et al. Early-onset severe rod-cone dystrophy in young children with RPE65 mutations. Invest Ophthalmol Vis Sci 2000;41:2735–2742.

16. Radu RA, Mata NL, Nusinowitz S, et al. Treatment with isotretinoin inhibits lipofuscin accumulation in a mouse model of recessive Stargardt's macular degeneration. Proc Natl Acad Sci USA 2003;100:4742–4747.

17. Gollapalli DR, Rando RR. The specific binding of retinoic acid to RPE65 and approaches to the treatment of macular degeneration. Proc Natl Acad Sci USA 2004;101:10030–10035.

18. Radu RA, Han Y, Bui TV, et al. Reductions in serum vitamin A arrest accumulation of toxic retinal fluorophores: a potential therapy for treatment of lipofuscin-based retinal diseases. Invest Ophthalmol Vis Sci 2005;46:4393–4401.

19. Maiti P, Kong J, Kim SR, et al. Small molecule RPE65 antagonists limit the visual cycle and prevent lipofuscin formation. Biochemistry 2006;45:852–860.

Steffen Schmitz-Valckenberg
Fred W. Fitzke

CHAPTER 5

Imaging Techniques of Fundus Autofluorescence

T he imaging of fundus autofluorescence (AF) phenomena in vivo, as discussed in Chapter 1, was first demonstrated in the early days of fluorescein angiography, when preinjection fluorescence of optic disc drusen and optic disc hamartomas in tuberous sclerosis, and within lesions of Best vitelliform macular dystrophy was detected (1–4). However, these observations were limited to a few patients with pathological accumulations of highly fluorescent material. By contrast, the naturally occurring intrinsic fluorescence of the ocular fundus is quite low—about 2 orders of magnitude lower than the background of a fluorescein angiogram at the most intense part of the dye transit (5). Absorption of excitation and emission light with partly additional generation of fluorescence by anatomical structures anterior to the retina further interferes with the detection of fundus AF. The main barrier is the crystalline lens, which has highly fluorescent characteristics in the short-wavelength range (excitation between 400 and 600 nm results in peak emission at 520 nm) (see also Chapter 3) (6). With increasing age and particularly the development of nuclear lens opacities, the fluorescence of the lens becomes even more prominent. Therefore, fundus AF imaging with a conventional fundus camera using the excitation and emission filters as applied for fluorescein angiography produces images with low contrast and high background noise in young persons (Fig. 5.1). In the elderly, the quality of the images drops even further and it becomes practically impossible to evaluate the distribution of fundus AF.

RECORDING FUNDUS AUTOFLUORESCENCE

To better record fundus AF, adjustments and modifications of existing camera systems or sophisticated new imaging devices are required. Such devices include the fundus spectrophotometer, the confocal scanning laser ophthalmoscope (cSLO), and the modified fundus camera.

Fundus Spectrophotometer

The fundus spectrophotometer developed by Delori and coworkers (5,7) was designed to measure and systematically analyze the excitation and emission spectra of the AF from small retinal areas (2 degrees diameter) of the fundus. By incorporating an image-intensifier-diode-array as detector, beam separation in the pupil, and confocal detection to minimize contribution of AF from the crystalline lens, this device allows absolute measurements of AF. Groundbreaking work by Delori et al. (5) demonstrated that lipofuscin is the dominant source of intrinsic fluorescence of the ocular fundus. However, the small field of view is not practical for recording fundus AF in large patient populations or in the clinical setting.

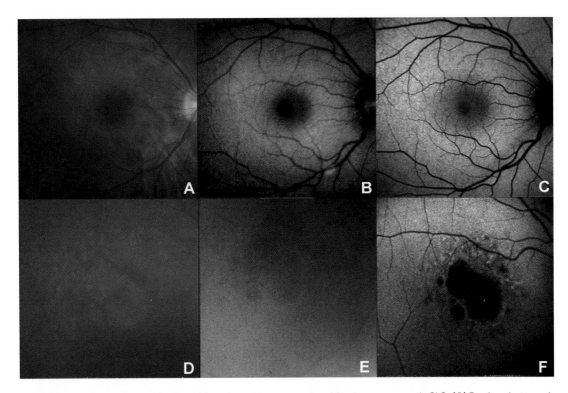

FIGURE 5.1.   Comparison of fundus AF imaging with a conventional fundus camera and cSLO. **(A)** Fundus photograph of a 29-year-old subject with no eye disease and clear media shows good quality, with small retinal vessels and foveal reflex visible. **(B)** Fundus AF imaging with the conventional fundus camera using the filters as applied for fluorescein angiography and maximum flash intensity (300 J) in the same subject produces a noisy image with low contrast. The optic nerve head appears to be artificially bright, which may be caused by scattered excitation light and therefore would be attributable to pseudofluorescence. **(C)** Fundus AF imaging with the cSLO, in contrast, results in a clear image with high image contrast and high sensitivity. **(D)** The quality of the fundus color photograph of this patient with geographic atrophy secondary to age-related macular degeneration (AMD) is slightly impaired as a result of concomitant nuclear sclerosis of the lens. **(E)** Corresponding fundus AF image obtained with a conventional fundus camera using the excitation and emission filters used for fluorescein angiography. The image is hazy and no retinal details are visible. **(F)** Fundus AF image obtained using a cSLO. The quality of the AF image is better than that obtained with the fundus camera, and macular abnormalities, including a central area of atrophy, are observed.

Confocal Scanning Laser Ophthalmoscopy

The use of a cSLO optimally addresses the limitations of the low intensity of the AF signal and the interference of the crystalline lens. It was used initially by von Rückmann and coworkers (8) in a clinical imaging system.

The cSLO projects a low-power laser beam on the retina that is swept across the fundus in a raster pattern (9). The intensity of the reflected light at each point, after it passes through the confocal pinhole, is registered by means of a detector and a two-dimensional image is subsequently generated. The use of confocal optics ensures that out-of-focus light (i.e., light originating outside the adjusted focal plane but within the light beam) is suppressed and thus the image contrast is enhanced. This suppression increases with distance from the focal plane, and signals from sources anterior to the retina, i.e., the lens or the cornea, are effectively reduced.

In contrast to the 2-degree discrete retinal field of the fundus spectrophotometer, the cSLO allows imaging over larger retinal areas. The standard image encompasses a retinal field of 30 degrees × 30 degrees. Additional lenses allow for imaging of a 55-degree field or, using the composite mode, imaging over even larger retinal areas. To reduce background noise and enhance image contrast, a series of several single images is usually recorded (8,10–13). For the final fundus AF image, a number of these frames (usually 4 to 32) are averaged and pixel values are normalized. Given the high sensitivity of the cSLO and the high frame rate of up to 16 frames per second, fundus AF imaging can be performed within seconds and at low excitation energies that are well below the maximum retinal irradiance limits of lasers established by the American National Standards Institute (14) and other international organizations.

Three different cSLOs have been widely used to obtain fundus AF images: the Heidelberg retina angiograph (HRA classic, HRA 2 and HRA Spectralis; Heidelberg Engineering, Dossenheim, Germany), the Rodenstock cSLO (RcSLO; Rodenstock, Weco, Düsseldorf, Germany), and the Zeiss prototype SM 30-4024 (ZcSLO; Zeiss, Oberkochen, Germany). For fundus AF imaging, all three use an excitation wavelength of 488 nm. Emitted light is detected above 500 nm for the HRA, above 515 nm for the RcSLO, and above 521 nm for the ZcSLO. Clinically useful fundus AF imaging has been reported with all three systems by several studies (8,10,12). A systematic comparison among the three systems by Bellmann and coworkers (15) in 2003 showed that both image contrast and image brightness were significantly higher with the ZcSLO and HRA classic compared to the RcSLO. Using a model eye, the highest background noise was measured with the ZcSLO and the lowest with the HRA classic. Since image contrast and brightness, and background noise are important indicators of image quality, Bellmann et al. (15) concluded that the observed differences might be of great importance when comparing fundus AF findings obtained with different imaging devices. Subsequent to their study, further developments led to the introduction of the HRA 2, which is currently the only commercially available cSLO for fundus AF imaging. This device allows real-time imaging, i.e., recording of the final mean and normalized image during acquisition. No time-consuming postacquisition processing of a movie is required. Thanks to an improved algorithm for automated image alignment to correct for eye movements during acquisition, a higher number of single frames can also be more easily captured, improving the signal-to-noise ratio and therefore possibly leading to better visualization of details. Recently, the combination of cSLO imaging with spectral-domain optical coherence tomography (OCT) in one instrument was made possible. This new imaging device enables simultaneous cSLO and OCT recordings, taking advantage of the registration of the fundus image and lateral eye movements by the cSLO system and synchronous topographic alignment to OCT scans. Several OCT scans can be averaged to reduce the background noise, and three-dimensional correlations of visible structural changes are possible.

MODIFIED FUNDUS CAMERA

Until recently, clinical applications of fundus AF imaging were limited to the cSLO, and in recent years the cSLO has gained increasing popularity and more widespread application. However, the major advantage of the cSLO—its sophisticated technical setup—also represents its major drawback: its considerable purchase and maintenance costs.

As mentioned above, fundus AF imaging with a conventional fundus camera operating in the same wavelength range as the cSLO has limitations due to the relatively low fundus AF signal, the absorption effects of the crystalline lens, and the nonconfocality, which makes the fundus camera prone to light scattering. Delori and coworkers (16) described the possibility of obtaining fundus AF images using a modified fundus camera. This included the insertion of an aperture in the illumination optics of the camera to minimize the loss of contrast caused by light scattering and fluorescence from the crystalline lens. However, this modification also resulted in the restriction of the angle of view to a 13-degree-diameter circle; this, together with the complex design, is the likely reason why this setup has not been further pursued and used by other groups or in a clinical setting to date. Spaide (17) reported his elegant idea of modifying a commercially available fundus camera by simply moving the excitation and emission wavelengths for fundus AF imaging toward the red end of the spectrum to bypass the fluorescence of the lens. The theoretically inexpensive purchase of an additional filter set, together with the broad availability of the fundus camera, may represent an attractive alternative. Figure 5.2 illustrates the excitation and emission filters of the modified fundus camera as introduced by Spaide in comparison with the cSLO for fundus AF imaging. Note that Spaide recently developed an additional modification of the filters (here called "modified fundus camera 2" as opposed to "modified fundus camera 1" for the first modification). Currently, there is only one commercially available modified fundus camera for fundus AF imaging (Topcon TRC-50IX; Topcon, Paramus, NJ), based on the modification by Spaide (modified fundus camera 2). Because only the filters are altered in the modified fundus camera, the other technical details remain unchanged compared to the conventional fundus camera, including the angle of coverage (up to 50 degrees) and possible range of flash light in-

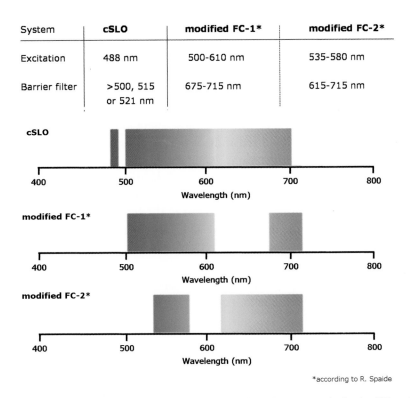

System	cSLO	modified FC-1*	modified FC-2*
Excitation	488 nm	500-610 nm	535-580 nm
Barrier filter	>500, 515 or 521 nm	675-715 nm	615-715 nm

*according to R. Spaide

FIGURE 5.2.   Overview of excitation and emission spectra of imaging systems for fundus AF imaging. The cSLO system is based on excitation of a blue laser beam ($\lambda = 488$ nm). Emission is detected with a cutoff filter ($\lambda \cong 500$ nm, depending on the system; see text). For the modified fundus camera, two bandwidth filters are applied (17,27), operating in a longer-wavelength range compared to the cSLO. Subsequent to the original modification (here called modified FC-1), Spaide recently introduced a second modification (here called modified FC-2).

tensities. Currently, fundus AF imaging with the modified fundus camera is based on excitation by one single flash and the immediate capture of a single image. After acquisition, the image brightness and contrast values of this single image are manually adjusted to better visualize the individual distribution of fundus AF intensities.

COMPARISON BETWEEN THE CSLO AND MODIFIED FUNDUS CAMERA FOR FUNDUS AF IMAGING

Both the cSLO and the modified fundus camera allow for fundus AF imaging in the clinical setting and both are commercially available. However, only one systematic comparison of different retinal pathologies is available. Theoretical considerations and preliminary observations suggest that fundus AF imaging with the modified fundus camera might not be entirely equivalent to the cSLO system. Table 5.1 summarizes the technical differences between both imaging devices, which are discussed in more detail below.

Excitation and Emission Spectra

Because of the broad excitation and emission spectra of ocular intrinsic fluorescence, it is conceivable that both systems, with their individual fluorescence settings, are able to detect fundus AF (5,7). However, fundus AF is made up of several fluorophores with different absorption and emission spectra as well as different amounts of fluorescence intensity (see also Chapters 1–3 and 8). For example, minor fluorophores of the fundus include $NAD-NADH^+$ (oxidized and reduced nicotinamidadenindinucleotide) and $FAD-FADH^2$ (oxidized and reduced flavinadeninucleotide) in mitochondria, advanced glycation end products (AGEs), collagen, and elastin (18–21). Furthermore, lipofuscin as the dominant fluorophore is composed of several molecules that may not only be disease-specific (and therefore may cause alteration of the spectrum), but also known to be characterized by a red shift of the emission with increasing excitation wavelength (22). These considerations would imply that the composition of the detected AF signal may vary between the cSLO and the modified fundus camera.

The different excitation and emission spectra may explain the different patterns of decreased intensity revealed by the two systems in the central macula in a normal subject (Fig. 5.3). Generally, the decreased AF signal in the macula of healthy individuals

TABLE 5.1	Summary of Technical Differences Between the cSLO and the Modified Fundus Camera for Fundus AF Imaging
cSLO	**Modified fundus camera**
One excitation wavelength (laser source)	Bandwidth filters for excitation and emission
Large emission spectrum (cutoff filter)	
Continuous scanning at low light intensities in a raster pattern	One single flash at maximum intensities
Confocal system	Entire cone of light
Laser power fixed by manufacturer, detector sensitivity adjustable	Flash light intensity, gain and gamma of detector adjustable
Image processing with averaging of single frames and pixel normalization	Manual contrast and brightness

Schmitz-Valckenberg S, Fleckenstein M, Göbel AP. Evaluation of autofluorescence imaging with the scanning laser ophthalmoscope and the fundus camera in age-related geographic atrophy. Am J Ophthalmol 2008;146(2):183–192.

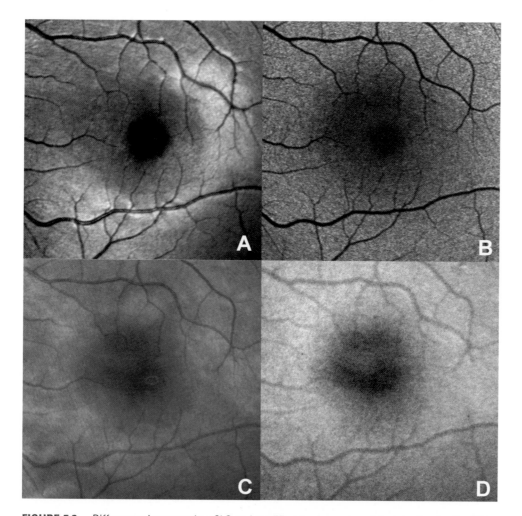

FIGURE 5.3.   Differences between the cSLO and modified fundus camera 1 in detecting fundus AF intensity in the central macular area. **(A–D)** High-magnification images of the same eye comparing the reflectance **(A)** and AF image **(B)** obtained with a cSLO, and the color fundus photograph **(C)** and the AF image obtained using the modified fundus camera **(D)**. A decreased signal is detected in the center of the macula in both images obtained with the cSLO, suggesting absorption of the excitation light. In contrast to the cSLO images, an irregular area of decreased intensity and overall a small area of decreased intensity is seen in the AF image obtained with the fundus camera. Note also that the contrast for retinal blood vessels is less on the image obtained with the fundus camera compared to the cSLO, which enables better visualization of the perifoveal vasculature.

has been attributed to macular pigment absorption, increased melanin deposition, and lower density of lipofuscin granules in central retinal pigment epithelium (RPE) cells (5,23). In particular, the absorption of macular pigment (peak absorbance at 460 nm, marked reduction >510–540 nm [5,24]) should differ between the two systems.

Mode of Excitation and Detection

A major difference between both systems is embodied in the scanning mode and the use of confocal optics with the cSLO as opposed to the excitation by a single flash and the fluorescence exhibition within the entire cone of light at one single instance with the fundus camera. The latter mode is particularly prone to pseudofluorescence phenomena. This term was used in the early days of fluorescein angiogram photography with the fundus camera and refers to the generation of fluorescence by structures anterior and posterior to the retina, particularly the crystalline lens (25,26). This fluorescent light is scattered and reflected back toward the detector. Because of its longer wavelength compared to the original excitation light, it is not rejected by the emission filter and is subsequently imaged as an increased signal. If pseudofluorescence occurs, it is not possible to differentiate between pseudofluorescence and real AF by just looking at the AF image. By reviewing the corresponding reflectance image (same excitation wavelength, but no emission filter), however, one can identify most pseudofluorescence phenomena by an increased intensity in both the reflectance and the AF image.

Even when operating in the longer-wavelength ranges, the modified fundus camera may be still affected by lens absorption and lens fluorescence to a larger extent compared to a confocal system operating in the short-wavelength range. This lens fluorescence would be scattered inside the vitreous cavity. In particular, the optic nerve head, with its highly reflective properties, would be prone to send this light back toward the detector. Because of the longer wavelength range, this secondary reflectance would easily pass the barrier filter and contribute to the detected signal. By contrast, the scanning mode and confocal optics of the cSLO ensure that the amount of light and the area of exposure are much less at one instance. Out-of-focus reflective light from structures outside the focal plane is mostly blocked. Scattered, secondary reflectance light can still contribute to the detected signal with the cSLO, but only if the out-of-focus fluorescence light is directly scattered through the pinhole. The likelihood of these events occurring, together with the low exposure at one instance, would be less compared to the fundus camera scenario.

Pseudofluorescence phenomena should be differentiated from filter leakage. Such leakage can also result in an enhanced signal that is not (or at least not totally) derived from AF phenomena. The barrier filter should ensure that the reflective light in the range of the excitation light is rejected and only the longer-wavelength fluorescence light reaches the detector. For the HRA, the emission filter suppresses light at 488 nm by a factor of 10^{-6}, and the barrier filter for the modified fundus camera introduced by Spaide affords a rejection of at least 10^{-7} of the excitation light (10,27). The reflective light in the range of the excitation light is therefore not entirely blocked. Consequently, neither the cSLO nor the modified fundus camera is absolutely resistant against filter leakage, which can become an important issue in the case of very strong reflectance properties of retinal structures (such as exposed sclera).

In a comparison of fundus AF images acquired with the cSLO and the modified fundus camera, one prominent difference is the appearance of the retinal blood vessels and the optic nerve head. With cSLO fundus AF imaging, these structures have been described to exhibit a markedly reduced AF signal, which has been explained by absorption phenomena resulting from blood contents and lack of AF material, respectively. In contrast, the signal detected from these anatomic structures with the modified fundus camera is less decreased. The reduction in contrast of blood vessels compared to the normal background signal may also explain why small foveal vessels are much less visible than with cSLO imaging. One possible explanation for the less decreased signal involves the different excitation and emission wavelengths (27). The longer wavelength used with the modified fundus camera may not be affected as much by the absorption phenomena of blood, and the blood contents themselves may have some AF properties at these wavelengths (a sudden increase in fluorescence emission of blood is observed above 580 nm) (5). However, this does not quite explain the homogeneous, increased gray signal of the optic nerve. Preliminary observations indicate that the signal of the optic nerve head imaged with the modified fundus camera is not just

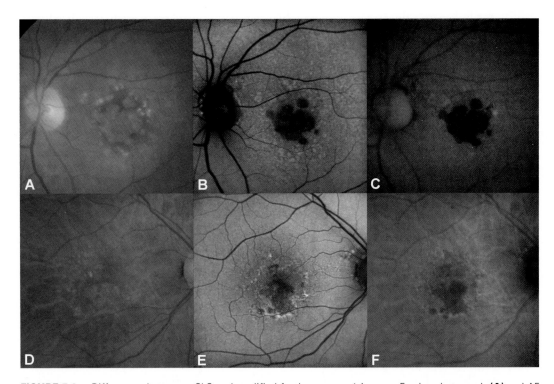

FIGURE 5.4.   Differences between cSLO and modified fundus camera-1 images. Fundus photograph **(A)** and AF images obtained using a cSLO **(B)** and modified fundus camera-1 **(C)** from two patients with advanced atrophic AMD. In the first example, the optic nerve head is characterized by a severely decreased signal on the cSLO image, as is generally the case **(B)**. By contrast, on the modified fundus camera image **(C)**, the optic disc exhibits a severely increased signal—not just a slightly increased one (as on all AF images obtained with the fundus camera images). Note that the crystalline deposits near the temporal-superior border of atrophy are hardly visible on the cSLO image, but show a marked increased signal on the corresponding fundus camera image. This difference in the signal could be explained by pseudofluorescence phenomena, as both the optic nerve head and crystalline deposits have highly reflective properties. In the second example **(D–F)**, the fundus photograph **(D)** shows prominent choroidal vessels. These large choroidal vessels are also visualized in the corresponding optimized AF image with the fundus camera **(F)** by increased intensity. Reading of abnormalities at the level of the RPE theoretically may be impaired in the presence of intrinsic fluorescence from choroidal vessels. By contrast, AF abnormalities of the RPE around the area of atrophy are clear in the cSLO image **(E)** and no underlying choroidal vessels are visible. Likely causes for these different observations include (alone or in combination) the nonconfocality of the fundus camera system and the long-wavelength reflectance signal that is generated by structures anterior to the retina and would pass the emission filter, finally contributing to the detected signal.

less decreased, but is characterized by almost maximum intensity in a few patients with advanced lens opacities (Fig. 5.4). When these particular images are reviewed, an uneven illumination of the signal and the appearance of glare, particularly at the optic nerve head or other structures in pathologic conditions (e.g., crystals) with high reflective properties, can be identified. Both the appearance of glare and the intense signal over highly reflective structures, which typically have no AF characteristics with the cSLO, suggest that the detected signal with the modified fundus camera is strongly influenced by pseudoautofluorescence phenomena in these subjects.

In other cases, the imaging mode of the fundus camera may represent an advantage. In exudative retinal disease (e.g., choroidal neovascularization or central serous retinopathy), fundus AF abnormalities adjacent to the primary lesion and inferior to the leakage on fluorescein angiography are usually much more easily visualized with the modified fundus camera. (It has been speculated that they represent areas with subretinal fluid and that their location is the result of gravity effects [28,29].) Another possible explanation is that short, dynamic AF changes due to photobleaching are more likely to occur with the continuous scanning mode as opposed to the short flash of the fundus camera. Furthermore, underlying choroidal blood vessels are sometimes seen with the modified fundus camera. The ability to image optic disc drusen, which are usually characterized by high AF, may be also be enhanced with the modified fundus camera, particularly if they are buried deeper in the optic nerve (30). These observations cannot be totally explained by pseudofluorescence phenomena. Two other reasons, alone or in combination, seem to be more likely: the different filter combination (e.g., detection of different fluorophores, including elastin and collagen within the blood vessel walls) and the nonconfocal setup (e.g., easier detection of out-of-focus fluorescence).

Image Acquisition

The cSLO scans the retina continuously and the actual image is immediately digitized and visualized on a computer screen. The orientation and position of the laser scanning camera, detector sensitivity, and refractive correction can be easily adjusted during the acquisition process and in real time by the operator. This practical and easily feasible mode of imaging is only possible because of the high sensitivity and relatively low light levels (intensity per retinal area) of the cSLO. Nevertheless, it is important to optimally adjust these three modifiable settings to achieve good image quality and gain reliable information from these recordings.

The acquisition mode with the fundus camera allows for modification of more settings. In addition to the orientation and position of the camera, gain of the detector, and focusing, the intensity of the flash of light and the gamma of the detector can be adjusted. These variations mean more choices for the user. However, it might be difficult or time-consuming to find the correct settings for an individual patient.

Image Processing

Compared to the cSLO, image processing with the modified fundus camera is easy and straightforward. To optimize the visualization of the distribution of intensities, image brightness and contrast are usually manually adjusted. However, this modification has not been standardized yet and it should be noted that, after manual adjustment of these image parameters, an absolute comparison of intensities within two images (even when taken with the same acquisition settings) is not possible.

Standard operating procedures for cSLO fundus AF imaging are available but have not found widespread use in many clinical centers (31). Postacquisition image processing with the cSLO allows for more modifications and is more time-consuming (unless the real-time mode is used) compared to the fundus camera. The key principle is that calculations of a mean and normalized image are required in order to overcome two major general drawbacks of fundus AF: noise and low sensitivity of the signal, with subsequent difficult visualization of the topographic distribution of intensities. As a result, these two modifications introduce two minor limitations: slight distortion of details (because of imperfect alignment of single frames) and inability to compare absolute intensities between images. In the following, the processing of cSLO fundus AF images is explained in more detail and compared with imaging by means of the modified fundus camera.

The noise of the signal within a single cSLO frame is significant. Noise is generally a random event and interferes with the actual signal. Image noise is reduced by a factor of $\sqrt{n}$, where n is the number of frames to be averaged. In practice, averaging a series of single frames can greatly improve the signal-to-noise ratio and therefore the visualization of details. The number of images to be processed is usually limited. For mathematical reasons (there is no linear relationship between the number of frames and the reduction of noise), the required number of frames increases by the square to achieve the same amount of noise reduction. For example, using four single frames reduces the noise by a factor of 2 ($\sqrt{4}$). To further decrease the noise by 2, one would need 16 ($\sqrt{16} = 4$) frames, not eight frames. Furthermore, other practical reasons limit the number of images used to calculate the mean image, including the exposure time to the laser beam needed to image the patient and the increasing difficulty of correcting for eye movements with more and more frames. The latter in particular can be troublesome and lead, when using a high number of frames (16–64, depending on the patient's stability of eye movements), to an increase in image noise and blurriness (fuzzy border of retinal structures) due to poor alignment of single frames. Therefore, in most cases it is more practical to use a reasonable number of single images to calculate the mean image. Compared to the cSLO, the modified fundus camera uses the maximum or near-maximum flash light intensities (200–300 J) for a single frame. This means that the number of images that can be safely taken is limited because of exposure levels. However, averaging even a small number of images has not yet been demonstrated to reduce noise and improve the visualization of details with the fundus camera AF imaging. Furthermore, to date, the commercially available software has not implemented averaging algorithms.

One additional factor affecting the number of frames required to calculate the mean image is the increase in sensitivity of the AF signal. A standard digital grayscale image is based on pixel values ranging from 0 to 255 units. However, with current devices, one AF image encompasses a band of approximately 20–40 units in most subjects (because of the low intensity of fundus AF). Therefore, a modification of the pixel histogram using all available values (0–255 units) greatly improves the visualization of the intensity distribution and therefore the visualization of more details, at the expense of losing a judgment on the absolute AF intensities. The easiest way to achieve this is to manually stretch the histogram and modify the contrast, as is done with the modified fundus camera. The more sophisticated cSLO method uses an automatic software algorithm with normalization of the histogram. Using the information of several frames, binary calculation allows for a smooth stretching of the pixel histogram. No gaps in between values occur (such as with the manual method using one image) and therefore the sensitivity of the signal is enhanced. Compared to the manual modification, such as with every computer software, the automatic normalization algorithm may not work properly. For example, incorrect settings during the acquisition process, particularly wrong detector settings, may not be seen on a normalized image at first glance and may lead to false interpretations. Therefore, it is prudent to review single images and always compare them with the mean normalized image. Furthermore, details within areas of very increased or very decreased signal intensities compared to most of the rest of the image may be also obscured on images by improper automatic normalization. In these cases, it is advisable not to use automatically generated normalized images and to adjust brightness and contrast values manually in the nonnormalized mean image.

It is very important to understand that neither automatic normalization nor manual adjustment of image contrast and brightness allows for the quantitative assessment of absolute AF intensities. Such image processing merely facilitates visualization of the topographic differences of AF intensities within one image, and thus the interpretation of localized alterations in the distribution of fundus AF in one eye at the time of acquisition. Because of the artificial change of the absolute pixel values and their relation to each other, an absolute comparison of normalized images among eyes of different patients, as well as images of the same eye obtained at different time points, is not possible. The software of modern cSLO imaging systems permits users to easily deactivate the normalization of mean images. However, to date, the absolute quantification of intensities remains a challenge. No reliable method for quantifying AF in small areas has been demonstrated. It is again the influence of the lens (as discussed at length above) that appears to be the major limiting factor for absolute quantification of AF intensities using the current commercially available systems.

REFERENCES

1. Schatz H, et al. Preinjection fluorescence. Disc leak. In: Schatz H, et al., eds. Interpretation of Fundus Fluorescein Angiography. St. Louis, MO: C.V. Mosby, 1978:251–259, 514–537.
2. Wessing A, Veränderungen der Papille M-SG. Papillenschwellung. In: Wessing A, Veränderungen der Papille M-SG, eds. Fluoreszenzangiographie der Retina. Lehrbuch und Atlas. Stuttgart: Georg Thieme Verlag, 1968:166–172.
3. Mustonen E, Nieminen H. Optic disc drusen—a photographic study. I. Autofluorescence pictures and fluorescein angiography. Acta Ophthalmol (Copenh) 1982;60:849–858.
4. Neetens A, Burvenich H. Autofluorescence of optic disc-drusen. Bull Soc Belge Ophtalmol 1977;179:103–110.
5. Delori FC, et al. In vivo fluorescence of the ocular fundus exhibits retinal pigment epithelium lipofuscin characteristics. Invest Ophthalmol Vis Sci 1995;36:718–729.
6. Bessems GJ, et al. Non-tryptophan fluorescence of crystallins from normal and cataractous human lenses. Invest Ophthalmol Vis Sci 1987;28:1157–1163.
7. Delori FC. Spectrophotometer for non-invasive measurement of intrinsic fluorescence and reflectance of the ocular fundus. Appl Optics 1994;33:7429–7452.
8. von Rückmann A, Fitzke FW, Bird AC. Distribution of fundus autofluorescence with a scanning laser ophthalmoscope. Br J Ophthalmol 1995;79:407–412.
9. Webb RH, Hughes GW, Delori FC. Confocal scanning laser ophthalmoscope. Appl Optics 1987;26:1492–1499.
10. Bellmann C, et al. [Topography of fundus autofluorescence with a new confocal scanning laser ophthalmoscope]. Ophthalmologe 1997;94:385–391.
11. Jorzik JJ, et al. Digital simultaneous fluorescein and indocyanine green angiography, autofluorescence, and red-free imaging with a solid-state laser-based confocal scanning laser ophthalmoscope. Retina 2005;25:405–416.
12. Solbach U, et al. Imaging of retinal autofluorescence in patients with age-related macular degeneration. Retina 1997;17:385–389.
13. Bindewald A, et al. [cSLO digital fundus autofluorescence imaging]. Ophthalmologe 2005;102:259–264.
14. American National Standard for the Safe Use of Lasers: ANSI Z136.1. Laser Institute of America. Orlando, FL: A.N.S. Institute, 2000.
15. Bellmann C, et al. Fundus autofluorescence imaging compared with different confocal scanning laser ophthalmoscopes. Br J Ophthalmol 2003;87:1381–1386.
16. Delori FC, et al. Autofluorescence distribution associated with drusen in age-related macular degeneration. Invest Ophthalmol Vis Sci 2000;41:496–504.
17. Spaide RF. Fundus autofluorescence and age-related macular degeneration. Ophthalmology 2003;110:392–399.
18. Schweitzer D, et al. In vivo measurement of time-resolved autofluorescence at the human fundus. J Biomed Opt 2004;9:1214–1222.
19. Schweitzer D, et al. Towards metabolic mapping of the human retina. Microsc Res Tech 2007;70:410–419.
20. Nelson DA, et al. Special report: noninvasive multi-parameter functional optical imaging of the eye. Ophthalmic Surg Lasers Imaging 2005;36:57–66.
21. Winkler BS, et al. Metabolic mapping in mammalian retina: a biochemical and 3H-2-deoxyglucose autoradiographic study. Exp Eye Res 2003;77:327–337.
22. Sparrow J. Lipofuscin of the retinal pigment epithelium. In: Holz FG, et al., eds. Atlas of Fundus Autofluorescence Imaging. Berlin, Heidelberg: Springer, 2007:1–16.
23. Weiter JJ, et al. Retinal pigment epithelial lipofuscin and melanin and choroidal melanin in human eyes. Invest Ophthalmol Vis Sci 1986;27:145–152.

24. Hammond Jr BR, Wooten BR, Snodderly DM. Density of the human crystalline lens is related to the macular pigment carotenoids, lutein and zeaxanthin. Optom Vis Sci 1997;74:499–504.

25. Machemer R, et al. Pseudofluorescence—a problem in interpretation of fluorescein angiograms. Am J Ophthalmol 1970;70:1–10.

26. Lemke L, Tilgner S, Jutte A. [Sources of error in fluorescence-photography]. Ophthalmologica 1967;153: 349–354.

27. Spaide RF. Autofluorescence imaging with the fundus camera. In: Holz FG, et al., eds. Atlas of Autofluorescence Imaging. Berlin, Heidelberg: Springer, 2007:49–53.

28. Dandekar SS, et al. Autofluorescence imaging of choroidal neovascularization due to age-related macular degeneration. Arch Ophthalmol 2005;123:1507–1513.

29. Spaide RF, Klancnik Jr JM. Fundus autofluorescence and central serous chorioretinopathy. Ophthalmology 2005;112:825–833.

30. Holz FG, Schmitz-Valckenberg S, Spaide RF, et al, eds. Atlas of fundus autofluorescence imaging. Berlin: Springer-Verlag, 2007:313–327.

31. Schmitz-Valckenberg S, et al. How to obtain the optimal fundus autofluorescence image with the cSLO. In: Holz FG, et al., eds. Atlas of Autofluorescence Imaging. Berlin, Heidelberg: Springer, 2007:37–48.

Ulrich Kellner
Simone Kellner

Near-Infrared Fundus Autofluorescence

Fundus autofluorescence (FAF) derived from lipofuscin and its major fluorophor, A2E, has developed into an important noninvasive imaging technique in the last decade. When interpreting images in normal and disease states, one must keep in mind that several different fluorophores are present within the retina and the retinal pigment epithelium (RPE) (see also Chapters 1–3) (1,2). A specific selection of the wavelength for excitation of AF and the wavelength of the cutoff filter for emitted light could provide additional possibilities for noninvasive imaging of the RPE.

Near-infrared autofluorescence (NIA) imaging, which uses the same excitation light and cutoff filters employed for indocyanine-green (ICG) angiography, is widely available. NIA was first described as pseudofluorescence prior to ICG angiography (3). The intensity of the emitted AF is about 60–100 times lower compared to that of AF (2), but imaging can be reliably repeated.

NIA imaging was first reported in 2006, and has been applied in several recently published studies (2,4–15). This chapter describes the imaging technique, the origin of the NIA signal, the distribution of NIA in the healthy eye, and the clinical findings in selected retinal diseases and their implications.

IMAGING TECHNIQUE

Imaging of NIA can be done using a confocal scanning laser ophthalmoscope (cSLO, Spectralis HRA; Heidelberg Engineering, Heidelberg, Germany) (2). Different camera objectives provide either a 30-degree or wide-angle field-of-view mode. The image resolution is usually 768 × 768 pixels, but it can be varied. Focusing is achieved using the near-infrared reflectance mode at 815 nm. Diode laser light (787 nm) is used to excite AF. A band-pass filter with a cutoff at 800 nm included in the system is inserted in front of the detector. Six pictures per second are recorded and about 15 single images are averaged depending on the fixation of the patient (Fig. 6.1). Because of the lower-intensity signal, optimal imaging is performed with dilated pupils. Cideciyan et al. (5) reported a technique termed near-infrared reduced-illuminance AF imaging (NIR-RAFI). Although they reduced the illuminance for FAF in their HRA2, they used the same manufacturer settings for NIR-RAFI as described above.

NIA images are evaluated qualitatively on a computer monitor. Abnormalities of NIA distribution are documented and classified as either increased, reduced, or absent NIA compared to other areas within the same image. Interindividual differences in media transmission properties due to the presence or absence of cataract, after cataract, or moderate vitreous opacities, and the associated difficulties with normalization in a clinical setting preclude an easy quantification of NIA intensity. Image

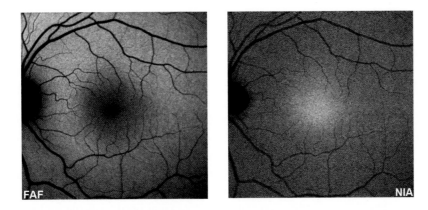

FIGURE 6.1.   Normal distribution of FAF as recorded using conventional AF imaging and NIA imaging. At the posterior pole, AF shows the highest intensity in the perifoveal area with a decrease toward the fovea. In contrast, NIA has a peak intensity in the foveal area with a decrease toward the periphery. More peripherally, AF and NIA distributions are homogeneous.

postprocessing with different programs and quantification of NIA images has been suggested in research settings (2,5).

ORIGIN OF THE NIA SIGNAL

The major fluorophore contributing to NIA is most likely melanin and its related compounds (melanolipofuscin, melanolysosomes, and oxidized melanin) in the RPE cells (2). A low-intensity signal is obtained from melanin in the deep choroid, which can be detected in areas denuded of RPE cells (i.e., geographic atrophy).

The notion that the NIA signal derives from melanin is based on the following evidence: The distribution of NIA seems to correspond to that of RPE melanin (16), although the contribution of choroidal melanin is evident (2). The severely reduced NIA signal in areas of RPE loss indicates that the major source for NIA is the RPE. The markedly increased NIA signal in choroidal nevi supports the view that NIA is derived predominantly from ocular melanin (see Chapter 15). Melanin absorption decreases with increasing wavelength (17,18). AF emission spectra of melanin granules of human RPE have been mostly examined for shorter wavelengths (17,19). At wavelengths used for conventional AF imaging (<500 nm), melanin AF is present but with much lower intensity compared to lipofuscin. For synthetic melanin and melanin in the skin, AF with a maximum at 870–900 nm was demonstrated after excitation at 785 nm (20). Melanin AF is increased with oxidation (18,21,22). Melanolipofuscin (melanin with a cortex of lipofuscin) and melanolysosomes (melanin with a cortex of enzyme-reactive material) accumulate with age and may represent melanin in the process of repair, modification, or degradation (23). The AF of melanolipofuscin is intermediate between melanin and lipofuscin (19). In summary, AF of melanin, oxidized melanin, and compound granules containing melanin contribute to the NIA signal.

Keilhauer and Delori (2) thoroughly discussed the possible contributions of other fluorophores to the NIA signal. Even for conventional AF imaging, only a few fluorophores within the lipofuscin complex (A2E, *cis*-isomers of A2E, and all-*trans*-retinal dimer conjugate [24–26]) have been clearly characterized (see also Chapter 3). Other fluorophores may be present, and the composition of fluorophores within the lipofuscin granules may differ among different diseases (1,26). Although the possibility that lipofuscin fluorophores contribute to the NIA signal cannot be ruled out, that is unlikely based on the different AF distributions observed in normal individuals and in patients with a variety of retinal disorders when imaged using conventional AF and NIA. Other possible fluorophores include collagen, elastin, and porphyrin. Porphyrins within the blood vessels do not emanate detectable AF, but a contribution to NIA in hemorrhages cannot be excluded (3,4). The emission spectra for collagen and elastin (27) have not been examined with near-infrared light. A major contribution of these other fluorophores to NIA is unlikely (2).

Histological examination of photoreceptors and RPE in retinal degenerative disease is of limited value for comparison with NIA images. First, primarily tissue obtained from patients with advanced stages of disease has been available for histological studies. Second, histological reports often focus on lipofuscin distribution, whereas melanin distribution is rarely mentioned. As discussed below, the available information on RPE melanin alterations in Stargardt disease, retinitis pigmentosa (RP), and age-related macular degeneration (AMD) are in accordance with NIA findings in these disorders.

NORMAL NIA

The optic disc and retinal vessels appear dark on normal NIA images (Fig. 6.1). The NIA signal remains relatively even from the mid-peripheral to the peripheral retina. At the posterior pole, the NIA signal is maximal, with a peak at the fovea and a marked decline of NIA intensity toward the perifoveal region. Large choroidal vessels are visible with NIA in about 5% of normal individuals. The distribution of NIA differs strongly from that obtained using conventional AF imaging (see also Chapters 3 and 9).

The distribution of NIA intensity varies among individuals. At present, the influence of aging on NIA imaging is unknown. An age-related decrease in the ratio of foveal to perifoveal NIA has been observed (2). Age changes are difficult to predict. The melanin content in the RPE cells decreases with age, but the fluorescence of melanin granules increases especially to longer wavelengths (17,19,28). With increasing age, pure melanin granules are increasingly transformed to melanolipofuscin or melanolysosomes, but melanin synthesis also occurs (28–30). It can be assumed that the result of these opposing age-related effects on melanin and its compounds may be variable.

ROLE OF MELANIN IN THE RPE

Melanin has a protective function in the RPE, sheltering the RPE from exposure to light scattering, radiation, oxidative stress, and light damage (31–33). Whereas lipofuscin is located in the basal portion of RPE cells (see also Chapter 2), melanin granules accumulate in the apical part of RPE cells, and a moderate decrease in the number of melanin granules is observed with age (34). Limited melanogenesis has been found in adults (29). The antioxidative properties of melanosomes decrease with age (35).

In vitro studies indicate that melanin is involved in the phagocytosis of photoreceptor outer segments (36). In one study (37), subretinal injection of rod outer segments induced melanogenesis in rat eyes. Tyrosinase activity, a key enzyme for melanin formation, can be induced in human adult RPE cells fed with rod outer segments in vitro (38,39). Melanin formation in human RPE has been observed in degenerative disease with degradation of rod outer segments (40).

MECHANISMS OF NIA ALTERATIONS

An increase in NIA signal could be caused by melanogenesis, formation of melanolysosomes or melanolipofuscin, or altered AF characteristics of melanin in disease processes. All of the above could occur as a response to increased phagocytotic activity due to photoreceptor cell degeneration (37). An increase of melanolysosomes and melanolipofuscin has been documented with age and in degenerative diseases (28,34,40). Alteration of melanin AF characteristics has been observed with age (11) or as a result of oxidation (18,21). In advanced RP, loss of pure melanin granules and a marked increase of melanolysosomes within the RPE have been documented in areas with preserved retinal function corresponding to cones with residual outer segments and intact cone synaptic pedicles (41–44). An anterior displacement of melanin in enlarged RPE cells, as observed in Stargardt disease, could also contribute to increased NIA (Fig. 6.2) (45,46). Increased melanolipofuscin formation has been observed adjacent to geographic atrophy in AMD (47). Increased NIA signal is also observed in choroidal nevi (see Chapter 15).

Reduced NIA appears to correspond to a reduced melanin content in RPE cells, which may correspond to lower melanin content or reduced melanin phagocytotic activity. In advanced RP, RPE cells in the perifovea or near the optic disc underlying cone cell bodies without outer segments and synaptic pedicles lose their melanin and contain no melanolysosomes (41,48). In addition, dissolution of melanin granules in enlarged RPE cells or, intriguingly (see above), posterior displacement of melanin granules in the RPE cells, as described in Stargardt disease, could contribute to reduced NIA (46,49). Reduced NIA can also be caused by blockage by vitreous opacities.

Absent NIA can be the result of blockage (e.g., by retinal vessels or hemorrhages) or the absence of RPE cells. Loss of RPE cells (e.g., in geographic atrophy) is indicated by an absent NIA signal as well as by an absent signal when imaging with conventional AF (see also Chapter 10C), although the atrophic areas often appear larger

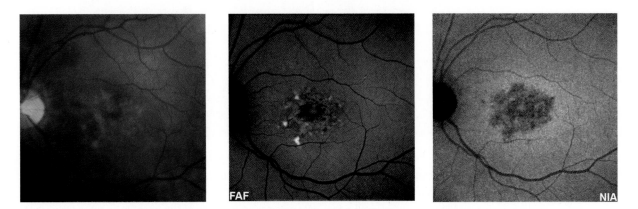

FIGURE 6.2.   Stargardt disease. More flecks are detected with conventional FAF imaging than on color fundus photographs. NIA is reduced in an area slightly larger than that detected with conventional AF.

on NIA compared to conventional AF. When there is no detectable NIA from RPE cells, a low-intensity NIA signal from the deep choroid can be detected between dark choroidal vessels.

CLINICAL FINDINGS

Given that NIA is a very new imaging technique, there are scarce data (to date) on the distribution of NIA in various retinal diseases, its clinical usefulness, and its implications for the understanding of pathophysiologic mechanisms of disease. Herein, we will describe only those conditions in which sufficient data are currently available.

ABCA4-Gene Related Stargardt Disease and Cone-Rod Dystrophy

In Stargardt disease and cone-rod dystrophies associated with mutations in the ABCA4 gene, characteristic NIA findings have been reported (5,8,11). Abnormalities in the distribution of NIA, as it occurs with conventional AF abnormalities (see also Chapter 11G) (50,51), may be limited to the posterior pole or progress beyond the vascular arcades. Whereas foci of increased AF are frequently seen when using conventional AF imaging, foci of increased NIA signals are rare. NIA is frequently reduced in patchy or confluent areas (Fig. 6.3); of interest, in these areas, foci of increased AF are frequently detected in conventional AF imaging. Areas of NIA abnormalities appear to be larger than those observed on conventional AF images, which may indicate that NIA alterations precede conventional AF abnormalities. Atrophic areas have absent NIA. The relative peripapillary sparing observed using conventional AF imaging (see also Chapter 11G) is also present on NIA imaging.

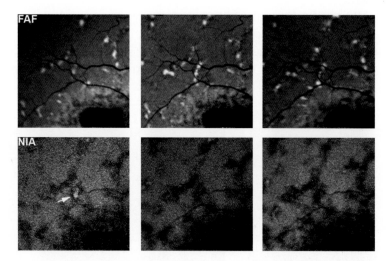

FIGURE 6.3.   Excerpts of conventional FAF and NIA images demonstrating progression of Stargardt disease. The images in the middle column were taken 6 months after the initial visit (*left*), and the images on the right were taken 6 months later. The lesion in the center of the image shows a spot of increased NIA at the initial visit (*arrow*), with progressive reduction of NIA intensity on subsequent visits. In contrast, in the same area, AF intensity increases from the initial to the second visit, but decreases at the last examination.

Follow-up on the above findings is limited. In a few documented cases, increased NIA preceded increased conventional AF, with a further increase in conventional AF as NIA decreased; the reduction in the NIA also preceded the reduction of conventional AF (Fig. 6.3). This sequence of events indicates that the initial increase in NIA signal may be the first sign of the pathological process that leads to RPE degeneration and loss.

The NIA findings in Stargardt disease are in accordance with histopathology findings (see Chapter 11G).

Retinitis Pigmentosa

NIA findings in RP are characteristic (Fig. 6.4). Typically, conventional AF shows a ring of increased AF in an area of relatively normal AF on both sides (see also Chapter 11A) (53,54). NIA is usually increased within this ring, with a sharp decline beyond this ring toward the periphery (9,12).

Marked abnormalities in the distribution of NIA and conventional AF have been observed in infants preceding ophthalmoscopic abnormalities. Thus, NIA and conventional AF imaging can be used as an important tool to establish the diagnosis of RP in small infants in whom electrophysiology and visual fields may be difficult to obtain.

The NIA findings in RP correspond to histological findings, which in previous reports showed absence of melanin in areas with nonfunctioning photoreceptors but preserved RPE cells (41,48), whereas melanin was present in areas with photoreceptors that kept their dendritic connections (41–44). As outlined above, rod outer segment phagocytosis induces melanogenesis (36,37). Thus, it could be speculated that the absent demand of phagocytosis leads to a decline of melanosomes after a period of increased phagocytosis because of photoreceptor degeneration.

It has been demonstrated that the ring of increased AF observed using conventional AF imaging corresponds to the peripheral border of preserved cone function in RP (see also Chapter 11A) (52,53). Combining the information from imaging and histology, one could speculate that the area of increased NIA encircled by a ring of increased AF, as observed using conventional AF imaging, indicates the area of preserved cone function, whereas the more peripheral area with markedly reduced NIA and normal AF corresponds to preserved RPE cells underlying defunct cones. More peripherally, the absence of NIA and AF signals indicates loss of RPE cells.

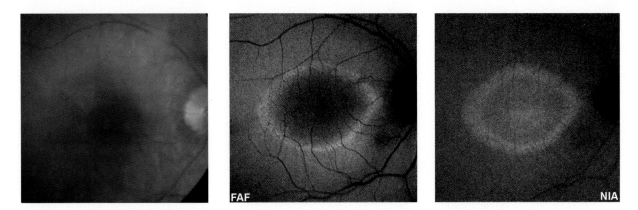

FIGURE 6.4.   Retinitis pigmentosa. A ring of increased signal with conventional FAF is observed corresponding to an area with increased NIA in a bull's-eye shape. AF and NIA alterations are not detectable in the color fundus photograph.

Age-Related Macular Degeneration

Abnormalities in the distribution of NIA have been described in patients with age-related maculopathy (ARM) and AMD (Kellner U; et al, IOVS 2008;49:ARVO E-Abstract 2235, paper submitted). In ARM (see also Chapter 10A), an increased signal on conventional AF imaging is detected more frequently than a reduced AF signal; however, increased and reduced NIA signals are seen with similar frequency. In the majority of eyes, the relative intensity of the AF signal as detected using conventional AF imaging is higher than that on NIA. When the relative intensity of NIA is higher than the AF signal observed on conventional AF imaging, usually these areas have increased NIA and normal AF. In geographic atrophy (see also Chapter 10C) and at the junctional zone, increased NIA is more frequently observed than increased AF (Fig. 6.5). This could correspond to increased melanolipofuscin in these areas (47). The area of geographic atrophy may be larger in NIA compared to AF in some patients; in no case have larger atrophic areas in AF compared to NIA been observed. In neovascular AMD (see also Chapter 10B), abnormalities are usually better detected with conventional AF imaging. Preservation of subfoveal RPE can be demonstrated with conventional AF and NIA; however, whether one of these methods has a better predictive value for functional outcomes remains to be seen (54).

NIA alterations have been observed preceding conventional AF changes, suggesting that abnormalities in the distribution of NIA could be the earliest morphologic sign of sight-threatening RPE dysfunction in ARM.

Chloroquine Retinopathy

An increased AF signal can be observed perifoveally by conventional AF imaging in early chloroquine retinopathy, prior to ophthalmoscopic or fluorescein angiographic changes (55). Once the disease progresses, areas of increased and reduced AF are seen on conventional AF imaging; areas of reduced AF correspond to areas of reduced NIA, whereas areas of increased NIA outline areas of increased AF. Of interest, in one case reported by Weinberger et al. (4) and two others observed by the authors, NIA was increased in an area superior to the fovea where conventional AF appeared normal (Fig. 6.6) (7). It is possible that areas with increased NIA may be destined to degenerate.

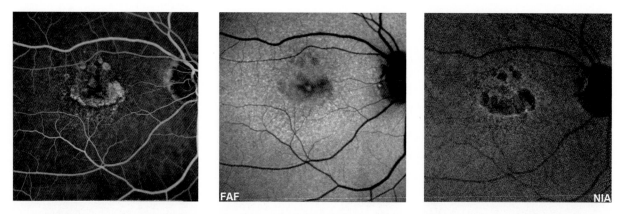

FIGURE 6.5.   AMD. Multiple spots of increased AF using conventional FAF imaging correspond to spot-like decreased NIA, but these alterations are better detectable with AF. The geographic atrophy is more clearly defined in the NIA image and corresponds to the fluorescein angiographic findings. Increased NIA is present adjacent to the area of geographic atrophy.

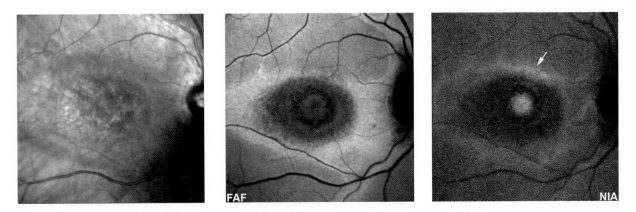

FIGURE 6.6.   Chloroquine retinopathy. Subfoveal preservation of AF, as determined by conventional FAF and NIA, and parafoveal reduced AF and NIA are observed. The more peripheral area of increased AF is outlined by increased NIA. NIA is especially increased superior to the fovea in an area with normal AF (*arrow*).

INTRAOCULAR TUMORS

The value of NIA in the differential diagnosis of intraocular tumors is reviewed in Chapter 15.

SUMMARY

NIA imaging is a noninvasive modality that allows evaluation of the RPE. Combined with conventional AF imaging, NIA imaging allows sophisticated monitoring of the RPE and provides insight into pathophysiological aspects of the degenerative processes of various retinal diseases. These noninvasive imaging techniques facilitate frequent follow-up examinations, which will be important for future therapeutic trials in children and adults as new treatment strategies for retinal disorders evolve.

In some disorders, abnormalities in the distribution of NIA precede those observed using conventional AF imaging, and represent the first detectable disease-associated morphologic change in the retina.

REFERENCES

1. Eldred GE, Katz ML. Fluorophores of the human retinal pigment epithelium: separation and spectral characterization. Exp Eye Res 1988;47:71–86.
2. Keilhauer CN, Delori FC. Near-infrared autofluorescence imaging of the fundus: visualization of ocular melanin. Invest Ophthalmol Vis Sci 2006;47:3556–3564.
3. Piccolino FC, Borgia L, Zinicola E, et al. Pre-injection fluorescence in indocyanine green angiography. Ophthalmology 1996;103:1837–1845.
4. Weinberger AW, Lappas A, Kirschkamp T, et al. Fundus near infrared fluorescence correlates with fundus near infrared reflectance. Invest Ophthalmol Vis Sci 2006;47:3098–3108.
5. Cideciyan AV, Swider M, Aleman TS, et al. Reduced-illuminance autofluorescence imaging in ABCA4-associated retinal degenerations. J Opt Soc Am A Opt Image Sci Vis 2007;24:1457–1467.
6. Sayanagi K, Ikuno Y, Tano Y. Different fundus autofluorescence patterns of retinoschisis and macular hole retinal detachment in high myopia. Am J Ophthalmol 2007;144:299–301.
7. Kellner U, Kellner S, Weinitz S. Chloroquine retinopathy: lipofuscin- and melanin-related fundus autofluorescence, optical coherence tomography and multifocal electroretinography. Doc Ophthalmol 2008;116:119–127.
8. Theelen T, Boon CJ, Klevering BJ, et al. Fundusautofluoreszenz bei erblichen Netzhauterkrankungen: Fluoreszenzmuster in zwei verschiedenen Wellenlangenbereichen. Ophthalmologe 2008;105:1013–1022.

9. Aleman TS, Cideciyan AV, Sumaroka A, et al. Retinal laminar architecture in human retinitis pigmentosa caused by rhodopsin gene mutations. Invest Ophthalmol Vis Sci 2008;49:1580–1590.
10. Kellner U, Kellner S. Klinik und Diagnostik der Zapfendystrophien. Ophthalmologe 2009;106:99–108.
11. Kellner S, Kellner U, Weber BHF, et al. Lipofuscin- and melanin-related fundus autofluorescence in patients with ABCA4-associated retinal dystrophies. Am J Ophthalmol 2009:Epub ahead of print.
12. Kellner U, Kellner S, Weber BH, et al. Lipofuscin- and melanin-related fundus autofluorescence visualize different retinal pigment epithelial alterations in patients with retinitis pigmentosa. Eye 2008:Epub ahead of print.
13. Herrera W, Aleman T, Cideciyan AV, et al. Retinal Disease in Usher Syndrome III Caused by Mutations in the Clarin-1 Gene. Invest Ophthalmol Vis Sci 2008;49:2651–2660.
14. Parodi MB, Iacono P, Pedio M, et al. Autofluorescence in adult-onset foveomacular vitelliform dystrophy. Retina 2008;28:801–807.
15. Ayata A, Tatlipinar S, Kar T, et al. Near-infrared and short-wavelength autofluorescence imaging in central serous chorioretinopathy. Br J Ophthalmol 2009;93:79–82.
16. Weiter JJ, Delori FC, Wing GL, et al. Retinal pigment epithelial lipofuscin and melanin and choroidal melanin in human eyes. Invest Ophthalmol Vis Sci 1986;27:145–152.
17. Boulton M, Docchio F, Dayhaw-Barker P, et al. Age-related changes in the morphology, absorption and fluorescence of melanosomes and lipofuscin granules of the retinal pigment epithelium. Vision Res 1990;30:1291–1303.
18. Kayatz P, Thumann G, Luther TT, et al. Oxidation causes melanin fluorescence. Invest Ophthalmol Vis Sci 2001;42:241–246.
19. Docchio F, Boulton M, Cubeddu R, et al. Age-related changes in the fluorescence of melanin and lipofuscin granules of the retinal pigment epithelium: a time-resolved fluorescence spectroscopy study. Photochem Photobiol 1991;54:247–253.
20. Huang Z, Zeng H, Hamzavi I, et al. Cutaneous melanin exhibiting fluorescence emission under near-infrared light excitation. J Biomed Opt 2006;11:34010.
21. Sarna T, Burke JM, Korytowski W, et al. Loss of melanin from human RPE with aging: possible role of melanin photooxidation. Exp Eye Res 2003;76:89–98.
22. Korytowski W, Pilas B, Sarna T, et al. Photoinduced generation of hydrogen peroxide and hydroxyl radicals in melanins. Photochem Photobiol 1987;45:185–190.
23. Boulton M. Melanin and the retinal pigment epithelium. In: Marmor MF, Wolfensberger TJ eds, The retinal pigment epithelium. New York: Oxford University Press; 1998:68–85.
24. Sparrow JR, Fishkin N, Zhou J, et al. A2E, a byproduct of the visual cycle. Vision Res 2003;43:2983–2990.
25. Sparrow JR, Parish CA, Hashimoto M, et al. A2E, a lipofuscin fluorophore, in human retinal pigmented epithelial cells in culture. Invest Ophthalmol Vis Sci 1999;40:2988–2995.
26. Kim SR, Jang YP, Jockusch S, et al. The all-trans-retinal dimer series of lipofuscin pigments in retinal pigment epithelial cells in a recessive Stargardt disease model. Proc Natl Acad Sci U S A 2007;104:19273–19278.
27. Wagnieres GA, Star WM, Wilson BC. In vivo fluorescence spectroscopy and imaging for oncological applications. Photochem Photobiol 1998;68:603–632.
28. Feeney-Burns L, Hilderbrand ES, Eldridge S. Aging human RPE: morphometric analysis of macular, equatorial, and peripheral cells. Invest Ophthalmol Vis Sci 1984;25:195–200.
29. Smith-Thomas L, Richardson P, Thody AJ, et al. Human ocular melanocytes and retinal pigment epithelial cells differ in their melanogenic properties in vivo and in vitro. Curr Eye Re. 15(11):1079–1091.
30. Schraermeyer U. Does melanin turnover occur in the eyes of adult vertebrates? Pigment Cell Res 1993;6:93–204.
31. Peters S, Lamah T, Kokkinou D, et al. Melanin protects choroidal blood vessels against light toxicity. Z Naturforsch (C) 2006;61:427–433.
32. Wang Z, Dillon J, Gaillard ER. Antioxidant properties of melanin in retinal pigment epithelial cells. Photochem Photobiol 2006;82:474–479.
33. Boulton M, Dayhaw-Barker P. The role of the retinal pigment epithelium: topographical variation and ageing changes. Eye 2001;15:384–389.
34. Feeney L. Lipofuscin and melanin of human retinal pigment epithelium. Fluorescence, enzyme cytochemical, and ultrastructural studies. Invest Ophthalmol Vis Sci 1978;17:583–600.
35. Burke JM, Henry MM, Zareba M, et al. Photobleaching of melanosomes from retinal pigment epithelium: I. Effects on protein oxidation. Photochem Photobiol 2007;83:920–924.
36. Schraermeyer U, Peters S, Thumann G, et al. Melanin granules of retinal pigment epithelium are connected with the lysosomal degradation pathway. Exp Eye Res 1999;68:237–245.
37. Peters S, Kayatz P, Heimann K, et al. Subretinal injection of rod outer segments leads to an increase in the number of early-stage melanosomes in retinal pigment epithelial cells. Ophthalmic Res 2000;32:52–56.
38. Schraermeyer U, Kopitz J, Peters S, et al. Tyrosinase biosynthesis in adult mammalian retinal pigment epithelial cells. Exp Eye Res 2006;83:315–321.
39. Julien S, Kociok N, Kreppel F, et al. Tyrosinase biosynthesis and trafficking in adult human retinal pigment epithelial cells. Graefes Arch Clin Exp Ophthalmol 2007;245:1495–1505.
40. Buchanan TA, Gardiner TA, Archer DB. An ultrastructural study of retinal photoreceptor degeneration associated with bronchial carcinoma. Am J Ophthalmol 1984;97:277–287.

41. Szamier RB, Berson EL. Retinal ultrastructure in advanced retinitis pigmentosa. Invest Ophthalmol Vis Sci 1977;16:947–962.
42. Szamier RB, Berson EL, Klein R, et al. Sex-linked retinitis pigmentosa: ultrastructure of photoreceptors and pigment epithelium. Invest Ophthalmol Vis Sci 1979;18:145–160.
43. Bunt-Milam AH, Kalina RE, Pagon RA. Clinical-ultrastructural study of a retinal dystrophy. Invest Ophthalmol Vis Sci 1983;24:458–469.
44. Szamier RB, Berson EL. Retinal histopathology of a carrier of X-chromosome-linked retinitis pigmentosa. Ophthalmology 1985;92:271–278.
45. Steinmetz RL, Garner A, Maguire JI, et al. Histopathology of incipient fundus flavimaculatus. Ophthalmology 1991;98:953–956.
46. Lopez PF. Autosomal-dominant fundus flavimaculatus. Clinicopathologic correlation. Ophthalmology 1990;97:798–809.
47. Sarks JP, Sarks SH, Killingsworth MC. Evolution of geographic atrophy of the retinal pigment epithelium. Eye 1988;2:552–577.
48. Milam AH, Jacobson SG. Photoreceptor rosettes with blue cone opsin immunoreactivity in retinitis pigmentosa. Ophthalmology 1990;97:1620–1631.
49. Eagle Jr RC, Lucier AC, Bernardino Jr VB, et al. Retinal pigment epithelial abnormalities in fundus flavimaculatus: a light and electron microscopic study. Ophthalmology 1980;87:1189–1200.
50. Delori FC, Staurenghi G, Arend O, et al. In vivo measurement of lipofuscin in Stargardt's disease—fundus flavimaculatus. Invest Ophthalmol Vis Sci 1995;36:2327–2331.
51. Lois N, Halfyard AS, Bird AC, et al. Fundus autofluorescence in Stargardt macular dystrophy-fundus flavimaculatus. Am J Ophthalmol 2004;138:55–63.
52. Robson AG, Saihan Z, Jenkins SA, et al. Functional characterisation and serial imaging of abnormal fundus autofluorescence in patients with retinitis pigmentosa and normal visual acuity. Br J Ophthalmol 2006;90:472–479.
53. Popovic P, Jarc-Vidmar M, Hawlina M. Abnormal fundus autofluorescence in relation to retinal function in patients with retinitis pigmentosa. Graefes Arch Clin Exp Ophthalmol 2005;243:1018–1027.
54. Vaclavik V, Vujosevic S, Dandekar SS, et al. Autofluorescence imaging in age-related macular degeneration complicated by choroidal neovascularization a prospective study. Ophthalmology 2008;115:342–346.
55. Kellner U, Renner AB, Tillack H. Fundus autofluorescence and mfERG for early detection of retinal alterations in patients using chloroquine/hydroxychloroquine. Invest Ophthalmol Vis Sci 2006;47:3531–3538.

Interpreting Fundus Autofluorescence

Interpretation of autofluorescence (AF) images with illumination at 488 nm (standard AF image) is based on the principle that the majority of the signal is derived from lipofuscin in the retinal pigment epithelium (RPE) (see Chapter 3) (1–3). Although there are many fluorophores in the retina, the signal from RPE lipofuscin is stronger than that from any other substance. The quantity of lipofuscin in the RPE is a balance between accumulation and clearance. Lipofuscin is formed of retinal and ethanolamine in the photoreceptor outer segment and is ingested by the RPE by phagocytosis of shed outer segment material (see Chapter 2) (4,5). Thus, accumulation of lipofuscin is driven by outer segment renewal. Clearance of lipofsucin may be due in part to discharge of long-term phagolysosomes by the RPE into the extracellular space (see Chapter 2) and in part to photodegradation (6), although the half life of the fluorophores is unknown. Thus, the "background" levels of AF in the normal healthy eye reflect a normal photoreceptor outer segment turnover and retinoid cycling. A reduction in the number of photoreceptors causes loss of AF over time. Increased levels of AF are caused by RPE dysfunction either because of an intrinsic failure of lipofuscin clearance or the presence of an abnormal metabolic load.

Imaging of AF depends on the clarity of the media. Extravascular blood internal to the RPE will prevent detection of the signal, and nuclear sclerosis will attenuate illumination. Under other circumstances, the variation reflects the lipofuscin content of the RPE. The image of a normal fundus with illumination at 488 nm shows homogeneous AF over most of the posterior pole (see Chapters 2 and 9) (2). The blood vessels and fovea are dark because of light absorption by blood and luteal pigment, respectively, since both absorb short wavelength light. The optic disc is dark because of the absence of a fluorophore. The AF level increases with age and tends to be highest at about 10 degrees of eccentricity (see also Chapter 3). Deviation from this pattern indicates outer retinal disease. Current imaging techniques with commercially available systems are very valuable for detecting abnormalities in the distribution of AF, but are relatively unreliable for measuring absolute levels of AF (see Chapter 5). Described below are the circumstances in which evaluation of fundus AF is the most valuable.

CONTINUITY OF AUTOFLUORESCENCE (NORMAL AUTOFLUORESCENCE PATTERN)

In the presence of unexplained loss of vision, the existence of normal AF with illumination of 488 nm usually implies that the loss of vision is unlikely to be due to outer retinal disease. However, there are certain circumstances in which normal AF is present in cases of outer retinal disease. This was observed in a study of patients with Leber congenital amaurosis (7) (see also Chapter 11D) (Fig. 7.1), in which it was concluded

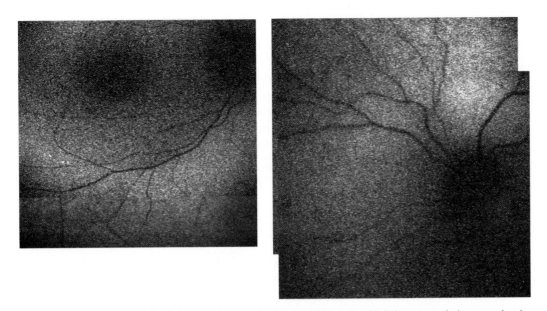

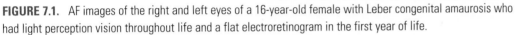

FIGURE 7.1.   AF images of the right and left eyes of a 16-year-old female with Leber congenital amaurosis who had light perception vision throughout life and a flat electroretinogram in the first year of life.

that photoreceptor cell dysfunction occurred without population loss. The loss of vision may be due to transduction failure or constant noise, i.e., the photoreceptor cells may behave as if they are in constant light, thus reducing signal-to-noise ratios. If it were possible to correct the metabolic abnormality, AF imaging suggests that such patients might be able to recover vision. A similar situation of loss of function with normal AF signal was found in acute zonal and occult outer retinopathy (AZOOR), at least in the first 5 years of disease, implying the possibility of spontaneous recovery (8). In some patients with retinitis pigmentosa (RP), there is a ring of increased AF at variable eccentricity around the fovea (see also Chapter 11A) (Fig. 7.2) (9,10). On either side of the ring of increased AF, AF is normal but scotopic function is markedly reduced; photopic function is also reduced in areas external to the ring of increased AF. There is no explanation as to why the function is poor in the presence of a normal pop-

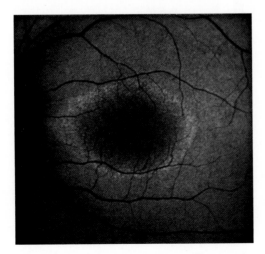

FIGURE 7.2.   AF image of a 32-year-old male with RP showing a ring of increased AF around the fovea and cystoid macular edema.

ulation of photoreceptor cells unless the half life of the fluorophores is very long. Curiously, near-infrared AF (NIA) coincides with function (see also Chapter 6).

AF is also very important for determining the integrity of the outer retina at the time of treatment of choroidal neovascularization (CNV). Until recently, poor visual acuity was interpreted as indicating loss of central photoreceptor cells, but recovery of visual acuity following intravitreal injection of antivascular endothelial growth factor (VEGF) agents implies that this is not the case. Further support for the concept that the outer retina may be physically intact comes from the observation of normal AF in such cases (see also Chapter 10B) (Fig. 7.3) (11,12). AF imaging would be of great value for assessing the likely therapeutic benefit of such treatments.

INCREASED AUTOFLUORESCENCE

In many disorders, pale areas appear at the level of the outer retina such as drusen and scarring. It is important to determine whether these areas represent lipofuscin in the

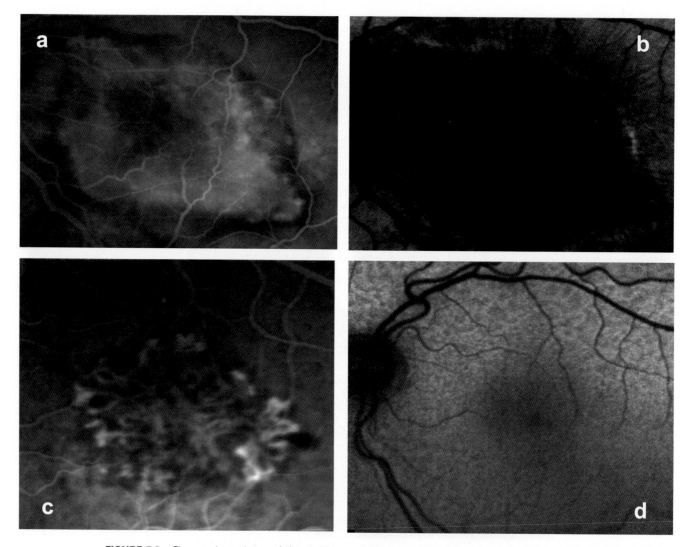

FIGURE 7.3. Fluorescein angiogram **(A)** and AF image **(B)** of a patient with an 8-month history of visual symptoms and a visual acuity of 6/36, showing CNV and absent AF centrally. Fluorescein angiogram **(C)** and AF image **(D)** of a patient with an 11-month history of visual symptoms and a visual acuity of 6/60, showing CNV and intact AF centrally.

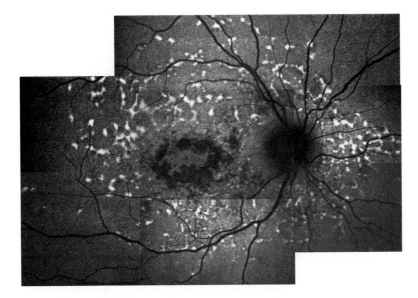

FIGURE 7.4. AF image of a 24-year-old female with Stargardt-fundus flavimaculatus and a visual acuity of 6/60, showing focal increased AF and discontinuous atrophy around the fovea.

RPE or in bloodborne macrophages. The distinction is easily made by determining whether these lesions autofluoresce on AF images.

The pattern of increased AF may be characteristic of a disorder. Macular dystrophies may present with focal lesions rather than continuous abnormalities. The former are characteristic of Stargardt disease (see also Chapter 11G) (Fig. 7.4), in which the initial change is discrete spots of increased AF that correspond with pale lesions seen on ophthalmoscopy, with totally normal AF elsewhere (13,14). As the disorder progresses, atrophy occurs at the sites of increased AF and new spots of increased AF appear. Focal increased AF with normal intervening levels is also seen in pattern dystrophies (see also Chapter 11E) (Fig. 7.5).

Increased AF seen in an area of the fundus that appears normal occurs in a variety of disorders and may be of diagnostic value. In bull's-eye macular dystrophies, a continuous ring of increased AF is seen early, followed by photoreceptor cell loss in a bull's-eye pattern (see also Chapter 11B) (Fig. 7.6) (13,15). There are

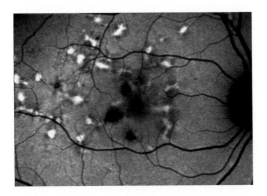

FIGURE 7.5. AF image of a 55-year-old female with 6/9 visual acuity and pattern dystrophy, showing focal increases of AF and normal intervening AF. Patches of reduced AF corresponding to areas of atrophy are also seen.

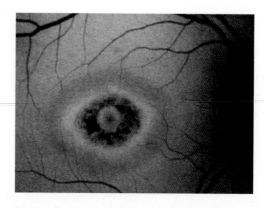

FIGURE 7.6. AF image of a 36-year-old male with bull's-eye maculopathy and a ring of atrophy around the fovea, and increased AF at the perimeter of the area of atrophy.

no ophthalmoscopic abnormalities that correspond with the ring of increased AF. In retinal degenerative disease resulting from the 172 *RDS* mutation, the central macula has increased AF at a time when there are no symptoms, the fundus is normal by ophthalmoscopy, and electrophysiological responses are normal (see also Chapter 11B and E) (Fig. 7.7).

In early age-related macular disease, focally increased AF occurs in some cases and appears to be indicative of a risk of geographic atrophy, rather than CNV, as a likely cause of visual loss (see also Chapter 10B and C) (16–18). In geographic atrophy, the presence of increased AF implies likely progression of the atrophy. Drusen in age-related macular disease do not fluoresce brightly (see also Chapter 10A), which is in marked contrast to drusen seen in the young or as part of a monogenic disorder such as Doyne honeycomb dystrophy (Fig. 7.8).

REDUCED AUTOFLUORESCENCE

Reduced AF indicates loss of photoreceptors—or at least their outer segments, or RPE loss. Outer retinal atrophy is not always obvious on biomicroscopy, but is unmistakably recognizable on AF imaging. It may have a distinctive distribution, such as in disease associated with an A3243G mitochondrial mutation in which the lesions are distributed and orientated in a circumferential fashion (see also Chapter 11H) (Fig. 7.9) (19). In Stargardt disease the atrophy is spotty (see also Chapter 11G) (Fig. 7.4), whereas it is continuous in bull's-eye lesions (Fig. 7.6).

IRREGULAR AUTOFLUORESCENCE

Diffusely irregular AF indicates disease at the level of the outer retina; it is seen in a variety of disease states and often has a distinctive distribution. The A3243G mitochondrial mutation (Fig. 7.9) and the 172 *RDS* mutation (Fig. 7.7) usually cause irregular AF associated with atrophy. Diffusely irregular AF also occurs in central serous retinopathy after the first 6 months of detachment (see also Chapter 13) (20). It is thought that this is due to outer segment shedding into the subretinal space that may collect inferiorly because of gravity and phagocytosis by the RPE or possibly other macrophages. Focal changes also occur that often correspond with the point of leakage on fluorescein angiography.

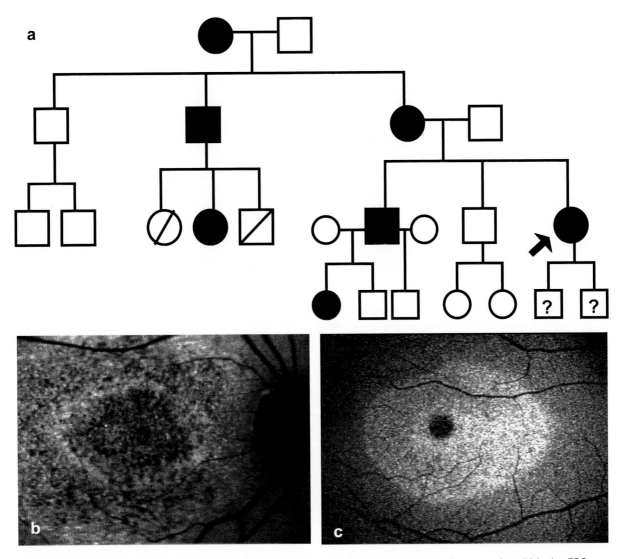

FIGURE 7.7. **(A)** Pedigree of a family with a dominantly inherited macular dystrophy resulting from mutation 172 in the *RDS* gene. **(B)** The proband had irregular AF occupying the whole of the posterior pole. Her 16-year-old son had no symptoms, and normal fundi and electrophysiological responses. **(C)** Increased AF centrally showed that he was affected by the disorder.

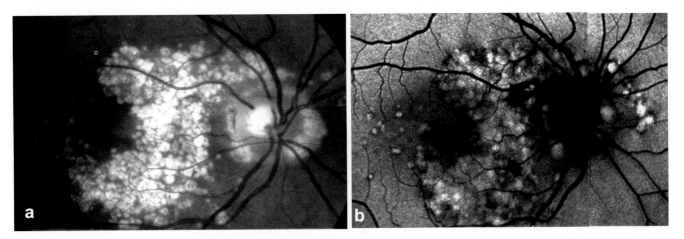

FIGURE 7.8. Reflectance **(A)** and AF images **(B)** of Doyne honeycomb dystrophy showing bright AF of drusen.

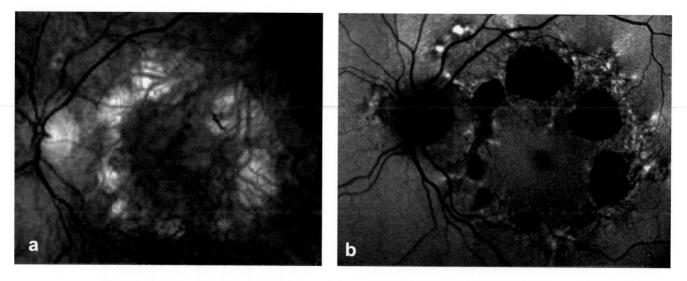

FIGURE 7.9. Reflectance **(A)** and AF **(B)** images of disease associated with an A3243G mitochondrial mutation in a 50-year-old female with deafness. Atrophy is associated with limited irregular AF.

SUMMARY

For the first time, it is possible to image changes at the level of the RPE that are integral to outer retinal diseases. Although experience with AF imaging is short, it is evident that the technique is clinically useful and at times can be an important factor in management decisions.

REFERENCES

1. Delori FC, Dorey CK, Staurenthi G, et al. In vivo fluorescence of the ocular fundus exhibits retinal pigment epithelium lipofuscin characteristics. Invest Ophthalmol Vis Sci 1995;36:718–719.
2. von Rückmann A, Fitzke FW, Bird AC. Distribution of fundus autofluorescence with a scanning laser ophthalmoscope. Br J Ophthalmol 1995;79:407–412.
3. Eldred GE, Katz ML. Fluorophores of the human retinal pigment epithelium: separation and spectral characterization. Exp Eye Res 1988;47:71–86.
4. Jang YP, Matsuda H, Itagaki Y, et al. Characterization of peroxy-A2E and furan-A2E photooxidation products and detection in human and mouse retinal pigment epithelial cell lipofuscin. J Biol Chem 2005;280:39732–39739.
5. Bui TV, Han Y, Radu RA, et al. Characterization of native retinal fluorophores involved in biosynthesis of A2E and lipofuscin-associated retinopathies. J Biol Chem 2006;281:18112–18119.
6. Fernandes AF, Zhou J, Zhang X, et al. Oxidative inactivation of the proteasome in retinal pigment epithelial cells: a potential link between oxidative stress and up-regulation of interleukin 2. J Biol Chem 2008; 283:20745–20753.
7. Scholl HPN, Chong NHV, Robson AG, et al. Fundus autofluorescence with Leber congenital amaurosis. Invest Ophthalmol Vis Sci 2004;45:2747–2752.
8. Schmitz-Valckenberg S, Holz FG, Bird AC, et al. Fundus autofluorescence imaging: review and perspectives. Retina 2008;28:385–409.
9. Robson AG, El-Amir A, Bailey C, et al. Pattern ERG correlates of abnormal fundus autofluorescence in patients with retinitis pigmentosa and normal visual acuity. Invest Ophthalmol Vis Sci 2003;44:3544–3550.
10. Robson AG, Egan CA, Luong VA, et al. Comparison of fundus autofluorescence with photopic and scotopic fine-matrix mapping in patients with retinitis pigmentosa and normal visual acuity. Invest Ophthalmol Vis Sci 2004;45:4119–4125.
11. Dandekar SS, Jenkins SA, Peto T, et al. An analysis of autoflorescence of choroidal neovascularization due to age-related macular disease. Arch Ophthalmol 2005;123:1507–1513.
12. Vaclavik V, Vujosevic S, Dandekar SS, et al. Autofluorescence imaging in age-related macular degeneration complicated by choroidal neovascularization: a prospective study. Ophthalmology 2008;115:342–346.

13. von Rückmann A, Fitzke FW, Bird AC. In vivo fundus autofluorescence in macular dystrophies. Arch Ophthalmol 1997;115:609–615.
14. Lois N, Holder GE, Bunce C, et al. Intrafamilial variation of phenotype in Stargardt macular dystrophy-fundus flavimaculatus. Invest Ophthalmol Vis Sci 1999;40:2668–2675.
15. Kurz-Levin MM, Halfyard AS, Bunce C, et al. Phenotypic assessment of bull's eye maculopathy. Arch Ophthalmol 2002;120:567–575.
16. von Rückmann A, Fitzke FW, Bird AC. In vivo fundus autofluorescence in age related macular degeneration. Invest Ophthalmol Vis Sci 1997;38:478–486.
17. Holz FG, Bellmann C, Margaritidis M, et al. Patterns of increased in vivo fundus autofluorescence in the junctional zone of geographic atrophy of the retinal pigment epithelium associated with age-related macular degeneration. Graefes Arch Clin Exp Ophthalmol 1999;237:145–152.
18. Holz FG, Bellman C, Staudt S, et al. Fundus autofluorescence and development of geographic atrophy in age-related macular degeneration. Invest Ophthalmol Vis Sci 2001;42:1051–1056.
19. Michaelides M, Jenkins SA, Bamiou DE, et al. Macular dystrophy associated with the A3243G mitochondrial DNA mutation: distinct retinal and associated features, disease variability, and characterization of asymptomatic family members. Arch Ophthalmol 2008;126:320–328.
20. von Rückmann A, Fitzke FW, Fan J, et al. Fundus autofluorescence in central serous retinopathy imaged with a laser scanning ophthalmoscope. Am J Ophthalmol 2002;133:780–786.

8

Dietrich Schweitzer

Quantifying Fundus Autofluorescence

INTRODUCTION

The investigation of endogenous fluorophores has the potential to aid in evaluating the metabolic status of tissues and thus detecting the early stages of disease (1,2). The redox pairs of fluorophores, the coenzymes NAD-NADH (oxidized and reduced forms of nicotinamide adenine dinucleotide) and FAD-FADH$_2$ (oxidized and reduced forms of flavin adenine dinucleotide) are electron transporters in the basic processes of cell metabolism (Fig. 8.1). NAD and FAD participate in reactions that occur in β-oxidation of fatty acids (acyl-CoA-dehydrogenase reaction), in glycolysis, in the citrate acid cycle (succinate dehydrogenase reaction), in the respiratory chain in complex I (NADH$^+$+H$^+$ ubichinone reductase) reactions, in the succinate dehydrogenase reaction in complex II reactions, and in the connection between the citrate acid cycle and the respiratory chain (3).

It appears that the dominant fluorophore of the fundus is the aging macular pigment lipofuscin, which appears to play an important role in the pathophysiology of several retinal diseases, including age-related macular degeneration (AMD) (see also Chapters 2 and 3). Other fluorophores include advanced glycation end-products (AGEs), which are involved in the pathogenesis of diabetes mellitus; elastin and collagen, which change during sclerotic processes and in glaucoma; pyridoxal phosphate, the prosthetic group of all amino transferases; protoporphyrin IX, a fluorophore in hem synthesis; and the amino acids tryptophan, kynurenin, and phenylalanine, which are strong fluorophores in connective tissues and the cornea, lens, and sclera (4) (see also Chapter 3).

Since an evaluation of the metabolic status of tissues requires information on single fluorophores, however, the separation of individual signals corresponding to each of these fluorophores from within the sum of the fundus autofluorescence (AF) signal represents a challenge. This chapter reviews possible methods to achieve that goal, as well as their limitations.

METHODS FOR DISCRIMINATION OF FLUOROPHORES

According to the chemical structure, there are three characteristic properties—the excitation spectrum, the emission spectrum, and the fluorescence lifetime after excitation by short pulses—that allow discrimination of fluorophores (5). In the eye, the spectral range for examination is limited to between 400 and 900 nm by the transmission of the ocular media in the short-wave range and the absorption of water in the long-wave range, respectively (6). The decrease in the ocular transmission, which occurs with increasing age, can be determined (7).

Redox pairs	Sufficient Oxygen	Lack of Oxygen
NAD - NADH ➡	no fluorescence	high fluorescence of NADH
FAD - FADH2 ➡	high fluorescence of FAD	no fluorescence

FIGURE 8.1.   Change of fluorescence of coenzymes NAD and FAD depending on the availability of oxygen.

Since specific excitation maxima are shorter than 400 nm, a differentiation of the fundus fluorophores is limited according to the excitation spectra. If the sample can be strongly excited and the fluorescence signal can be detected with a high signal-to-noise ratio, the contribution of single fluorophores can be recalculated in the sum emission spectrum. In such a fitting procedure, the spectral course of the emission spectra of each fluorophore must be known. Weighting factors are optimized until the approximation of the model function and the measured sum fluorescence spectrum are optimal. These weighting factors correspond to the contribution of each fluorophore to the sum spectrum. The signal-to-noise ratio is equal to the square root of the collected number of photons. To obtain a high number of photons, the irradiance must be high or the measuring time will be long. Generally, spectral intensity measurements suffer from absorption and scattering in nonfluorescent substances, which weaken the excitation light and change the spectral shape of the emission spectrum.

The fluorescence lifetime, the third parameter for discrimination of fluorophores, has some important advantages. The lifetime is independent of the absorption or scattering of neighboring substances. There is also no dependence on the concentration of fluorophores. Weakly emitting fluorophores can be separated from strongly emitting fluorophores if the lifetimes are sufficiently different. Only about one hundred photons are necessary for approximation of a monoexponential decay (8). Because the lifetime depends on pH value and viscosity, information can be found related to the cellular embedding matrix.

Limiting Conditions for Measuring Fundus Fluorophores

There are some limiting conditions that must be taken into account in two-dimensional (2D) measurements of fundus fluorophores in vivo:

1. The fundus fluorescence is covered by the strong fluorescence of the anterior segment of the eye. The techniques of aperture division and confocal laser scanning can reduce the influence of fluorescence of, cornea and lens (see also Chapters 3 and 5); a combination of both methods is advisable for accurate measurements (9). The emission spectra of the lens and cornea are minimal for wavelengths longer than 570 nm (10), and thus their influence will be reduced when long waves are used.
2. Endogenous fluorophores are present in all layers of the fundus.
3. The strong fluorescence of lipofuscin covers the weak fluorescence of other fluorophores.
4. Eye movement limits the time available for highly spatially resolved measurements.
5. The maximal permissible exposure (MPE) is the most important limitation for spectral measurements in the eye (11).

Fluorescence Lifetime Measurements

Lifetime measurements are best suited for detection and discrimination of fluorophores in images of the fundus. There are two methods for detecting fluorescence decay: measurement in the frequency domain or measurement in the time domain (5).

Fluorescence Lifetime Measurements in the Frequency Domain

In the frequency domain, the sample is excited by intensity-modulated light. The emitted fluorescence light is also modulated. There is a phase shift between excitation and emission light because of the delay between absorption and emission. This phase shift depends on the modulation frequency. The modulation in the fluorescence light is also weaker than the excitation light and decreases with increasing modulation frequency.

From the phase shift, the fluorescence lifetime τp is determined according to the following equation:

$$\tau_p = \frac{\tan \Phi}{\omega} \qquad [1]$$

where Φ = phase shift and ω = modulation frequency.

The lifetime τ_m, as determined from demodulation measurements, is calculated by:

$$\tau_m = \frac{\sqrt{\frac{1}{m^2} - 1}}{\omega} \qquad [2]$$

where m = demodulation.

The demodulation m is determined by the ratio of maximal and minimal intensity in the emitted light, divided by the ratio of the maximal and minimal intensity in the excitation light. The same values ($\tau_p = \tau_m$) are determined in monoexponential decay, but in multiexponential decay they are $\tau_p < \tau_m$. In the case of multiexponential decay, the decay times are calculated according to the complicated set of formulas (12):

$$\tan \Phi(\omega) = \frac{Z(\omega)}{N(\omega)} \qquad [3]$$

$$m(\omega) = \sqrt{N(\omega)^2 + Z(\omega)^2} \qquad [4]$$

$$Z(\omega) = \frac{\sum_{i=1}^{n} \frac{\alpha_i \cdot \omega \cdot \tau_i^2}{1 + \omega^2 \cdot \tau_i^2}}{\sum_{i=1}^{n} \alpha_i \cdot \tau_i} \qquad [5]$$

$$N(\omega) = \frac{\sum_{i=1}^{n} \frac{\alpha_i \cdot \tau_i^2}{1 + \omega^2 \cdot \tau_i^2}}{\sum_{i=1}^{n} \alpha_i \cdot \tau_i} \qquad [6]$$

The lifetimes τ_i and the pre-exponential factors α_i of the component i are calculated iteratively, not analytically.

In principle, one can determine the fluorescence lifetimes simultaneously for all image pixels by illuminating the whole image and detecting phase shift or demodulation using a detector matrix. Sequential excitation of all image pixels can be achieved with the use of a scanning system with only one detector. A combination of both methods is also possible.

Fluorescence Lifetime Measurements in the Time Domain

Fluorescence lifetime measurements are performed in the time domain by exciting the sample by pulses having a short full width at half maximum (FWHM), e.g., in the pico- or femtosecond range. Because the decay of the fluorescence is too short for direct measures to be obtained, the fluorescence intensity is detected during multiple excitations in a number of time windows, in a single variable time window (boxcar principle), or by time-correlated single photon counting (TCSPC). In TCSPC, the sample is excited by weak light pulses. The intensity is so low that only one photon will be detected in a sequence of about 10 excitation pulses. Each fluorescence photon will be accumulated in time channels according to the detection time after the excitation pulses. After a sufficient measuring time, the content of all time channels represents the probability density function of the decay process. The principle of TCSPC, technical details, and practical applications were previously explained by Becker (13).

The process is mostly assumed as an exponential decay, which can be approximated by a sum of e-functions:

$$\frac{I(t)}{I_0} = \sum_{i=1}^{p} \alpha_i \cdot e^{\frac{t}{\tau_i}} + b \tag{7}$$

where α_i = preexponential factor of exponent i or amplitude, τ_i = lifetime of exponent i, b = background, and p = degree of exponential function.

Because the excitation is not a Dirac pulse, the measured decay of fluorescence is the convolution of excitation pulse with the decay process. Therefore, the criterion for the fitting process is the minimization of χ_r^2:

$$\chi_r^2 = \frac{1}{n-q} \cdot \sum_{j=1}^{n} \frac{[N(t_j) - N_c(t_j)]^2}{N(t_j)} \tag{8}$$

In this equation, $N(t_j)$ is the measured number of photons in the time channel j; $N_c(t_j)$ is the number of expected photons, which are calculated by the convolution of the instrumental response function and the model function; n is the number of time channels; and q is the number of free parameters (α_i, τ_i, b).

If the detection of photons is a Poisson process, the mean square root error between detected photons and calculated photons is equal to the square root of the detected events:

$$Noise = \sqrt{[N(t_j) - N_c(t_j)]^2} = \sqrt{N(t_j)} \tag{9}$$

Thus, the ratio in the sum of Eq. [8] is one for each time channel and the sum is n. This means that the limiting value of χ_r^2 is one. The algorithm is independent of the degree of exponential function, but the calculation time increases with the number of exponents. The time between two excitation pulses should be about five times the longest expected decay time.

The separation of fluorophores can be improved by global analysis (14). In this analysis, at least two data sets are considered that contain the same fluorophores, characterized by the decay time, but have different contributions α_i.

In addition to discrete e-functions, other models can describe the distribution of lifetime in complex systems, including the lifetime distribution (15), stretched e-function (16), time-resolved area-normalized emission spectroscopy (17), and Laguerre expansion techniques (18).

For evaluation of lifetime measurements, in addition to the single amplitudes and lifetimes, the parameters mean lifetime τ_{mean} and relative contribution Q_i are helpful. Here the mean lifetime is defined as:

$$\tau_{mean} = \frac{\sum_{i=1}^{p} \alpha_i \cdot \tau_i}{\sum_{i=1}^{p} \alpha_i}$$

[10]

The relative contribution Q_i of the component i corresponds to the area under the decay curve, determined by the component i. This value is calculated according to:

$$Q_i = \frac{\alpha_i \cdot \tau_i}{\sum_{i=1}^{p} \alpha_i \cdot \tau_i}$$

[11]

Two-dimensional lifetime measurements can be performed in scanning systems, with a pulse laser used as the light source. In contrast to applications in microscopy, the movement of the object eye must be detected and compensated for. The correct relation between detected photons and the position in the sample can be determined by the control signals, the frame and line clocks, and the (line) timer signal. The time between the excitation pulse (sync signal) and the detection time of the first and unique photon is used for allocation in the time channel. If there are multiple detectors in different spectral channels, differences in the fluorescence spectra can be used for further differentiation of fluorophores, e.g., by global fitting. In addition, fluorescence spectra can be reconstructed from the photons detected in each spectral channel.

Starting from the MPE of the eye, lifetime measurements in the time domain were optimally suited for measuring the dynamic AF of the fundus (19). Only a weak excitation power is required for detection of signal in TCSPC. This technique offers the most sensitive detection of light. To ensure a high number of photons, which is required for a good signal-to-noise ratio, the photons are added from a series of single image measurements after image registration.

STUDIES ON ISOLATED FLUOROPHORES

Excitation and Emission Spectra of Expected Fundus Fluorophores

Knowledge of the specific excitation and emission of expected fluorophores is required for selected investigation and interpretation of time-resolved AF images. In addition, the transmission of the ocular media must be taken into account, transforming this spectral information for studies at the fundus. In the study described below, ocular transmission data from a 20-year-old person were used. The excitation and emission spectra were measured with a Fluorolog (SPEX; Jobin Yvon Longjumeau Cedex, France) after the absorbancy of the substances was adjusted to about 0.08.

In the excitation spectrum of NAD, the maximum is at 350 nm and the emission is maximal at 450 nm. Although NADH is a strong fluorophore in human tissue, the ocular transmission blocks nearly all excitation at the fundus, and thus the detection of NADH in living human fundus is unlikely. In contrast, in the excitation spectrum of FAD (Fig. 8.2) there are two maxima at 370 nm and 446 nm. The excitation at 350 nm results in maxima of fluorescence at 441 nm and 520 nm. For investigation of the fundus, only the excitation around 446 nm is relevant.

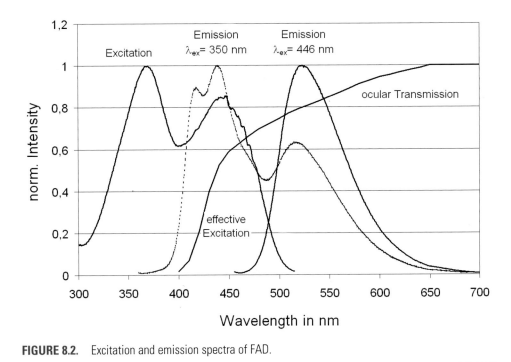

FIGURE 8.2. Excitation and emission spectra of FAD.

Excitation at both 446 nm and 468 nm results in the same maximal emission spectrum at 526 nm. The area under excitation spectrum and ocular transmission is large enough to excite FAD at the fundus in living eyes.

Lipofuscin is the most intensive emitting fundus fluorophore in elderly humans (20,21) (see also Chapter 3). It consists of 10 fluorophores (22) (see also Chapter 2). The component VIII has been identified as N-retinylidene-N-retinylethanolamine (A2E) (23), a by-product of the visual cycle that accumulates in the retinal pigment epithelium (RPE) throughout life (24) (see also Chapter 2). Figure 8.3 shows the

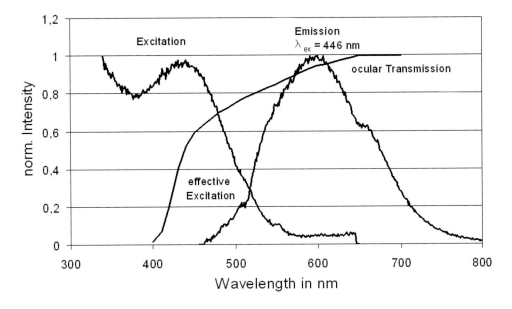

FIGURE 8.3. Excitation and emission spectra of A2E in relation to the ocular transmission.

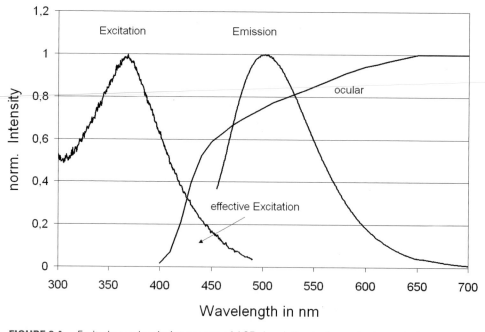

FIGURE 8.4. Excitation and emission spectra of AGEs in relation to the ocular transmission.

excitation and emission spectra of A2E (12.8 mM, dissolved in ethanol), synthesized according to Parish et al. (25). In the visible spectral range, the maximum excitation of A2E is at 441 nm. An excitation at 446 nm results in maximal fluorescence at 600 nm. Because the area is large under the curves of excitation and ocular transmission, A2E can be excited at the fundus, which confirms practical experiences in AF measurements.

AGEs are a mixture of different glycolyzed proteins. In a human sample (Fig. 8.4), excitation at 446 nm resulted in an emission maximum at 502 nm. The extended area under the excitation curve and ocular transmission make the in vivo excitation possible. A comparison of the excitation spectrum of melanin in relation to the transmission of the ocular media shows that the in vivo excitation of detectable melanin fluorescence at the fundus is unlikely (Fig. 8.5).

Ocular structures contain connective tissue composed of collagens and elastin, among other structures. Taking into account the strong increase of the ocular transmission starting from 400 nm, the detection of fluorescence of connective tissue cannot be excluded at the fundus, which is excited in the visible spectrum (Fig. 8.6).

Considering the excitation spectra of isolated substances in relation to the transmission of the ocular media, the effective excitation spectrum should be calculated as a product of the excitation spectrum and spectral ocular transmission. It is done for the fluorophores with the highest excitation probability (A2E, FAD, and AGE). In this way, a certain discrimination of fundus fluorophores can be achieved according to the spectral range of excitation (Fig. 8.7). Furthermore, endogenous fundus fluorophores can be discriminated according to the emission spectra (Fig. 8.8).

Fluorescence Lifetime of Expected Fundus Fluorophores

In addition to the excitation and emission spectra, the fluorescence lifetime is a distinguishing feature. The lifetimes of different fluorophores, estimated using a published

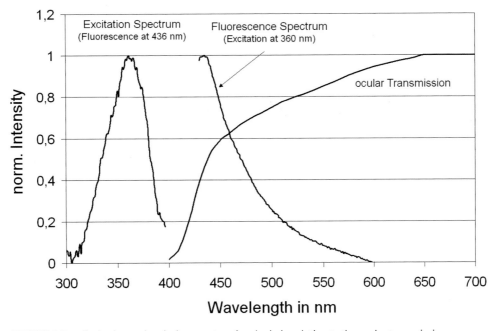

FIGURE 8.5. Excitation and emission spectra of melanin in relation to the ocular transmission

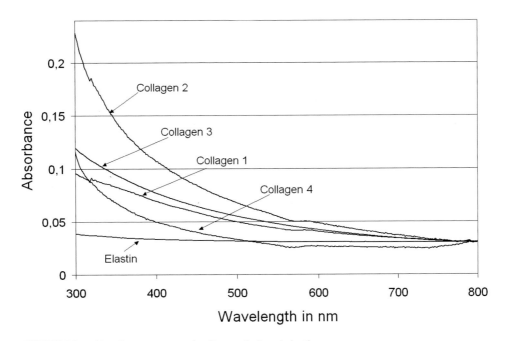

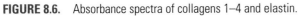

FIGURE 8.6. Absorbance spectra of collagens 1–4 and elastin.

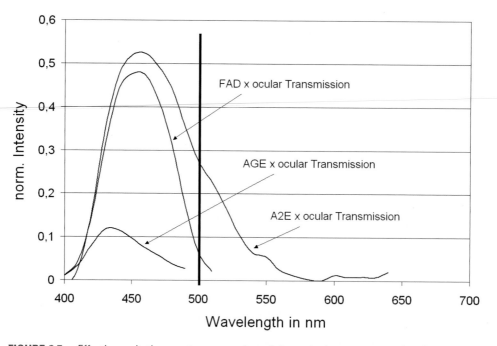

FIGURE 8.7. Effective excitation spectra as a product of the excitation spectrum and ocular transmission for A2E, FAD, and AGE. A2E, FAD, and AGE are excited by light in the short-wave range between 400 nm and 500 nm; predominantly A2E is excited by wavelengths longer than 500 nm.

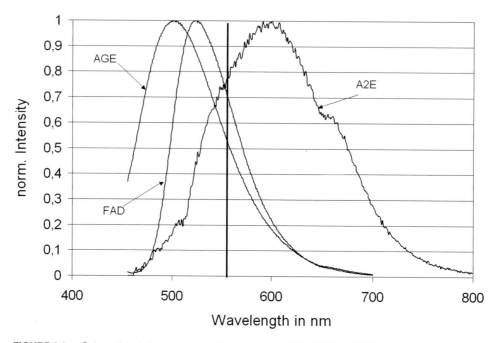

FIGURE 8.8. Selected emission ranges for discrimination of A2E, FAD, and AGE. In the short-wave emission range between 450 nm and 560 nm, AGE, FAD, and A2E are detectable, but the emission range above 560 nm is dominated by A2E.

TABLE 8.1	Lifetimes and Amplitudes of Isolated Fluorophores Expected at the Fundus			
Substance	τ_1 in ps	α_1 in %	τ_2 in ps	α_2 in %
Collagen 1	670	68	4040	32
Collagen 2	470	64	3150	36
Collagen 3	345	69	2800	31
Collagen 4	740	70	3670	30
Elastin	380	72	3590	28
A2E	170	98	1120	2
Melanin	280	70	2400	30
FAD	330	18	2810	82
AGE	865	62	4170	28
NADH	387	73	3650	27

method (26), are given in Table 8.1. This property (lifetime) is especially interesting for investigations of the macula behind the absorbing macular pigment. The absorption of macular pigment changes both the intensity and the spectrum of emitted light originating from the RPE. In contrast, the lifetime of the RPE fluorescence stays unchanged. Because the lifetime depends on viscosity and pH, information related to properties of the embedding matrix in the tissue can be obtained. In a less viscous environment, the molecules display internal rotation and charge transfer, which results in radiationless decay. As a result, the quantum yield and the lifetime depend on viscosity. Fluorophores can have both a protonated and a deprotonated form. Both forms have different lifetimes. The average lifetime is related to the equilibrium of both forms, which depends on the pH of the local environment.

STUDIES ON OCULAR TISSUES

Excitation and Emission Spectra of Ocular Tissues

To evaluate the excitation and emission spectra of ocular tissues, the cornea, aqueous humor, lens, vitreous, neuronal retina, retinal pigment epithelium, choroid, and sclera obtained from porcine eyes were separated and the absorption spectra were measured with a Lambda 2 UV/VIS spectrometer (PerkinElmer, Waltham, MA). With excitation in the absorbance maxima, fluorescence spectra were measured with an LS 5 spectrometer (PerkinElmer). With illumination at 45 degrees, the fluorescence was detected in reflection under 0 degrees. To measure the fluorescence in aqueous humor and in vitreous, the absorbance was adjusted to 0.05. This adjustment was not possible in any other opaque or scattering ocular structures. The excitation spectra of ocular tissues, detected at 460 nm, are shown in Figure 8.9.

To check FAD, the excitation spectra of ocular tissues were determined by measuring changes in the fluorescence intensity at 524 nm when excited at single wavelengths between 310 nm and 490 nm (Fig. 8.10).

Fluorescence Lifetime of Ocular Tissues

Considerable differences among different ocular structures in histograms of mean lifetime τ_{mean} (Fig. 8.11) are observed in biexponential approximation.

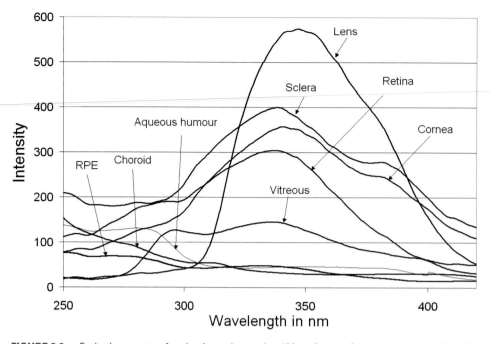

FIGURE 8.9. Excitation spectra of ocular tissue detected at 460 nm (mean of measurements obtained from 10 ocular samples). Excitation maxima around 350 nm were detectable from lens, sclera, and cornea as well as from retina, and to a certain degree also from vitreous. In the RPE this excitation maximum is only weakly detectable. No clear excitation maximum at 350 nm was detected from choroid and aqueous humor. An additional shoulder in the excitation spectra was detectable at 380 nm from lens, sclera, and cornea.

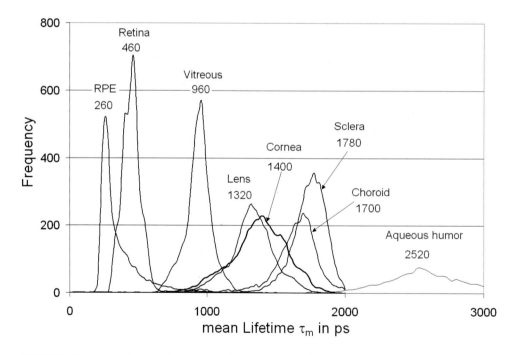

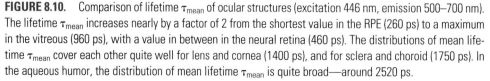

FIGURE 8.10. Comparison of lifetime τ_{mean} of ocular structures (excitation 446 nm, emission 500–700 nm). The lifetime τ_{mean} increases nearly by a factor of 2 from the shortest value in the RPE (260 ps) to a maximum in the vitreous (960 ps), with a value in between in the neural retina (460 ps). The distributions of mean lifetime τ_{mean} cover each other quite well for lens and cornea (1400 ps), and for sclera and choroid (1750 ps). In the aqueous humor, the distribution of mean lifetime τ_{mean} is quite broad—around 2520 ps.

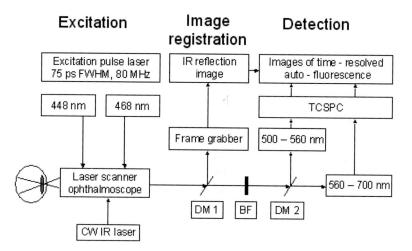

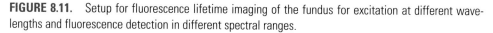

FIGURE 8.11.   Setup for fluorescence lifetime imaging of the fundus for excitation at different wavelengths and fluorescence detection in different spectral ranges.

In histograms of the amplitude α_1, the decay of AF is dominated by the short component in RPE ($\alpha_1 = 95\%$) and in neuronal retina ($\alpha_1 = 88\%$). In the choroid, lens, cornea, and sclera, the amplitude is much smaller and are nearly the same (α_1 about 70%).

The lifetimes and amplitudes of ocular structures are given in Table 8.2. Individual deviations from these values are on the order of 10%.

EXPERIMENTAL SETUP FOR FLUORESCENCE LIFETIME MEASUREMENTS IN THE HUMAN EYE

Technical Description

At our institution, a scanning laser ophthalmoscope (SLO) was developed for 2D measurements of time-resolved AF of the fundus (Fig. 8.11). It works in the time domain. In this device, the parameters required for discrimination of fluorophores are combined; therefore, two wavelengths can be used for excitation, and the time-resolved fluorescence can be measured in two spectral emission ranges.

TABLE 8.2   **Lifetimes and Amplitudes of Ocular Tissue of Porcine Eyes in Biexponential Approximation (Excitation 446 nm, Emission 500–700 nm)**

Tissue	τ_1 in ps	α_1 in %	τ_2 in ps	α_2 in %
RPE	200	95	1800	4
Retina	240	88	2560	10
Choroid	530	70	3400	30
Lens	460	69	3200	31
Cornea	470	70	3600	30
Sclera	620	64	3640	36
Vitreous	260	78	3200	22

The basic device is a commercially available SLO (HRA 2, Heidelberg Engineering, Heidelberg, Germany). Two pulse lasers can be used for excitation, emitting at 446 nm or 468 nm (Lasos, Jena, Germany; Becker & Hickl, Berlin, Germany; or Picoquant, Berlin, Germany). These lasers deliver pulses of 75 ps FWHM at a repetition rate of 80 MHz. The average radiation power is less than 100 μW in the cornea plane. The fundus is irradiated by an infrared (IR) laser at 820 nm simultaneously with the excitation light. Since the acquisition time is short for single images, it is unlikely that eye movements will interfere with the measurements. The contrast is high in each IR image but very weak in the AF image. Subsequent images are registered in relation to this IR reference image. The calculated image transformation is also used for the registration of the lifetime images. Thus, each photon will be added at the right position in the correct time channel for lifetime measurement. Images are automatically excluded if not enough structure is found for registration, such as in the case of blinking and eye movement resulting in doubling of vessel structures or fixation outside of one-half of the reference image. The IR light is separated from the fluorescence light by a dichroic filter (DM 1). Additionally, the fluorescence light is detected in a short-wave spectral range (490–560 nm) and a long-wave range (560–700 nm). A dichroic filter (DM 2) separates both beams. In both spectral ranges, the fluorescence will be detected by a multichannel-photomultiplier (MCP-PMT, HAM-R 3809U-50; Hamamatsu, Herrsching, Germany) with jitter <50 ps. The fluorescence decay is detected in the TCSPC technique by a SPC 150 board (Becker & Hickl). This board works in the first-in/first-out mode and has direct memory access. A HRT41 router (Becker & Hickl) separates the photons from both spectral channels. During measurement, online registration is performed in both channels.

The measurements last until a certain number of photons are collected at each pixel in the fluorescence image. Practical measuring times are realized with a spatial resolution of 40×40 μm^2. Since the number of detected photons increases with the pixel area, the measuring time can be reduced if the spatial resolution is not so high.

Experimental Results

Images and Histograms of Parameters of Dynamic Fluorescence in a Healthy Subject

In the following examples, results are presented that can be calculated from measurements of time-resolved fundus AF. The first example is the dynamic fundus AF of a 63-year-old healthy subject. The fundus was excited at 468 nm by a pulse laser. The dynamic fluorescence at each pixel was approximated by a biexponential model function using the program SPCImage 2.9.1 (Becker & Hickl). As result of the fit, images of the fluorescence intensity, lifetimes, and amplitudes, as well as histograms of these parameters, can be demonstrated. By comparing the intensity images of channels 1 and 2 (Fig. 8.12), one can see that the contrast of the vessel structure is higher in the long-wave emission range than in the short-wave one. This means that the main part of long-wave fluorescence light originates from behind the vessels. Also, almost no long-wave fluorescence light is detected from the dark optic disc, whereas in the short-wave range the contrast is weak and fluorescence light is also detected from the optic disc. Therefore, the short-wave fluorescence light also contains signal originating in front of the vessels. In lifetime images, τ_{mean} differs considerably between the two spectral channels (Fig. 8.13; in the color range, red means τ_{mean} = 150 ps, and

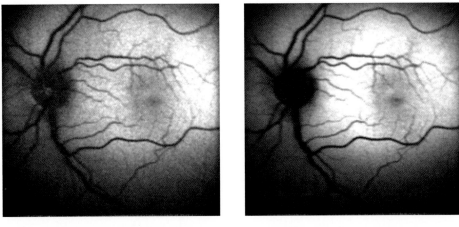

500 nm- 560 nm   **560 nm – 700 nm**

FIGURE 8.12.   Images of fluorescence intensity of healthy fundus in different spectral channels (excitation 468 nm). *Left*: Short-wave channel K1. *Right*: Long-wave channel K2.

blue τ_{mean} = 300 ps). The longest lifetime is detectable from the optic disc. This long decay originates from connective tissue (collagen, elastin, and cholesterol) (27). Especially in the short-wave range, the macula exhibits the shortest lifetime (RPE), and in the papillomacular range the lifetime τ_{mean} is in between them. In contrast, in the long-wave channel, this range exhibits nearly the same long lifetime as the optic disk. Clear differences in lifetime distribution of τ_{mean} exist for the fluorescence in both channels (Fig. 8.14).

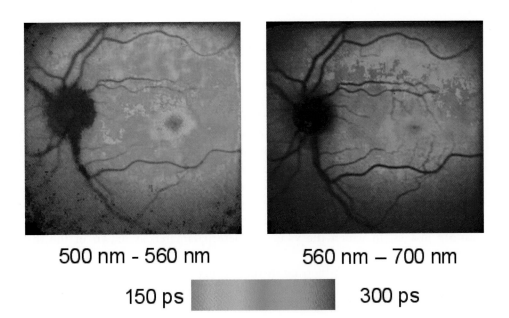

500 nm - 560 nm   **560 nm – 700 nm**

150 ps   **300 ps**

FIGURE 8.13.   Images of fluorescence lifetime τ_{mean} in the short-wave channel (*left*) and the long-wave channel (*right*).

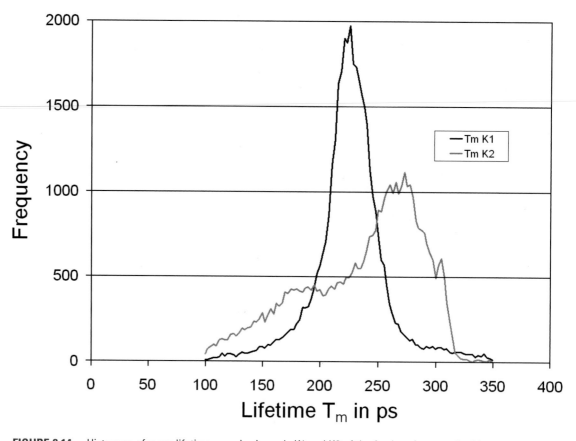

FIGURE 8.14. Histogram of mean lifetime τ_{mean} in channels K1 and K2 of the fundus of a normal subject.

The amplitude α_1 is generally higher in the short-wave channel K1 (94.4%) than in K2 (85.6%). In the optic disc in K1, α_1 is quite low, which means that the influence of the component corresponding to τ_1 is considerably reduced in the optic disc.

Quasi-3D Images in Early Age-Related Maculopathy

Investigations of dynamic fluorescence are of special interest in early stages of AMD. Here, the advantage of lifetime measurements is evident. The RPE fluorescence can be studied with no interference from the macular pigment.

In addition to 2D images or histograms of lifetimes τ_i, amplitudes α_i, and relative contribution Q_i, cluster diagrams of τ_i vs. τ_j, or α_i vs. α_j, are well suited for detection and interpretation of pathological alterations. Of special interest are quasi-3D images, in which the value of these parameters is drawn in the third coordinate.

Contrary alterations in lifetime in the macula are detectable in both spectral channels. As demonstrated in nonexudative AMD (Fig. 8.15), in the short-wave channel τ_3 is increased in an extended range temporal the optic disc, excluding the macula, where low values of τ_3 are determined. In this macular range, the lifetime τ_3 is increased up to 4 ns in the long-wave channel. According to the emission in the long-wave range, a component of lipofuscin may be detected with a long decay time. For comparison, the lifetime of A2E (component VIII) was determined with 170 ps.

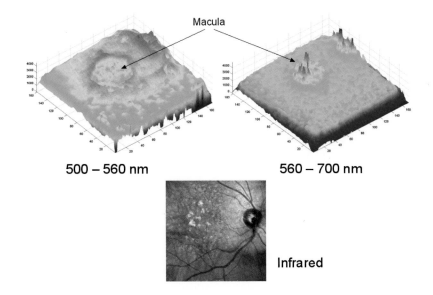

FIGURE 8.15.   Complementary macular lifetime τ_3 in short- and long-wave channels in nonexudative AMD. *Left*: τ_3 in the short-wave channel. *Right*: τ_3 in the long-wave emission channel. *Blue*: Short lifetime τ_3; *red*: long lifetime τ_3. *Below*: IR fundus image for comparison. The encircled macular range of enlarged lifetime τ_3 only in the long-wave emission channel points to the accumulation of a component of lipofuscin with a long fluorescence decay time.

SUMMARY

Quantitative, independent evaluation of fundus fluorophores seems to be possible. For this purpose and in the clinical setting, fundus images demonstrating local distribution of fluorophores would be of great value. However, various problems can be encountered, such as the variety of fluorophores contributing to the measurable fluorescence, and the weak fluorescence of interesting fluorophores, such as FAD, which is covered by the strong fluorescence of lipofuscin, the predominant fluorophore of the ocular fundus. Furthermore, the fluorescence of the crystalline lens should be eliminated. A good separation between fluorescence from RPE and neuroretina on one hand and fluorescence from the crystalline lens on the other hand can be achieved by fluorescence lifetime measurements. Lifetime measurements can effectively be performed in the time domain with the use of pulse lasers in confocal SLOs and by detecting the dynamic fluorescence in the TCSPC technique. A nearly complete elimination of lens fluorescence can be achieved in fluorescence measurements of the fundus by combining the confocal technique with division of the aperture diaphragm.

The combination of fluorescence lifetime measurements with selected excitation wavelengths and simultaneous detection of fluorescence in separate spectral ranges is an optimal method for characterizing fluorophores in fundus images.

Because several fluorophores are excited at the fundus simultaneously, the interpretation of such measurements is challenging. For such interpretation, knowledge of the excitation and emission spectra as well as the fluorescence lifetimes of expected fluorophores is required (28). Equivalent measurements on ocular tissue and comparisons with the anatomy of the eye point to the origin of the measured fluorescence (10). The performance of different methods must be evaluated for analysis of dynamic fluorescence measurements. Model studies on cell and tissue cultures (29–31) make it possible to compare spectrometric measurements with the results of other analytical methods, such as high-performance liquid chromatography, mass spectrometry, nuclear magnetic resonance, and surface-enhanced Raman scattering (32).

In clinical practice, the interpretation of fluorescence lifetime measurements can be improved by metabolic provocation tests. Measurements on eyes with known anatomical or functional defects would enable a simple interpretation of the lifetime information.

In addition to investigation of endogenous fluorophores, studies on exogenous fluorophores are interesting because lifetimes may change between the free and protein-bond states, and such studies may facilitate further understanding of clinical findings.

REFERENCES

1. Niesner R, Peker B, Schluesche P, et al. Noniterative biexponential fluorescence lifetime imaging in the investigating of cellular metabolism by means of NAD(P)H autofluorescence. Chem Phys Chem 2004;5: 1141–1149.
2. Wu Y, Zheng W, Qu JY. Sensing cell metabolism by time-resolved autofluorescence. Optics Letters 2006;31:3122–3124.
3. Stryer L. Biochemie. Spektrum Akad. Heidelberg, Berlin, New York: Verlag, 1991.
4. Berman ER. Biochemistry of the eye. In: Blakemore C, ed. Perspectives in Vision Research. New York: Plenum Press, 1991.
5. Lakowicz JR. Principles of Fluorescence Spectroscopy. 2nd ed. New York: Kluwer Academic/Plenum, 1999.
6. Geeraets WJ, Berry ER. Ocular characteristic as related to hazards from laser and other light sources. Am J Ophthalmol 1968;66:15–20.
7. van de Kraats J, van Norren D. Optical density of the aging human ocular media in the visible and the UV. J Opt Soc Am A 2007;24:1842–1857.
8. Koellner M, Wolfrum J. How many photons are necessary for fluorescence lifetime measurements? Chem Phys Lett 1992;200:2.
9. Schweitzer D, Hammer M, Schweitzer F. Grenzen der konfokalen Laser Scanning Technik bei Messungen der zeitaufgelösten Autofluoreszenz am Augenhintergrund. Biomedizinische Technik 2005;50:263–267.
10. Schweitzer D, Jentsch S, Schenke S, et al. Spectral and time-resolved studies on ocular structures. SPIE-OSA 2007;6628:662807-1–662807-12.
11. American National Standard for the Safe Use of Lasers. ANSI Z 136.1-2000. Orlando, FL: Laser Institute of America, 2000.
12. Clegg RM, Schneider PC. Fluorescence lifetime-resolved imaging microscopy: a general description of lifetime-resolved imaging measurements. In: Fluorescence Microscopy and Fluorescence Probes. New York: Plenum Press, 1996:15–25.
13. Becker W. Advanced time-correlated single photon counting techniques. Springer Series in Chemical Physics 81. Berlin, Heidelberg, New York: Springer, 2005.
14. Knutson JR, Beechem JM, Brand L. Simultaneous analysis of multiple fluorescence decay curves: a global approach. Chem Phys Lett 1983;102:501–507.
15. Alcala JR, Gratton E, Prendergast FG. Fluorescence lifetime distribution in proteins. Biophys J 1987;51: 597–604.
16. Lee BKC, Siegel J, Webb SED, et al. Application of stretched exponential function to fluorescence lifetime imaging. Biophys J 2001;81:1265–1274.
17. Koti ASR, Krishna MMG, Periasami N. Time-resolved area-normalized emission spectroscopy (TRANES). A novel method for confirming emission from two excited states. J Phys Chem A 2001;105: 1767–1771.
18. Jo JA, Marcu L, Fang Q, et al. New methods for time-resolved fluorescence spectroscopy data analysis based on the Laguerre expansion technique—applications in tissue diagnosis. Methods Inf Med 2007; 46:206–211.
19. Schweitzer D, Kolb A, Hammer M, et al. Tau-mapping of the autofluorescence of the human ocular fundus. Proc SPIE 2000;4164:79–89.
20. Feeney-Burns L, Berman ER, Rothman H. Lipofuscin of human retinal pigment epithelium. Am J Ophthalmol 1980;90:783–791.
21. Delori FC, Dorey CK, Staurenghi G, et al. In vivo fluorescence of the ocular fundus exhibits retinal pigment epithelium lipofuscin characteristics. Invest Ophthalmol Vis Sci 1995;36718–36729.
22. Eldred GE, Katz ML. Fluorophores of the human retinal pigment epithelium: separation and spectral characterization. Exp Eye Res 1988;47:71–86.
23. Eldred GE, Lasky MR. Retinal age—pigments generated by self-assembling lysosomotropic detergents. Nature 1993;361:724–726.

24. Sparrow JR, Fishkin N, Zhou J, et al. A2E, a by-product of the visual cycle. Vision Res 2003;43: 2983–2990.
25. Parish CA, Hashimoto M, Nakanishi K, et al. Isolation and one step preparation of A2E and iso-A2E, fluorophores from human retinal pigment epithelium. Proc Natl Acad Sci USA 1998;95:14609–14613.
26. Schweitzer D, Hammer M, Schweitzer F, et al. In vivo measurement of time-resolved autofluorescence at the human fundus. J Biomed Optics 2004;9:1214–1222.
27. Marcu L, Grundfest WS, Maarek JML. Photobleaching of arterial fluorescent compounds: characterization of elastin, collagen and cholesterol time-resolved spectra during prolonged ultraviolet irradiation. Photochem Photobiol 1999;69:713–712.
28. Schweitzer D, Schenke S, Hammer M, et al. Towards metabolic mapping of the human retina. Microsc Res Tech 2007;70:410–419.
29. Cubeddu R, Taroni P, Hu DN, et al. Photophysical studies of A2E, putative precursor of lipofuscin, in human retinal pigment epithelial cells. Photochem Photobiol 1999;70:172–175.
30. Doccio F, Boulton M, Cubeddu R, et al. Age-related changes in the fluorescence of melanin and lipofuscin granules of the retinal pigment epithelium: a time-resolved fluorescence spectroscopy study. Photochem Photobiol 1991;54:247–253.
31. Bui TV, Han Y, Roxana A, et al. Characterization of native retinal fluorophores involved in biosynthesis of A2E and lipofuscin-associated retinopathies. J Biol Chem 2006;281:18112–18119.
32. Kneipp K, Kneipp H, Kneipp J. Surface-enhanced Raman scattering in local optical fields of silver and gold nanoaggregates—from single-molecule Raman spectroscopy to untrasensitive probing in live cells. Acc Chem Res 2006;39:443–450.

SECTION **II**

Clinical Science
Fundus Autofluorescence in the Healthy Eye

CHAPTER 9

R. Theodore Smith

The Normal Distribution of Fundus Autofluorescence

Τhis chapter concentrates on the image of the normal fundus itself and its analysis. In particular, it first discusses images obtained from the most widely used and available systems, the Heidelberg Retinal Angiograph (HRA; Heidelberg Engineering, Dossenheim, Germany) and its latest model, the HRA2. These confocal scanning laser ophthalmoscopes (cSLOs) use an excitation wavelength of 488 nm and a barrier filter of 500 nm to provide fundus autofluorescence (AF) imaging in vivo (see also Chapter 5) (1,2). A discussion on the variations in such images when acquired with longer-wavelength excitation systems follows.

AF images acquired by the HRA consist of 30-degree field-of-view laser scans, 512×512 pixels in size, centered on the macula. The resolution of the HRA2 is 768×768 pixels. As explained in Chapter 5, several scans with a relatively low signal-to-noise ratio are registered and then averaged to improve the signal-to-noise ratio. The resulting image is then histogram-stretched by the HRA software to increase contrast for viewing. These details serve to remind us that the final images are not pixel-by-pixel representations of absolute AF levels, such as would be obtained by spectrophotometry; rather, they show the *relative* AF intensities of neighboring pixels. Further, just as in fundus photography, even the relative intensities of widely separated pixels are affected by intrinsic variability in the acquisition process. In other words, illumination may vary gradually from one portion of a photograph or AF scan to another, with a resulting effect on measured intensities that is purely photographic, not physiologic. Nonetheless, a wealth of qualitative information may be gleaned from these images, properly interpreted, as reviewed throughout this book. Furthermore, it is possible, as will be discussed in this chapter, to take these qualitative data back to quantitative interpretation by demonstrating that (i) a large portion of the variability observed in the background AF of a normal AF image has a smooth and regular structure, (ii) this structure can be mapped by an appropriate mathematical model, and (iii) this model of a normal AF image naturally provides a framework for the interpretation and quantification of AF abnormalities as variations from the normal model.

NORMAL DISTRIBUTION OF FUNDUS AUTOFLUORESCENCE

In vivo spectrophotometric recording of fundus AF was described by Delori et al. (3), who showed that AF arose predominantly from lipofuscin in the retinal pigment epithelium (RPE; see Chapter 3). Thus, the intensity of fundus AF mostly parallels the amount and distribution of lipofuscin (subject to exceptions noted further below). Lipofuscin is derived, in large part, from phagocytosis of outer segment discs containing bisretinoid by-products of light absorption (see Chapters 1 and 2). The emission of lipofuscin has a broad band ranging from 500 nm to 750 nm (3) (see Chapter 3).

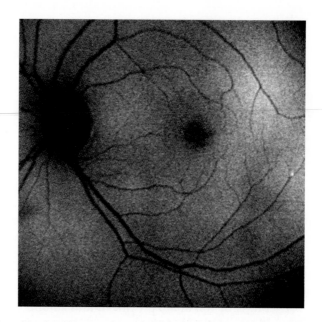

FIGURE 9.1.   Normal fundus AF pattern from the HRA. The optic disc and retinal blood vessels are dark. The background pattern is mildly variable, with lighter and darker areas throughout, and with greatest intensity roughly surrounding the fovea. The central macula is particularly dark due to absorption of the blue excitation light by luteal pigments. There is a tiny "speck" of increased AF temporally, which probably represents a small druse in this normal 54-year-old woman.

In the normal fundus AF pattern, diffuse AF is most intense between 5 and 15 degrees from the fovea. However, mild variability throughout the fundus is the rule in a normal AF image, with lighter and darker areas due at least in part to the image acquisition process, much as can be seen in a normal fundus photograph (Fig. 9.1). The optic disc and retinal blood vessels have a low (dark) autofluorescent signal, and the blood vessels mask the RPE beneath them. However, these findings are not determined by the AF of lipofuscin alone, a fact that complicates their interpretation. One of the complicating factors is the absorption of the 488 nm blue light by macular pigments, especially the carotenoids lutein and zeaxanthin (see also Chapter 3) (4,5). On fundus photographs and under visual observation, these pigments are characterized by strong yellow coloration (6). Their absorption is greatest in the center of the macula. This absorption markedly diminishes the foveal AF signal (Fig. 9.1), which would otherwise approximate the remainder of the macular background. There is also some absorption of the 488 nm light by melanin granules located in the RPE (7). Further, cone photopigments will be incompletely bleached after an approximately 15- to 30-second exposure to the HRA in AF mode (8); hence, absorption by these structures will also diminish the AF signal centrally. On the other hand, an advantage of the HRA system is that the AF that is recorded is dominated by lipofuscin. In particular, AF from melanin, which can be recorded in the near infrared (IR) (9) (see Chapter 6), does not affect the HRA signal.

NORMAL DISTRIBUTION OF FOVEAL AUTOFLUORESCENCE

Normal AF fundus images of the fovea are affected the most by the anatomic distribution of fluorescent lipofuscin and blue light attenuating pigments; hence, the structure of such an image deserves separate and detailed consideration. Our approach to demonstrating the structure of a foveal image is as follows: Noise is first removed with a fine Gaussian filter, and then the image is further contrast-enhanced for visualization of the resulting contours of isoautofluorescence (Fig. 9.2). These contours are referred to as isobars. The resulting normal foveal AF images exhibit finely resolved concentric elliptical isobars of AF, with AF increasing outward along any radius from a least-fluorescent center. Further, these elliptical foveal patterns are consistent with the known anatomic distribution of lipofuscin, luteal pigment, cone pigment, and RPE thickening in the center of the fovea. A two-zone elliptic quadratic polynomial model provides an accurate fit for foveal data and can be used to reconstruct the entire foveal data from small subsets of data (8). The fine structure of the foveal AF is illustrated in two examples in Figure 9.2.

Conversely, the imaging data are evidence for anatomic regularity in the normal eye. That is, the extraordinary geometric regularity and precise isobar resolutions

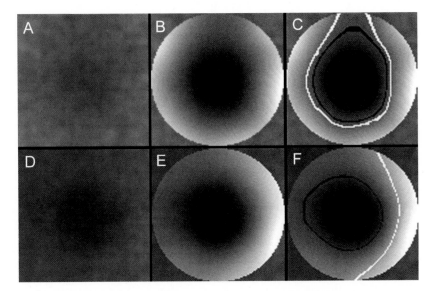

FIGURE 9.2.   Normal foveal AF images and isobar patterns. The foveal regions of interest from two normal AF images have been filtered (Gaussian filter, radius 36 μm) on a small scale for noise reduction. The central fovea has on the average reduced AF, but no pattern is yet apparent **(B,E)**. The fovea (1500-μ-diameter disk) has been further filtered (Gaussian, radius 180 μm) to establish a very regular shading pattern of concentric elliptical isobars of isoautofluorescence. Contrast enhancement has also been applied to emphasize the geometry of the pattern **(C)**. The individual isobars in **B** are still too fine to be discernible, so three are highlighted with black (AF = 112), gray (AF = 120), and white (AF = 123), respectively. There are 30 distinct isobars in this pattern that fill the 750 μm radius, yielding an average isobar resolution of 750 μm/30 = 25 μm. The isobars illustrated are even finer, mostly one pixel (15 μm) in width. In this typical pattern, the central isobars are nearly circular, with the more peripheral isobars becoming more vertically elongated until the last ones are only partial annuli. **(F)** A similar demonstration of the isobar pattern in **E**. In **E** we see that the temporal fovea has a slightly more increased AF signal than that of other quadrants, and the reduced AF at the center appears somewhat elongated horizontally. These features are dramatically more evident in the individual isobars in **F**, where isobars are highlighted in black (AF = 62), gray (AF = 75), and white (AF = 97), respectively. The ellipses in this less-typical pattern become more elongated horizontally and an increased AF signal arc appears temporally. There are 36 isobars in all in this pattern, yielding an average isobar resolution of 21 μm. The isobars shown are 1 pixel (15 μm) in width, with occasional single-pixel discontinuities.

demonstrated by the foveal AF patterns suggest that the normal anatomic spatial variations of luteal and RPE pigment and lipofuscin have similar elliptic regularity and equally fine resolution.

MATHEMATICAL MODEL FOR AUTOFLUORESCENCE IMAGES IN THE 6000-μ REGION

To make quantitative assessments of abnormal AF relative to the image background, and to perform these measurements efficiently and uniformly in the setting of significant background variability, it is desirable to "level" the AF image to an image with a uniform background. Then areas of reduced or increased AF will appear against a "level playing field" or basal level of fluorescence and can be calculated with a uniform threshold. To accomplish this, Hwang et al. (10) extended the foveal model of AF background described above to a 12-zone quadratic polynomial mathematical model of the background in the 6000-μ region of a normal AF image. The model was tested and fit to normal AF scans, as described below.

Four inner zones were defined: a 600-μ central disc and three annular zones (600–1000, 1000–2000, and 2000–3000 μ diameter), and two outer annular zones (3000–4500 μ and 4500–6000 μ). The two outer zones were each subdivided into four quadrants (superior, nasal, inferior and temporal), giving eight outer zones, which with the 4 inner zones gave 12 zones in all. The two innermost zones were those used for the foveal model described previously. The two-threshold Otsu method (11) was used throughout to define candidate regions in each zone with increased and decreased AF, and local quadratic polynomials were fit to the remaining normal, or background, pixel values, as described in a previously published study (12). Precisely, the candidate regions were C_0 (nonbackground sources with decreased AF, e.g., vessels), C_1 (background AF), and C_2 (areas of increased AF). For each zone, there was an initial choice of background, C_1, for input to the quadratic polynomial background model. The resulting global model was formed from the 12 local models with appropriate radial and angular cubic spline interpolations at interfaces.

This model of macular background was fit to 10 normal AF images from 10 subjects with normal dilated retinal examinations. The average absolute errors were 3.8% $\pm$ 3.5% of net image range. The mean local standard deviations of the original images in each zone (exclusive of the pixels with increased and reduced AF) ranged from 3.0% to 4.1% over the 10 images. Thus, if these mean local standard deviations were taken as representative of noise in the image, it follows that the errors of the model were of the same magnitude as the noise in the original data. This demonstrated that the model was an excellent fit to normal AF data. Finally, each AF image was then leveled by subtracting its background model (with an offset of 125 gray levels to center the brightness of the resulting image within the usual [0, 255] range), and the mean and standard deviation σ of the leveled image (excluding vessels) was calculated. It was found that the leveled image fell within 2.0 σ of the mean for 99.7% of pixels in each of the images (Fig. 9.3).

Because such a consistently small fraction of pixels in a normal leveled image fell 2.0 σ above the image mean, it seemed reasonable to propose this as a working definition of focally increased AF (FIAF) in a normal image, i.e., not more than 0.3% of pixels may have a gray level greater than 2.0 σ above the image mean, after the image has been leveled by the model. The same terminology can then be used as the working definition of FIAF in an abnormal image: all those pixels whose gray level is greater than 2.0 σ above the image mean, after the image has been leveled by the model.

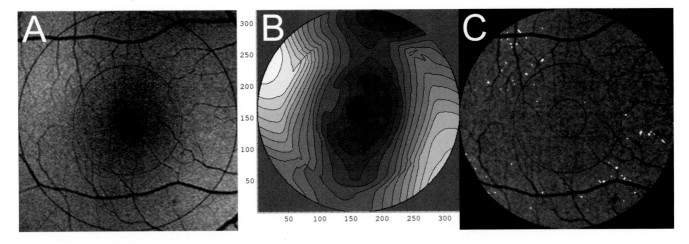

FIGURE 9.3.   Mathematical model and segmentation of a normal AF scan (6000-μ region). **(A)** Normal AF scan of the right eye of 54-year-old female. Note significant background variability and foveal decreased AF due largely to luteal pigment. The 12-zone mathematical model of the AF background in **A** is presented in **B** as a contour graph. Note how the model captures the background variability of the original scan. It is essentially smooth throughout, with the exception of a residual mild discontinuity superotemporally in this blend zone. The contour lines are closer together in the fovea, where the background is more highly variable. **(C)** The image in **A** leveled by subtracting the model in **B**. The background of the leveled image is now quite homogeneous, with mean gray level 126 and standard deviation 11.6. The global threshold of 2.0 standard deviations above the mean defining increased AF was therefore 149.2, which was applied to the entire leveled image and yielded the increased AF shown in white (0.28% of the 6000-μ zone). Comparison of the increased AF with the original image **(A)** demonstrates a very reasonable selection. By contrast, the use of any single threshold in the unleveled image **(A)** to define increased AF would cause major errors due to the image background variability.

The leveling of an abnormal AF image is beyond the scope of this chapter. For details and applications, the interested reader is referred to published work on AF in geographic atrophy (10) and drusen (13). Note that this also allows great flexibility in the definition of abnormal FIAF: in a given circumstance, and because there is as yet no absolute consensus on the definition of FIAF, a definition based on 1.5 σ or 2.5 σ of deviation from image mean could equally well be used. Focally decreased AF can be defined similarly, with the understanding that normal retinal vessels will always fall in this category.

Longer Wavelengths

Spaide et al. (14) demonstrated fundus AF using a fundus camera-based system with a band-pass filter for the excitation light of 580 nm and a barrier filter of 695 nm to avoid AF from the crystalline lens (lens AF is rejected by the confocal optics of the SLO systems) (see Chapter 5). An advantage of the camera-based system is that the longer excitation wavelength is minimally absorbed by the luteal and photopigments. Hence, the central macular AF signal is only slightly diminished (by the higher RPE melanin concentration) relative to the remaining background signal, so central macular increased or reduced AF may be easier to interpret. On the other hand, melanin itself, which fluoresces in the near IR (9), could contribute to the total detected AF above 695 nm. When there is attenuation of a normally uniform RPE melanin, the melanin in the choroid may be imaged in a banded pattern. This could complicate interpretation, as well as any attempt to model the normal AF background from such images.

SUMMARY

A precise mathematical description of the normal AF image will be useful in the quantitative interpretation of focally increased or decreased AF in AF images obtained from eyes with pathological fundus changes.

REFERENCES

1. von Ruckmann A, Fitzke FW, Bird AC. In vivo fundus autofluorescence in macular dystrophies. Arch Ophthalmol 1997;115:609–615.
2. Holz FG, Bellmann C, Margaritidis M, et al. Patterns of increased in vivo fundus autofluorescence in the junctional zone of geographic atrophy of the retinal pigment epithelium associated with age-related macular degeneration. Graefes Arch Clin Exp Ophthalmol 1999;237:145–152.
3. Delori FC, Dorey CK, Staurenghi G, et al. In vivo fluorescence of the ocular fundus exhibits retinal pigment epithelium lipofuscin characteristics. Invest Ophthalmol Vis Sci 1995;36:718–729.
4. Bone RA, Landrum JT, Cains A. Optical density spectra of the macular pigment in vivo and in vitro. Vis Res 1992;32:105–110.
5. Handelman GJ, Snodderly DM, Adler AJ, et al. Measurement of carotenoids in human and monkey retinas. Methods Enzymol 1992:220–230.
6. Gellerman W, Bernstein PS. Noninvasive detection of macular pigments in the human eye. J Biomed Optics 2004;9:75–85.
7. Bindewald A, Jorzik JJ, Loesch A, et al. Visualization of retinal pigment epithelial cells in vivo using digital high-resolution confocal scanning laser ophthalmoscopy. Am J Ophthalmol 2004;137:556–558.
8. Smith RT, Koniarek JP, Chan JK, et al. Autofluorescence characteristics of normal foveas and reconstruction of foveal autofluorescence from limited data subsets. Invest Ophthalmol Vis Sci 2005;46:2940–2946.
9. Keilhauer CN, Delori FC. Near-infrared autofluorescence imaging of the fundus: visualization of ocular melanin. Invest Ophthalmol Vis Sci 2006;47:3556–3564.
10. Hwang JC, Chan J, Chang S, et al. Predictive value of fundus autofluorescence for development of geographic atrophy in age-related macular degeneration. Invest Ophthalmol Vis Sci 2006;47:2655–2661.
11. Otsu N. A threshold selection method from gray-level histograms. IEEE Trans Syst Man Cybernet 1979;9:62–66.
12. Smith RT, Chan JK, Nagasaki T, et al. Automated detection of macular drusen using geometric background leveling and threshold selection. Arch Ophthalmol 2005;123:200–206.
13. Smith RT, Chan JK, Busuoic M, et al. Autofluorescence characteristics of early, atrophic, and high-risk fellow eyes in age-related macular degeneration. Invest Ophthalmol Vis Sci 2006;47:5495–5504.
14. Spaide RF. Fundus autofluorescence and age-related macular degeneration. Ophthalmology 2003;110:392–400.

Clinical Science

Fundus Autofluorescence in the Diseased Eye

Almut Bindewald-Wittich
Robert P. Finger
Frank G. Holz

CHAPTER 10A

Fundus Autofluorescence in Age-Related Maculopathy

A ge-related macular degeneration (AMD) has become the most common cause of severe visual loss in industrialized countries (1–3). AMD is a multifactorial, complex disease with genetic and environmental risk factors that affect the central photoreceptors, retinal pigment epithelium (RPE), Bruch's membrane, and choriocapillaris. The underlying pathophysiological mechanisms are still incompletely understood (4,5).

The phenotypic characteristics of early AMD include drusen and focal hypo- and hyperpigmentation. Drusen were first described by Donders (6) and Wedl (7) in 1855 and 1854, respectively. Although patients with drusen and pigment irregularities usually have good central vision, minor symptoms may be present, such as prolonged dark adaptation and problems under low-luminance conditions. The term "age-related maculopathy" (ARM) was introduced by the International ARM Epidemiological Study group to describe the presence of drusen and RPE abnormalities in the absence of neovascular or atrophic manifestations of AMD (8).

PATHOLOGY OF DRUSEN IN AGE-RELATED MACULOPATHY

Drusen, a hallmark of ARM, are extracellular deposits between the RPE and the inner collagenous layer of Bruch's membrane. Drusen cause a lateral stretching of the RPE and physical displacement of the RPE from its immediate vascular supply, the choriocapillaris. Therefore, they are thought to interfere with the physiological metabolite diffusion between the neurosensory retina and the choroid.

The molecular composition of drusen is complex and includes lipids and various matrix proteins, such as vitronectin, as well as constituents of the inflammatory pathways (9–11). The latter include complement activators and inhibitors, activation-specific complement fragments, and terminal pathway components, including the lytic membrane attack complex (9,12,13). Hageman and coworkers (15) showed that factor H (HF1), the major inhibitor of the alternative complement pathway, accumulates within drusen and is synthesized by the RPE. Variants in the complement factor H gene have been shown to be associated with an increased risk for AMD (14–19).

Ophthalmoscopically, focal drusen appear as small, roundish, yellowish lesions underneath the RPE. Various drusen classifications have been proposed (20–23), depending on their size, shape, appearance, and topographic distribution. Well-delineated drusen with a diameter of less than 64 μm are referred to as "hard" drusen. Drusen with a diameter of 64–124 μm are classified as "intermediate," and those larger than 125 μm are considered "large." The former may occur as part of the normal aging process and do not appear to increase the risk of advanced AMD. Over a 5-year period in patients with many small drusen or few intermediate drusen, the risk for progression to advanced AMD was shown to be 1.3% (24). In contrast, the risk for progression to advanced AMD in patients with many intermediate or large drusen was 18% in the Age Related Eye Disease Study (AREDS) (24). "Soft" drusen describes the presence of amorphous and poorly demarcated lesions in the presence of thickening of the inner aspects of Bruch's membrane. "Confluent" drusen refers to contiguous boundaries between several soft drusen. Eyes with soft, confluent drusen are more likely to progress to late-stage AMD (15.1%) (25).

The so-called "reticular drusen" have been described as a variant of soft drusen with unique features (21,26,27). The prevalence of reticular drusen seems to be higher in AMD patients than in age-matched subjects without the disease (21,26,27). Reticular drusen seem to represent an important risk factor for the development of neovascular AMD (28), although a subgroup analysis of AREDS found a higher rate of progression to geographic atrophy than to choroidal neovascularization in the presence of reticular drusen (29). Klein and colleagues (30) recently described a 15-year cumulative incidence of reticular drusen (3.0%) in a population-based (n = 4926) prospective study. Eyes with reticular drusen had a higher risk to progress to geographic atrophy (cumulative incidence 21%) or to exudative AMD (cumulative incidence 20%) than those with soft indistinct drusen. From histopathological findings in one eye with reticular drusen, it appeared that fundus changes did not correlate with the extracellular material deposited in the inner aspect of Bruch's membrane, but did correlate with choroidal alterations; therefore, the term "pseudodrusen" was proposed (27). However, the precise histopathological changes in reticular drusen is yet unknown.

In addition to the above drusen types, a different type of material can be found deposited between the RPE cell plasma membrane and its basement membrane. This complex composite of granular electron-dense material, coated membrane bodies, and fibrous collagen was initially termed "basal *linear* deposit" (31,32). Based on light and electron microscopy, the deposit was later renamed "basal *laminar* deposit," whereas the term "basal linear deposit" was introduced to describe vesicular material underneath the basement membrane of the RPE. Because of this confusing terminology, Loeffler and Lee (33) suggested the terms "basement membrane deposit" (BMD) for material located between the RPE cell and its basement membrane, and "basal laminar deposit" (BLD) for vesicular material located within Bruch's membrane. However, these deposits are detected only by light and electron microscopy and remain invisible by slit-lamp biomicroscopy. Apart from these ophthalmoscopically invisible deposits, Bonanomi et al. (34) and Gass et al. (35) described basal laminar *drusen* in association with pseudovitelliform lesions that angiographically appear as "stars in the sky." Histologically, these basal laminar drusen correspond to nodular, hyaline thickening of the basement membrane of the RPE (35).

Over time, drusen may be subject to dynamic changes: (i) hard drusen may enlarge and turn into soft drusen (36), (ii) soft confluent drusen may lead to a drusenoid retinal pigment epithelial detachment, (iii) drusen material may show signs of calcification, and (iv) drusen may regress with the occurrence of a corresponding area of geographic atrophy (37).

IMAGING TECHNIQUES IN ARM

Fluorescein Angiography

During fluorescein angiography (FA), drusen may appear hyper-, iso-, or hypofluorescent (Fig. 10A.1). Particularly soft drusen may be hypofluorescent in early phases and hyperfluorescent due to staining in late phases of the angiogram. These angio-

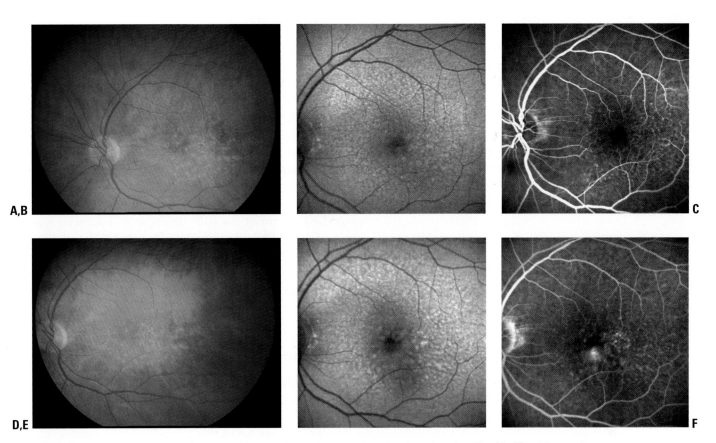

FIGURE 10A.1.   Left eye of a patient with soft and reticular drusen at the posterior pole at baseline **(A–C)** and 2 years later **(D–F)**. Funduscopically visible drusen **(A,D)** demonstrate increased fundus AF **(B,E)** with enlargement and multiplication of areas of increased AF over time. FA **(C,F)** shows hyperfluorescence in the presence of drusen and development of a small choroidal neovascularization over time **(F)**.

graphic features are thought to depend on the chemical composition of drusen. Hyperfluorescent drusen contain mainly polar phospholipids, whereas hypofluorescent drusen are formed by neutral lipids (11). In contrast, areas of focal hyperpigmentation at the level of the RPE are characterized by hypofluorescence due to blockage phenomena (38). FA is used only to evaluate patients with ARM when neovascular AMD is suspected.

Indocyanine Green Angiography

Hard drusen are very difficult to distinguish on indocyanine green (ICG) angiography. Larger soft drusen appear mostly hypofluorescent throughout the ICG angiogram. ICG angiography does not usually reveal essential diagnostic/prognostic information in eyes with ARM. As for FA, ICG angiography is only used in patients with ARM when certain forms of neovascular AMD, including polypoidal choroidal vasculopathy and retinal angiomatous proliferation, are suspected.

Optical Coherence Tomography

Optical coherence tomography (OCT) allows for cross-sectional imaging of the retina in vivo with a micron resolution, helping to precisely evaluate the anatomical localization of pathological processes (39). OCT imaging of drusen shows various microstructural alterations, including focal elevations and irregularities at the level of the RPE, which normally appears as a continuous highly reflective straight layer. Drusen may lead to a focal irregularity as well as to disruption of the RPE signal. In the case of soft confluent drusen, OCT allows detection of drusenoid RPE detachments.

High-resolution, spectral domain OCT has revealed further details of anatomical alterations (40). Using ultrahigh-resolution (UHR) OCT with a 3 μm axial image resolution, the external limiting membrane appears to be intact in the presence of ARM, whereas in the presence of drusen, irregularities in the RPE and the inner and outer segments of the photoreceptors can be seen in the OCT images (41). Pieroni and coworkers (42) described three patterns of drusen in the presence of ARM: (i) distinct RPE excrescences, (ii) a sawtoothed pattern of the RPE (multiple excrescences, suggesting a wrinkling or bunching of the RPE), and (iii) nodular drusen. OCT and spectral-domain OCT help to identify RPE changes with or without RPE cell migration into the overlying neurosensory retina (Fig. 10A.2). Furthermore, high-resolution OCT may help to detect early exudative changes, i.e., extracellular fluid, that may not be visible on funduscopy or FA (42).

Fundus Autofluorescence Imaging

AF imaging is not only of interest to help understand the pathophysiological processes of ARM; it can be also used to precisely diagnose and monitor phenotypic changes. Recently, variations in AF have been demonstrated in eyes with ARM (43–45). It was noted that alterations in the AF signal do not necessarily correspond with funduscopically or angiographically visible changes (43).

Hyperpigmentation and pigment mottling are usually associated with an increased AF signal, which is thought to derive from melanolipofuscin, whereas hypo- and depigmentation are characterized by loss of AF signal due to degenerated RPE or absence of viable RPE. Of interest, hyperpigmentation may be present in the vicinity of drusen associated with focal and linear increased AF (46). The AF signal from individual drusen may be slightly increased, normal, or decreased compared to normal background AF. Therefore, drusen may or may not be identified in AF images (47). The composition of drusen (including possible autofluorescent constituents), drusen size, and alterations of the overlying RPE may be responsible for the variation in the AF pattern. In general, larger drusen are more frequently associated with extensive AF abnormalities compared to smaller drusen. Crystalline

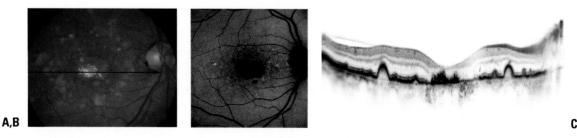

A,B   C

FIGURE 10A.2. Fundus photograph **(A)**, fundus AF image **(B)**, and optical coherence tomography **(C)** of a patient with drusen and geographic atrophy with crystalline material in the atrophic area. In addition to lack of AF due to pigment epithelial atrophy, fundus AF irregularities outside the atrophic patch are seen. **(B)** Drusen show very mildly increased AF. Optical coherence tomography reveals several "bumps" in the RPE due to drusen under the RPE.

drusen typically show a corresponding area of decreased AF signal. In contrast, large soft and confluent drusen with drusenoid RPE detachments are characterized by a moderately increased and patchy AF signal (43,44,48). Such drusenoid detachments have been found to be associated with increased risk of choroidal neovascularization (CNV) (49).

Delori and colleagues (50) demonstrated another distinct variation of the AF signal associated with drusen consisting of decreased AF in the center of the druse with a surrounding annulus of increased AF signal. Possible explanations for this pattern are that (i) the RPE may be stretched over the druse with a subsequent reduction on the density of LF granules; (ii) the druse makes the central overlying RPE release lipofuscin granules, which are phagocytosed by RPE cells at the margin of the druse, creating reduced central AF surrounded by an annulus of increased AF; and (iii) drusen occur in incipient RPE cell atrophy.

Reticular drusen (see above) or "pseudodrusen" are readily identified on AF images. They show a unique reticular AF pattern with multiple small rounded or elongated areas of decreased AF surrounded by an interlacing network of normal AF. The preferential localization of reticular drusen is superior and superotemporal to the macula, but they may also spread toward the mid-periphery as well as nasally to the optic disc. As explained above, it was assumed that "pseudodrusen" would represent an attenuated choroidal venous layer with regression of the choriocapillaris and broadening of intercapillary pillars due to fibrous replacement. Based on fundus AF images together with funduscopic findings, deposition of abnormal material underneath the RPE in the inner aspect of Bruch's membrane appears more likely to be the substrate for this phenotypic change. The yellowish appearance similar to soft drusen could hardly be explained if the alterations were in the choroidal layer. A decreased AF intensity as seen in correspondence with these yellowish lesions would be expected to result from changes in the RPE cell layer or from a somehow stretched RPE. However, a decrease in AF intensity cannot be explained by broadened intercapillary pillars, since the location in an anatomical layer posterior to the RPE would not conceivably induce an attenuation of the AF signal derived from the RPE.

Classification of Fundus AF Patterns in ARM

Recently, a classification system for AF changes associated with ARM was proposed by an international consensus group (43). AF findings in patients with ARM indicate more widespread abnormalities and diseased areas than assumed by fundus examination or fundus photography. The proposed ARM AF classification system includes eight different AF patterns in ARM, as described below.

Normal Pattern
A normal AF pattern (see also Chapter 9) with homogeneous background AF with a gradual decrease AF at the fovea can be seen in patients with ARM. This pattern is commonly seen in the presence of hard drusen (Fig. 10A.3).

Minimal Change Pattern
Very limited irregular increased or decreased background AF without an obvious topographic pattern in the presence of few hard drusen and pigment abnormalities (Fig. 10A.4).

Focal Increased Pattern
The presence of at least one well-defined spot (<200 μm diameter) of markedly increased AF, which is much brighter than the surrounding background AF. Some areas

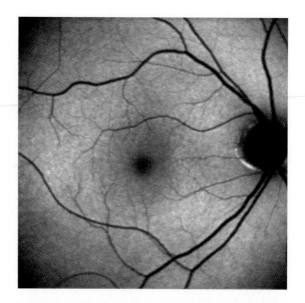

FIGURE 10A.3. Fundus AF image with a homogeneous background fluorescence and a gradual decrease in the inner macula toward the foveola due to the masking effect of macular pigment (normal pattern). Only small hard drusen were seen clinically. (Reprinted from Bindewald A, Bird AC, Dandekar, et al. Classification of fundus autofluorescence patterns in early age-related macular disease. Invest Ophthalmol Vis Sci 2005;46:3309–3314, with permission.)

of focal increased AF may be surrounded by a darker appearing halo. These areas of focal increased AF, such as focal hyperpigmentation or drusen, may or may not correspond to visible alterations on color fundus photographs (Fig. 10A.5).

Patchy Pattern

The presence of at least one larger area (>200 μm diameter) of markedly increased AF that is brighter than the surrounding background AF. The borders of these areas

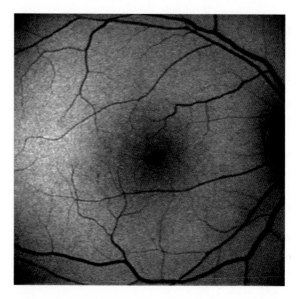

FIGURE 10A.4. Fundus AF image with only minimal variations from the normal background FAF (minimal change pattern) due to multiple small hard drusen, clinically visible. (Reprinted from Bindewald A, Bird AC, Dandekar, et al. Classification of fundus autofluorescence patterns in early age-related macular disease. Invest Ophthalmol Vis Sci 2005;46:3309–3314, with permission.)

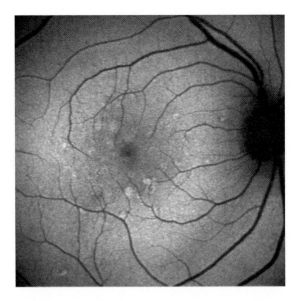

FIGURE 10A.5.   Fundus AF image showing the focal increased pattern with several well-defined spots of markedly increased AF. Multiple hard and soft drusen were detected on slit-lamp biomicroscopy. (Reprinted from Bindewald A, Bird AC, Dandekar, et al. Classification of fundus autofluorescence patterns in early age-related macular disease. Invest Ophthalmol Vis Sci 2005;46:3309–3314, with permission.)

are typically ill defined. Increased AF corresponds to large soft drusen that may be accompanied by hyperpigmentations (Fig. 10A.6).

Linear Pattern

The presence of at least one linear area with well-demarcated, markedly increased AF. These linear structures of increased AF usually correspond to hyperpigmented lines on color fundus photographs (Fig. 10A.7).

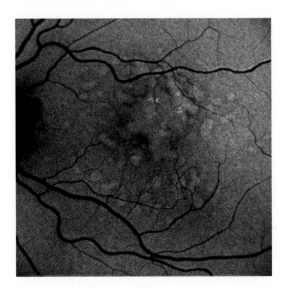

FIGURE 10A.6.   Fundus AF image showing multiple large areas of increased AF (patchy pattern) corresponding to large soft drusen and/or hyperpigmentation clinically. (Reprinted from Bindewald A, Bird AC, Dandekar, et al. Classification of fundus autofluorescence patterns in early age-related macular disease. Invest Ophthalmol Vis Sci 2005;46:3309–3314, with permission.)

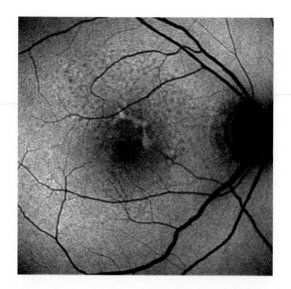

FIGURE 10A.7. The linear pattern is characterized by the presence of at least one linear area with a markedly increased fundus AF. A corresponding hyperpigmented line was visible clinically. (Reprinted from Bindewald A, Bird AC, Dandekar, et al. Classification of fundus autofluorescence patterns in early age-related macular disease. Invest Ophthalmol Vis Sci 2005;46:3309–3314, with permission.)

Lace-Like Pattern

Multiple branching linear structures of increased AF forming a lace-like pattern. The borders may be difficult to define because a gradual decrease of AF is occasionally observed from the center of the linear areas toward the surrounding background. This lace-like pattern of increased AF may correspond to hyperpigmentation or to no visible abnormality (Fig. 10A.8).

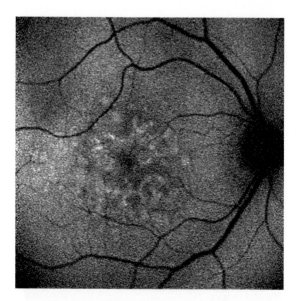

FIGURE 10A.8. Fundus AF image demonstrating multiple branching linear structures of increased AF in a lace-like pattern. This lace-like pattern corresponds to hyperpigmentation on fundus examination. (Reprinted from Bindewald A, Bird AC, Dandekar, et al. Classification of fundus autofluorescence patterns in early age-related macular disease. Invest Ophthalmol Vis Sci 2005;46:3309–3314, with permission.)

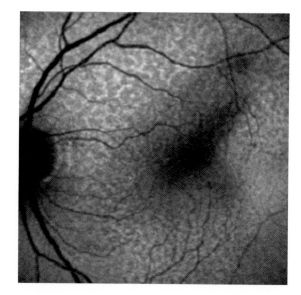

FIGURE 10A.9.   Multiple specific small areas of decreased AF with brighter lines in between character-ize the reticular pattern. There may be visible reticular drusen on fundoscopy. (Reprinted from Bindewald A, Bird AC, Dandekar, et al. Classification of fundus autofluorescence patterns in early age-related mac-ular disease. Invest Ophthalmol Vis Sci 2005;46:3309–3314, with permission.)

Reticular Pattern

The presence of multiple small areas (<200 μm diameter) of decreased AF with mild in-creased AF around them. The reticular pattern occurs not only in the macular area but also in a superotemporal location. This pattern may be associated with funduscopically visible reticular drusen (Fig. 10A.9).

Speckled Pattern

The simultaneous presence of a variety of AF abnormalities in a larger area of the AF image. The corresponding abnormalities visible on color fundus photographs include pigment abnormalities and multiple (sub-) confluent drusen (Fig. 10A.10).

This phenotypic classification may help to (i) identify prognostic determinants in longitudinal studies, (ii) better evaluate the progression of the disease, and (iii) allow phenotype/genotype correlations to be established. Similar longitudinal studies in at-rophic AMD have identified the prognostic relevance of different AF patterns in the junctional zone of geographic atrophy (51,52). In the case of ARM, more longitudinal data are needed to evaluate the impact of distinct AF patterns on disease progression.

DIFFERENTIAL DIAGNOSIS

Apart from normal aging, a variety of retinal diseases may mimic ARM. In the case of idiopathic central serous chorioretinopathy (ICSC) (see also Chapter 13), age, ab-sence of drusen, and the occurrence of distinct small serous retinal detachments may be helpful in differentiating this disease entity from ARM. However, chronic ICSC may present with phenotypic alterations reminiscent of ARM and occult choroidal neovascularization. Pattern dystrophy can mimic ARM (see also Chapter 11E); how-ever, the high-intensity AF signal corresponding to the yellow deposits seen in pattern dystrophy is not observed in ARM. Similarly, autosomal-dominant (AD) drusen,

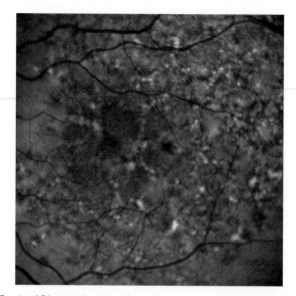

FIGURE 10A.10. Fundus AF image showing AF abnormalities in a large area (speckled pattern). Less extensive changes are seen in these cases on slit-lamp biomicroscopy. (Reprinted from Bindewald A, Bird AC, Dandekar, et al. Classification of fundus autofluorescence patterns in early age-related macular disease. Invest Ophthalmol Vis Sci 2005;46:3309–3314, with permission.)

which typically occur at a younger age than ARM, demonstrate a high AF signal, in contrast to drusen in ARM. Toxic maculopathies, such as chloroquine and thioridazine, can be excluded by history.

SUMMARY

ARM is characterized by various drusen phenotypes and pigment irregularities in the macula. Fundus AF imaging in patients with ARM may reveal typical patterns of AF. Areas of abnormal AF may extend beyond ophthalmoscopically visible fundus changes. AF imaging provides information in addition to that gathered by other imaging techniques and therefore aids in accurately phenotyping patients with ARM. AF imaging is very helpful in differentiating ARM from other simulating diseases, such as pattern dystrophy and AD drusen. Ongoing longitudinal studies will address the potential prognostic relevance of different AF patterns in ARM.

REFERENCES

1. Bird AC. Age-related macular disease. Br J Ophthalmol 1996;80:1–2.
2. Bressler NM, Bressler SB. Preventative ophthalmology. Age-related macular degeneration. Ophthalmology 1995;102:1206–1211.
3. Klaver CCW, van Leeuwen R, Vingerling JR, et al. Epidemiology of age-related maculopathy. In: Holz FG, Pauleikhoff D, Spaide RF, Bird AC, eds. Age-Related Macular Degeneration. Berlin, Heidelberg, New York: Springer, 2003.
4. Haddad S, Chen CA, Santangelo SL, et al. The genetics of age-related macular degeneration: a review of progress to date. Surv Ophthalmol 2006;51:361–363.
5. Holz FG, Pauleikhoff D, Spaide RF, et al. Age-Related Macular Degeneration. Berlin: Springer, 2004.
6. Donders FC. Die Metamorphose der Pigmentschicht der Choroidea. Arch Ophthalmol 1855;1:107.
7. Wedl C. Rudiments of Pathological Histology. London: Busk, 1854:282.
8. International ARM Epidemiology Study Group. An international classification and grading system for age-related maculopathy and age-related macular degeneration. Surv Ophthalmol 1995;39:365–374.

9. Anderson DH, Mullins RF, Hageman GS, et al. A role for local inflammation in the formation of drusen in the aging eye. Am J Ophthalmol 2002;134:411–431.
10. Hageman GS, Mullins RF, Russell SR, et al. Vitronectin is a constituent of ocular drusen and the vitronectin gene is expressed in human retinal pigmented epithelial cells. FASEB J 1999;13:477–484.
11. Pauleikhoff D, Zuels S, Sheraidah GS, et al. Correlation between biochemical composition and fluorescein binding of deposits in Bruch's membrane. Ophthalmology 1992;99:1548–1553.
12. Hageman GS, Mullins RF. Molecular composition of drusen as related to substructural phenotype. Mol Vis 1999;5:28.
13. Mullins RF, Russell SR, Anderson DH, et al. Drusen associated with aging and age-related macular degeneration contain proteins common to extracellular deposits associated with atherosclerosis, elastosis, amyloidosis, and dense deposit disease. FASEB J 2000;14:835–846.
14. Edwards AO, Ritter 3rd R, Abel KJ, et al. Complement factor H polymorphism and age-related macular degeneration. Science 2005;308:421–424.
15. Hageman GS, Anderson DH, Johnson LV, et al. A common haplotype in the complement regulatory gene factor H (HF1/CFH) predisposes individuals to age-related macular degeneration. Proc Natl Acad Sci USA 2005;102:7227–7232.
16. Haines JL, Hauser MA, Schmidt S, et al. Complement factor H variant increases the risk of age-related macular degeneration. Science 2005;308:419–421.
17. Klein RJ, Zeiss C, Chew EY, et al. Complement factor H polymorphism in age-related macular degeneration. Science 2005;308:385–389.
18. Scholl HP, Fleckenstein M, Charbel Issa P, et al. An update on the genetics of age-related macular degeneration. Mol Vis 2007;13:196–205.
19. Seddon JM, Santangelo SL, Book K, et al. A genomewide scan for age-related macular degeneration provides evidence for linkage to several chromosomal regions. Am J Hum Genet 2003;73:780–790.
20. Bressler NM, Silva JC, Bressler SB, et al. Clinicopathologic correlation of drusen and retinal pigment epithelial abnormalities in age-related macular degeneration. Retina 1994;14:130–142.
21. Klein R, Davis MD, Magli YL, et al. The Wisconsin Age-Related Maculopathy Grading System. Ophthalmology 1991;98:1128–1134.
22. Kliffen M, van der Schaft TL, Mooy CM, et al. Morphologic changes in age-related maculopathy. Microsc Res Tech 1997;36:106–122.
23. Spraul CW, Grossniklaus HE. Characteristics of Drusen and Bruch's membrane in post-mortem eyes with age-related macular degeneration. Arch Ophthalmol 1997;115:267–273.
24. Age-Related Eye Disease Study Research Group. A randomized, placebo-controlled, clinical trial of high-dose supplementation with vitamins C and E, beta carotene, and zinc for age-related macular degeneration and vision loss: AREDS report no. 8. Arch Ophthalmol 2001;119:1417–1436.
25. Klein R, Klein BE, Tomany SC, et al. Ten-year incidence and progression of age-related maculopathy: the Beaver Dam Eye Study. Ophthalmology 2002;109:1767–1779.
26. Arnold JJ, Sarks SH, Killingsworth MC, et al. Reticular pseudodrusen. A risk factor in age-related maculopathy. Retina 1995;15:181–193.
27. Maguire MG, Fine SL. Reticular pseudodrusen. Retina 1996;16:167–168.
28. Cohen SY, Dubois L, Tadayoni R, et al. Prevalence of reticular pseudodrusen in age-related macular degeneration with newly diagnosed choroidal neovascularization. Br J Ophthalmol 2007;91:354–359.
29. Armstrong JR, Davis MD, Danis Jr RP, et al. Reticular drusen as a baseline risk factor for progression to advanced AMD in AREDS. Invest Ophthalmol Vis Sci 2005;46:E-Abstract 220.
30. Klein R, Meuser SM, Knudtson MD, et al. The epidemiology of reticular drusen. Am J Ophthalmol 2008;145:317–326.
31. Loeffler KU, Lee WR. Basal linear deposit in the human macula. Graefes Arch Clin Exp Ophthalmol 1986;224:493–501.
32. Sarks SH. New vessel formation beneath the retinal pigment epithelium in senile eyes. Br J Ophthalmol 1973;57:951–965.
33. Loeffler KU, Lee WR. Terminology of sub-RPE deposits: do we all speak the same language? Br J Ophthalmol 1998;82:1104–1105.
34. Bonanomi MT, Maia Júnior OO, Lower LM, et al. [Vitelliform macular detachment associated with basal laminar drusen: case report]. Arq Bras Oftalmol 2006;69:269–272.
35. Gass JDM, Jallow S, Davis B. Adult vitelliform macular detachment occurring in a patient with basal laminar drusen. Am J Ophthalmol 1985;99:445.
36. Sarks SH, Van Driel D, Maxwell L, et al. Softening of drusen and subretinal neovascularization. Trans Ophthalmol Soc UK 1980;100:414–422.
37. Sarks S. Laser treatment of soft drusen in age-related maculopathy. Br J Ophthalmol 1996;80:4.
38. Spaide RF. Fluorescein angiography. In: Spaide RF, ed. Diseases of the Retina and Vitreous. Philadelphia: W.B. Saunders, 1999:29–38.
39. Costa RA, Skaf M, Melo Jr LA, et al. Retinal assessment using optical coherence tomography. Prog Retin Eye Res 2006;25:325–353.
40. Fleckenstein M, Charbel Issa P, Helb HM, et al. High resolution spectral domain OCT imaging in geographic atrophy associated with age-related macular degeneration. Invest Ophthalmol Vis Sci 2008; 49:4137–4144.
41. Ko TH, Fujimoto JG, Schuman JS, et al. Comparison of ultrahigh- and standard-resolution optical coherence tomography for imaging macular pathology. Ophthalmology 2005;112:1922.e1–e15.

42. Pieroni CG, Witkin AJ, Ko TH, et al. Ultrahigh resolution optical coherence tomography in non-exudative age related macular degeneration. Br J Ophthalmol 2006;90:191–197.

43. Bindewald A, Bird AC, Dandekar, et al. Classification of fundus autofluorescence patterns in early age-related macular disease. Invest Ophthalmol Vis Sci 2005;46:3309–3314.

44. Lois N, Owens SL, Coco R, et al. Fundus autofluorescence in patients with age-related macular degeneration and high risk of visual loss. Am J Ophthalmol 2002;133:341–349.

45. Spaide RF. Fundus autofluorescence in age-related macular degeneration. Ophthalmology 2003;110:392–399.

46. von Rückmann A, Fitzke FW, Bird AC. Fundus autofluorescence in age-related macular disease imaged with a laser scanning ophthalmoscope. Invest Ophthalmol Vis Sci 1997;38:478–486.

47. von Rückmann A, Fitzke FW, Bird AC. Autofluorescence imaging of the human fundus. In: Marmor MF, Wolfensberger TJ, eds. The Retinal Pigment Epithelium. Oxford: Oxford University Press, 1998:224–234.

48. Smith RT, Chan JK, Busuoic M, et al. Autofluorescence characteristic of early, atrophic, and high-risk fellow eyes in age-related macular degeneration. Invest Ophthalmol Vis Sci 2006;47:5495–5504.

49. Einbock W, Moessner A, Schnurrbusxch UE, et al. Changes in fundus autofluorescence in patients with age-related maculopathy. Correlation to visual function: a prospective study. Graefes Arch Clin Ophthalmol 2005;243:300–305.

50. Delori FC, Fleckner MR, Goger DG, et al. Autofluorescence distribution associated with drusen in age-related macular degeneration. Invest Ophthalmol Vis Sci 2000;41:496–504.

51. Holz FG, Bindewald-Wittich A, Fleckenstein M, et al. Progression of geographic atrophy and impact of fundus autofluorescence patterns in age-related macular degeneration. Am J Ophthalmol 2007;143:463–472.

52. Schmitz-Valckenberg S, Bindewald-Wittich A, Dolar-Szczasny J, et al. Correlation between the area of increased autofluorescence surrounding geographic atrophy and disease progression in patients with AMD. Invest Ophthalmol Vis Sci 2006;47:2648–2654.

Ehab Abdelkader
Vikki McBain
Noemi Lois

CHAPTER 10B

Fundus Autofluorescence in Neovascular Age-Related Macular Degeneration

Neovascular or exudative age-related macular degeneration (AMD) is the most common cause of visual loss in patients with AMD (1,2). It is defined by the presence of any of the following (3): (i) retinal pigment epithelium (RPE) detachment(s), which may be associated with a neurosensory retinal detachment; (ii) subretinal or sub-RPE choroidal neovascularization (CNV); (iii) epiretinal (with exclusion of idiopathic macular puckers), intraretinal, subretinal, or sub-RPE scar/glial tissue or fibrin-like deposits; (iv) subretinal hemorrhages not related to other retinal vascular disease; and (v) hard exudates (lipids) within the macular area related to any of the above and not related to other retinal vascular disease.

In addition to the typical neovascular AMD caused by the occurrence of CNV, two additional phenotypes have been recognized: (i) so-called retinal angiomatous proliferation (RAP) and (ii) idiopathic polypoidal choroidal vasculopathy (IPCV). In RAP the neovascular process starts in the retina and extends into the subretinal and sub-RPE space. RAP appears to represent about 20% of exudative AMD cases (4). IPCV affects the inner choroid and is characterized by a dilated network of vessels and multiple terminal aneurysmal dilations in a polypoidal configuration (5). IPCV represents 4%–23% of exudative AMD and is more frequent in Asian populations (6,7).

The prevalence of neovascular AMD in people 50 years of age and older ranges between 0.1% and 7.4%; it is more common in Caucasians and its frequency increases with increasing age (1,8–16).

Patients with neovascular AMD usually present with distortion or loss of central vision. On slit-lamp biomicroscopy, there is usually a serous or hemorrhagic detachment of the neurosensory retina and/or RPE with or without hard exudation. Drusen and RPE changes are often present in the affected eye or in the fellow eye.

Until recently, laser photocoagulation and photodynamic therapy (PDT) were the only treatments shown through randomized controlled trials (RCTs) to be effective in a small group of patients with exudative AMD (17,18). However, new antivascular endothelial growth factor (VEGF) therapies are now available and provide benefit to the majority of patients with active exudative AMD (19,20).

HISTOPATHOLOGY AND PATHOGENESIS

The process of CNV formation starts with the growth of blood vessels from the choroid, which then extends through the Bruch membrane under the RPE (sub-RPE CNV) (21). The CNV may then extend further into the subretinal space (22). This abnormal neovascular process leads to serous or hemorrhagic detachment of the RPE and/or neurosensory retina. Eventually, if untreated, scarring will ensue and degeneration of photoreceptors and RPE and subsequent loss of central vision will occur (23).

The signals that stimulate the invasion of choroidal vessels through Bruch's membrane are not completely understood. Under normal circumstances the RPE secretes VEGF at its basolateral surface, which helps to maintain the fenestrations in the choriocapillaris (24). With aging, accumulation of lipofuscin in the RPE and deposition of material (predominantly lipid) and subsequent thickening in Bruch's membrane occurs (25,26). These events result in reduced oxygen transmission from the choriocapillaris into the outer retina with outer retinal hypoxia and subsequent upregulation of VEGF secretion by the RPE (27), which could lead to CNV formation. It is thought that the neovascular complex in these cases provides nutrients and oxygen to the ischemic RPE/outer retina, which is expressing VEGF (28,29). Activated macrophages may migrate from the choroid into Bruch's membrane with the goal of removing the waste material deposited in this layer, with the possible creation of channels in Bruch's membrane through which blood vessels could then invade the retina (30). It has been shown that the RPE can produce monocyte-chemoattractant-protein and IL8 during the active phase of CNV development, which would stimulate the migration of monocytes (macrophages) from the choriocapillaris into the outer surface of Bruch membrane (31). Macrophages obtained from surgically removed CNVs and from whole postmortem eyes with CNV showed increased expression of many inflammatory cytokines by these cells (31). Increased expression of many growth factors, specifically VEGF, in the RPE and photoreceptors, as well as recruited macrophages and proliferation of vascular endothelium from choriocapillaris, has been demonstrated in specimens obtained from patients with neovascular AMD (28,29,31,32).

Gass (33) suggested that CNV in AMD grows predominantly under the RPE (so-called type 1 CNV), although in some patients it can extend mainly into the subretinal space (type 2 CNV). Several histopathology studies have shown that in CNVs angiographically classified as occult, the growth of new vessels occurred predominantly underneath the RPE (22,34–38). In contrast, lesions classified angiographically as classic CNVs contained a subretinal neovascular component, with or without a sub-RPE component (22,34). A combination of both types has also been found (39). CNVs are classified as classic on fluorescein angiography (FA) when they demonstrate early, well-defined hyperfluorescence and late leakage blurring the margins, and as occult when ill-defined, late, stippled hyperfluorescence or late leakage of undetermined source is present (2).

Histopathology studies of surgically excised RAP lesions showed an intraretinal neovascular mass in all cases; in some specimens, an additional CNV was also found (40,41). Immunohistochemistry in these cases demonstrated expression of hypoxia-induced growth factors and macrophages, suggesting that ischemia and inflammation may be involved in the pathogenesis of RAP (41). Histopathology studies in enucleated eyes of patients with IPCV showed large, thin-walled choroidal vessels underneath the RPE with choroidal capillary proliferation (42,43).

CLINICAL FINDINGS AND IMAGING STUDIES

Slit-Lamp Biomicroscopy

On slit-lamp biomicroscopy, patients with exudative AMD may demonstrate (i) a subretinal grayish lesion (CNV), an intraretinal reddish lesion (RAP), or a round, reddish lesion at the RPE level or deeper (IPCV); (ii) subretinal or intraretinal fluid, including cystoid macular edema (CME); or (iii) intraretinal, subretinal, or sub-RPE blood, and serous or vascularized pigment epithelial detachment (PED), including hemorrhagic PED, hard exudation, and, at the end stage of the neovascular process, disciform scarring. Drusen and RPE changes or disciform scarring are commonly present in the fellow eye. In IPCV, the fellow eye may demonstrate no abnormalities. CME and intraretinal hemorrhages are typically seen associated with RAP. Large serous or hemorrhagic PEDs are commonly observed in IPCV, typically affecting the peripapillary area and the macula, but they can also be found in the peripheral fundus (44,45).

Fluorescein Angiography

FA remains the most valuable tool in the diagnosis of exudative AMD. In addition, it allows phenotyping of the disease, i.e., by determining the type of CNV (classic, minimally classic, or occult) or, in many cases, whether there is a RAP or possibly IPCV (although RAP and IPCV may be better imaged by indocyanine green angiography [ICG] [see below]), and the location of the neovascular process with respect to the fovea and its size. FA is also important to establish whether the neovascular process is actively leaking or mainly inactive, by demonstrating active leakage of dye in the former or only staining in the latter. This is of particular importance when treatment is considered.

Precise localization of the neovascular process with respect to the fovea (extra-, juxta-, or subfoveal) is very important when deciding treatment options. Argon laser photocoagulation may still be considered appropriate for patients with extrafoveal neovascularization, whereas for those with subfoveal lesions anti-VEGF therapies are now the treatment of choice. Similarly, the size of the CNV is important when choosing a suitable therapy. This is especially relevant when considering treatment with argon laser photocoagulation or photodynamic therapy (PDT) (e.g., a small extra or juxtafoveal lesion could be treated with argon laser, but a large lesion on the same location might not be treated in this manner because of the resulting scotoma that would occur following treatment).

Knowing which type of CNV is present is crucial when considering the effective treatment options for each patient. Classic CNV can be treated by argon laser photocoagulation, PDT, or intravitreal injections of anti-VEGF therapy. The treatment of choice is based on the site and size of the lesion and the patient's preference. On the other hand, argon laser photocoagulation and PDT are not effective for occult CNV; to date, anti-VEGF therapy is the most successful form of treatment for such cases (20). The classification of neovascular AMD (classic, minimally classic, predominantly classic, or occult), however, is subjective. Interobserver and intraobserver agreement has been shown to be only moderate, in most studies >0.7 (using kappa statistics) (46–49). It should be taken into account that previous studies on inter- and intraobserver agreement of FA classification in exudative AMD were conducted without stereoangiography. Stereoscopic assessment of FA allows the observer to better appreciate the level of the lesion, whether deep or superficial, in relation to the RPE, as well as any elevation in the RPE, and is now common practice in most retinal clinics.

The main disadvantage of FA imaging is that it is invasive and occasionally can result in reactions to the dye, ranging from itching (in 0.5%) and nausea (in 2.9%) to anaphylactic reactions (in 0.2%) (50).

Indocyanine Green Angiography

Indocyanine green (ICG) angiography is an important adjunct in the evaluation of patients with exudative AMD, especially those with IPCV and RAP.

In cases of occult CNV, ICG angiography can sometimes be useful to delineate the neovascular complex (51). Occult CNV can appear on ICG as a plaque or an area with focal hyperfluorescence, or a combination of both (52). ICG may be helpful for identifying the CNV in predominantly hemorrhagic lesions (53).

In the cases of IPCV, the lesion is usually classified on FA as occult. ICG demonstrates the presence of polyps, which appear as small areas of hyperfluorescence in mid to late phases of the ICG angiogram (54–56). The identification of polyps, and their site and size, helps to guide argon laser or PDT (55,57).

On FA, RAP lesions appear as areas of hyperfluorescence that are usually classified as minimally classic or occult. On ICG, RAP lesions appear as a well-defined area of hyperfluorescence. ICG, therefore, allows physicians to confirm the diagnosis and accurately localize the lesion, which is important if laser treatment or PDT is being considered alone or in combination with other therapies (58,59).

Optical Coherence Tomography

Optical coherence tomography (OCT) appears to be useful for detecting CNV in patients in whom the diagnosis of exudative AMD is suspected clinically; under these circumstances, a sensitivity of 96–97% and a specificity of 59–66% have been reported in comparison with FA (60–62). OCT also appears to be useful for differentiating classic (predominantly above the RPE) and occult (predominantly underneath the RPE) CNV (63,64). In our experience, however, this differentiation is often difficult to achieve if only OCT is used. OCT may be helpful in identifying RAP lesions by demonstrating intraretinal areas of high reflectivity with intraretinal fluid (65,66).

Recently, it was suggested that OCT could be used to monitor the activity of exudative AMD specifically to monitor the response to anti-VEGF therapies and guide retreatment (62,67–72). However, the sensitivity and specificity of OCT to detect active exudative AMD in comparison with FA in this context remain to be elucidated.

Fundus Autofluorescence

Fundus autofluorescence (AF) is emerging as a useful tool for the evaluation of patients with exudative AMD (48,73–82). This is highlighted by the fact that this imaging technique is now being included, together with FA and OCT, as part of the routine investigations in RCTs assessing the effectiveness of new treatments for this disease.

Several observations seem to suggest that the integrity of the RPE layer is preserved early on during the course of the disease in patients with exudative AMD. Thus, in patients with a CNV of recent onset, a normal or minimally abnormal distribution of fundus AF at the macula is often observed (77). Furthermore, when small CNVs are present, the abnormalities on fundus AF seem to be restricted to the area of the lesion, with a preserved, homogeneous AF detected outside the area involved by the neovascular process in most cases (Fig. 10B.1) (74). Moreover, a normal or near-normal distribution of fundus AF has been recorded in fellow eyes of patients with exudative AMD in whom age-related maculopathy changes were detected (74). In addition, no or minimal changes on the distribution of fundus AF, specifically a lack of increased AF signal, have been detected before the development of CNV at the site of the lesion (Fig. 10B.2) (74). The above findings have important implications. First, and as suggested by a recent study (75) in which a continuous and predominantly preserved AF pattern at the macula was correlated with better VA, fundus AF may be a useful prognostic tool in exudative AMD. Second, it is plausible that a relatively preserved RPE may be needed for initiation of the neovascular process. In this regard, and as discussed

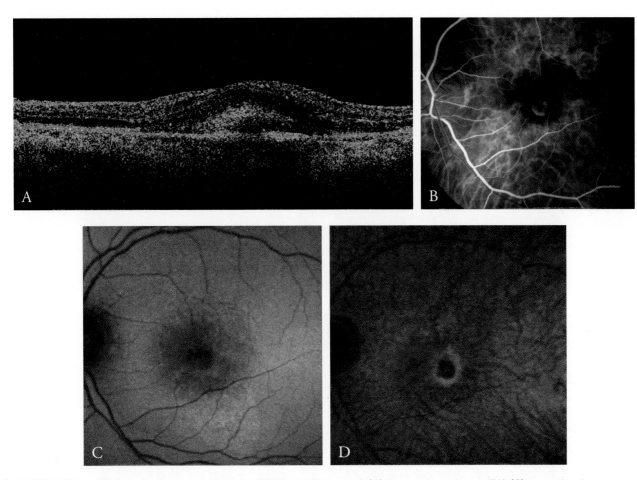

FIGURE 10B.1. **(A)** Optical coherence tomography (OCT) (axis 330 degrees), **(B)** fluorescein angiogram (FA), **(C)** conventional fundus autofluorescence (AF), and **(D)** near-infrared autofluorescence (NIA) obtained from a patient with a classic subfoveal choroidal neovascular membrane (CNV). **(A)** OCT demonstrates a highly reflective lesion above the RPE surrounded by subretinal fluid. **(B)** Early hyperfluorescence in observed on FA. **(C)** A decreased AF signal at the site of the CNV is seen on conventional AF imaging; the neighboring RPE appears to be preserved. **(D)** On NIA there is reduced signal corresponding to the area of the CNV; this reduced signal is surrounded by a ring on increased signal. Note the lack of the normal pattern of increased AF signal at the center of the macula on NIA (see text for details).

above (see histopathology and pathogenesis section), the RPE is a major source of VEGF, the key molecule in the development of neovascularization. This is also supported by the reduced incidence of CNV in patients with geographic atrophy, and by the fact that under the latter circumstances the CNV seems to develop in areas of relatively preserved fundus AF rather than in those showing abnormal and increased AF (personal observation) (Fig. 10B.3).

Although, as discussed above, the distribution of fundus AF in patients with recent-onset exudative AMD is minimally abnormal in many cases when studied by conventional AF imaging (wavelength of 488 nm), this does not seem to be the case when near-infrared autofluorescence (NIA) is used (personal observation) (Figs. 10B.1 and 10B.2). The typical increased NIA signal at the center of the macula (see Chapter 6) is often lacking in patients with exudative AMD. Given that the NIA signal appears to emanate predominantly from melanin in the RPE (83,84), conventional and NIA findings seem to indicate that a loss or depletion of melanin in a relatively intact RPE may be an

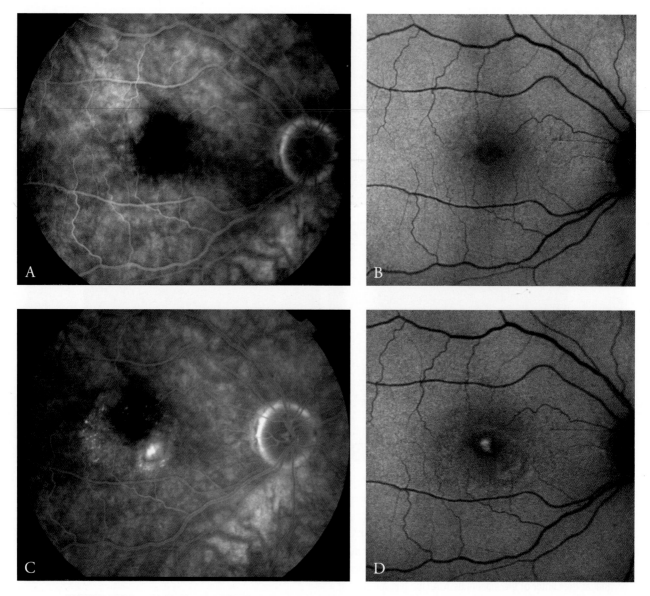

FIGURE 10B.2.   FA **(A,C)** and AF **(B,D)** images obtained from a patient before **(A,B)** and after **(C,D)** the development of a minimally classic CNV. **(C)** The CNV developed at a site where no changes on the distribution of AF had been previously detected. The blocked fluorescence and the fovea on FA **(C)** and the increased AF signal at the fovea **(D)** appear to correspond clinically to an area of resolving blood.

initial step in the sequence of events that lead to neovascularization. In this regard, melanin is recognized as a protective substance by its photo-screening effect (85) and, more importantly, by its biochemical effect in reducing photooxidative damage (86). The melanin content of the RPE, as well as its protective effect, was found to decrease with age (87–89). It was also found that aging melanosomes in the RPE contain degraded melanin that could be phototoxic to the RPE and could aid in the pathogenesis of AMD (90). However, NIA is a very newly developed imaging technique and further work is needed to support these preliminary observations.

It has been shown that the area of abnormal AF signal in most cases of exudative AMD is larger than the total area seen on FA (77). This finding is also supported by some histopathology data (91) and may have implications for assessing the size of the lesion to be treated and possibly the outcomes following treatment.

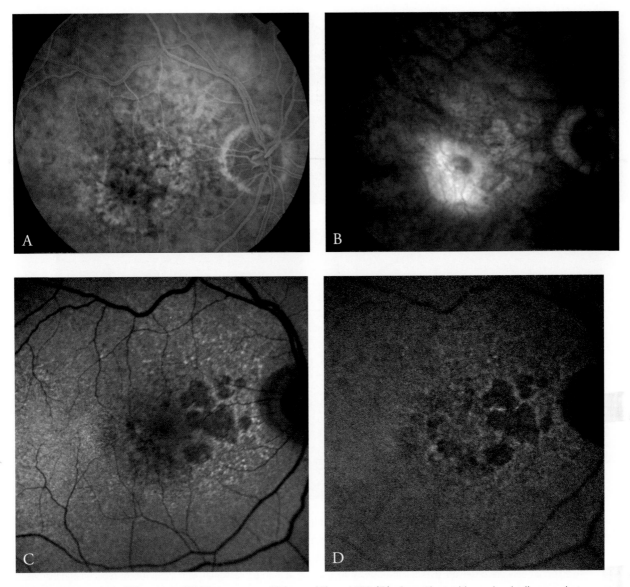

FIGURE 10B.3.   Early **(A)** and late **(B)** FA frames, an AF image **(C)**, and NIA **(D)** of a patient with previously diagnosed atrophic AMD and a newly developed classic CNV. Foci of increased AF signal are seen surrounding well-defined areas of reduced AF (RPE atrophy); these are not present at or around the site of the CNV. Note how the preservation of the foveal RPE is more readily detected by AF and NIA compared to FA.

Differences in the distribution of fundus AF have been described in eyes with classic, occult, and mixed CNV (74). A reduced AF signal at the site of classic CNV has been observed in most cases (79–90%) (Fig. 10B.1) (73,74). In cases of occult CNV, multiple foci of low AF signal at the site of the CNV are commonly seen (Fig. 10B.4). Recent observations using combined AF and OCT imaging in patients with newly developed classic CNV suggest that the reduced AF signal at the site of classic CNV does not indicate loss/damage of RPE, but rather, as previously hypothesized (74), masking of the RPE-AF signal by the CNV growing in the subretinal space (personal observation) (Fig. 10B.1). In contrast, it is likely that the foci of reduced AF signal observed in cases of occult CNV could represent small areas of RPE loss or a more irregular pattern of growth followed by the CNV (Fig. 10B.4).

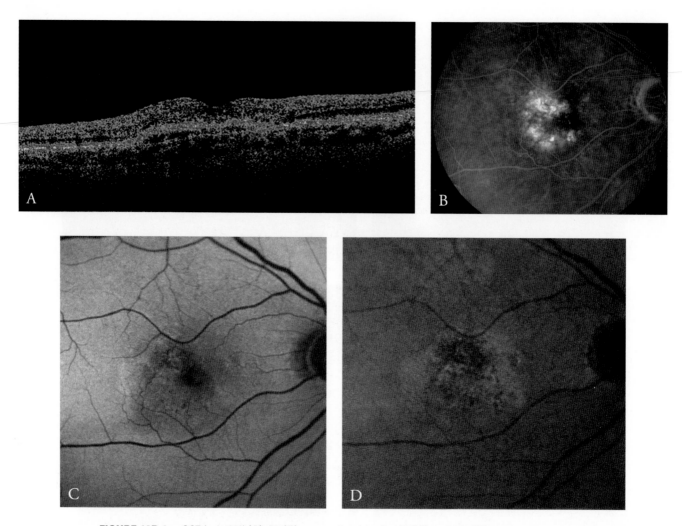

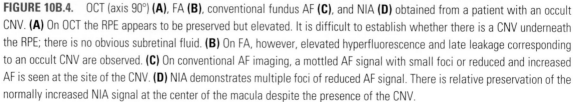

FIGURE 10B.4.   OCT (axis 90°) **(A)**, FA **(B)**, conventional fundus AF **(C)**, and NIA **(D)** obtained from a patient with an occult CNV. **(A)** On OCT the RPE appears to be preserved but elevated. It is difficult to establish whether there is a CNV underneath the RPE; there is no obvious subretinal fluid. **(B)** On FA, however, elevated hyperfluorescence and late leakage corresponding to an occult CNV are observed. **(C)** On conventional AF imaging, a mottled AF signal with small foci or reduced and increased AF is seen at the site of the CNV. **(D)** NIA demonstrates multiple foci of reduced AF signal. There is relative preservation of the normally increased NIA signal at the center of the macula despite the presence of the CNV.

AF imaging is useful for following the behavior of the CNV and the status of the RPE following treatment. Framme et al. (73) found that 2–3 months after PDT the majority of classic lesions became better defined, as evidenced by increased AF signal around the lesion compared to before treatment (73). This could be related to proliferation of RPE cells at the margin of the lesion, which may result from laser activation of the RPE or laser damage to the central RPE with more activity of the RPE at the perimeter of the CNV (73). This agrees with the observations by Gass (92) that proliferation of RPE occurs at the edge of classic CNV induced by the separation of the neurosensory retina from the RPE and in an attempt to engulf the new vessels.

It was recently shown that intact foveal AF is associated with better visual outcomes following anti-VEGF therapy (93). It has also been suggested that poorer visual outcomes after successful anti-VEGF therapy may be associated with atrophic RPE changes detected on AF (94).

SUMMARY

The above imaging techniques can be used by the clinician, in combination, to obtain a more accurate diagnosis and perform an in-depth evaluation of the status of the retina. They can also guide the clinician in the treatment and counseling of patients with exudative AMD.

FA remains, to date, the gold standard for establishing the diagnosis of exudative AMD and is also required to determine the location, type, size, and degree of activity of the exudative lesion. ICG angiography is often needed to confirm the diagnosis of RAP and IPCV. OCT can be used to determine the presence of sub- or intraretinal fluid, and it may be useful in the follow-up of patients after treatment. AF imaging provides information on the status of the RPE and indirectly of the photoreceptors; it may have a prognostic value for determining the natural history of exudative AMD and may help to predict visual outcomes after treatment. Fundus AF may also assist in determining the type of CNV (classic vs. occult) and the extent of the lesion. Like conventional AF, NIA provides a means of assessing the status of the RPE; it is likely that this imaging technique will be of value in predicting visual outcomes following treatment. Both AF and NIA are providing insights into the pathogenesis of exudative AMD.

REFERENCES

1. Friedman DS, Katz J, Bressler NM, et al. Racial differences in the prevalence of age-related macular degeneration: the Baltimore Eye Survey. Ophthalmology 1999;106:1049–1055.
2. Subfoveal neovascular lesions in age-related macular degeneration. Guidelines for evaluation and treatment in the macular photocoagulation study. Macular Photocoagulation Study Group. Arch Ophthalmol 1991;109:1242–1257.
3. Bird AC, Bressler NM, Bressler SB, et al. An international classification and grading system for age-related maculopathy and age-related macular degeneration. The International ARM Epidemiological Study Group. Surv Ophthalmol 1995;39:367–374.
4. Massacesi AL, Sacchi L, Bergamini F, et al. The prevalence of retinal angiomatous proliferation in age-related macular degeneration with occult choroidal neovascularization. Graefes Arch Clin Exp Ophthalmol 2008;246:89–92.
5. Yannuzzi LA, Sorenson J, Spaide RF, et al. Idiopathic polypoidal choroidal vasculopathy (IPCV). Retina 1990;10:1–8.
6. Sho K, Takahashi K, Yamada H, et al. Polypoidal choroidal vasculopathy: incidence, demographic features, and clinical characteristics. Arch Ophthalmol 2003;121:1392–1396.
7. Yannuzzi LA, Ciardella A, Spaide RF, et al. The expanding clinical spectrum of idiopathic polypoidal choroidal vasculopathy. Arch Ophthalmol 1997;115:478–485.
8. Kawasaki R, Wang JJ, Aung T, et al. Prevalence of age-related macular degeneration in a malay population: the Singapore Malay Eye Study. Ophthalmology 2008;115:1735–1741.
9. Andersen MV, Rosenberg T, la Cour M, et al. Prevalence of age-related maculopathy and age-related macular degeneration among the Inuit in Greenland. The Greenland Inuit Eye Study. Ophthalmology 2008;115:700–707.e1.
10. Mitchell P, Smith W, Attebo K, et al. Prevalence of age-related maculopathy in Australia. The Blue Mountains Eye Study. Ophthalmology 1995;102:1450–1460.
11. Vingerling JR, Dielemans I, Hofman A, et al. The prevalence of age-related maculopathy in the Rotterdam Study. Ophthalmology 1995;102:205–210.
12. Varma R, Fraser-Bell S, Tan S, et al. Prevalence of age-related macular degeneration in Latinos: the Los Angeles Latino eye study. Ophthalmology 2004;111:1288–1297.
13. Oshima Y, Ishibashi T, Murata T, et al. Prevalence of age related maculopathy in a representative Japanese population: the Hisayama Study. Br J Ophthalmol 2001;85:1153–1157.
14. Wong TY, Loon SC, Saw SM. The epidemiology of age related eye diseases in Asia. Br J Ophthalmol 2006;90:506–511.
15. Li Y, Xu L, Jonas JB, et al. Prevalence of age-related maculopathy in the adult population in China: the Beijing Eye Study. Am J Ophthalmol 2006;142:788–793.
16. Klein R, Peto T, Bird A, et al. The epidemiology of age-related macular degeneration. Am J Ophthalmol 2004;137:486–495.
17. Argon laser photocoagulation for idiopathic neovascularization. Results of a randomized clinical trial. Arch Ophthalmol 1983;101:1358–1361.

18. Photodynamic therapy of subfoveal choroidal neovascularization in age-related macular degeneration with verteporfin: one-year results of 2 randomized clinical trials—TAP report. Treatment of Age-Related Macular Degeneration with Photodynamic Therapy (TAP) Study Group. Arch Ophthalmol 1999;117: 1329–1345.

19. Brown DM, Kaiser PK, Michels M, et al. Ranibizumab versus verteporfin for neovascular age-related macular degeneration. N Engl J Med 2006;355:1432–1444.

20. Rosenfeld PJ, Brown DM, Heier JS, et al. Ranibizumab for neovascular age-related macular degeneration. N Engl J Med 2006;355:1419–1431.

21. Green WR. Histopathology of age-related macular degeneration. Mol Vis 1999;5:27.

22. Lafaut BA, Bartz-Schmidt KU, Vanden Broecke C, et al. Clinicopathological correlation in exudative age related macular degeneration: histological differentiation between classic and occult choroidal neovascularisation. Br J Ophthalmol 2000;84:239–243.

23. Green WR, Enger C. Age-related macular degeneration histopathologic studies. The 1992 Lorenz E. Zimmerman Lecture. Ophthalmology 1993;100:1519–1535.

24. Blaauwgeers HG, Holtkamp GM, Rutten H, et al. Polarized vascular endothelial growth factor secretion by human retinal pigment epithelium and localization of vascular endothelial growth factor receptors on the inner choriocapillaris. Evidence for a trophic paracrine relation. Am J Pathol 1999;155:421–428.

25. Holz FG, Sheraidah G, Pauleikhoff D, et al. Analysis of lipid deposits extracted from human macular and peripheral Bruch's membrane. Arch Ophthalmol 1994;112:402–406.

26. Peters S, Kayatz P, Kociok N, et al. Cellular transport of subretinal material into choroidal and scleral blood vessels: an electron microscopic study. Graefes Arch Clin Exp Ophthalmol 1999;237:976–983.

27. Schlingemann RO. Role of growth factors and the wound healing response in age-related macular degeneration. Graefes Arch Clin Exp Ophthalmol 2004;242:91–101.

28. Lopez PF, Sippy BD, Lambert HM, et al. Transdifferentiated retinal pigment epithelial cells are immunoreactive for vascular endothelial growth factor in surgically excised age-related macular degeneration-related choroidal neovascular membranes. Invest Ophthalmol Vis Sci 1996;37:855–868.

29. Kvanta A, Algvere PV, Berglin L, et al. Subfoveal fibrovascular membranes in age-related macular degeneration express vascular endothelial growth factor. Invest Ophthalmol Vis Sci 1996;37:1929–1934.

30. Penfold P, Killingsworth M, Sarks S. An ultrastructural study of the role of leucocytes and fibroblasts in the breakdown of Bruch's membrane. Aust J Ophthalmol 1984;12:23–31.

31. Grossniklaus HE, Ling JX, Wallace TM, et al. Macrophage and retinal pigment epithelium expression of angiogenic cytokines in choroidal neovascularization. Mol Vis 2002;8:119–126.

32. Kliffen M, Sharma HS, Mooy CM, et al. Increased expression of angiogenic growth factors in age-related maculopathy. Br J Ophthalmol 1997;81:154–162.

33. Gass JD. Biomicroscopic and histopathologic considerations regarding the feasibility of surgical excision of subfoveal neovascular membranes. Trans Am Ophthalmol Soc 1994;92:91–111; discussion 111–116.

34. Kang SJ, Schmack I, Benson HE, et al. Histopathological findings in postmortem eyes after photodynamic therapy for choroidal neovascularisation in age-related macular degeneration: report of two cases. Br J Ophthalmol 2007;91:1602–1606.

35. Grossniklaus HE, Wilson DJ, Bressler SB, et al. Clinicopathologic studies of eyes that were obtained postmortem from four patients who were enrolled in the submacular surgery trials: SST report no. 16. Am J Ophthalmol 2006;141:93–104.

36. Grossniklaus HE, Gass JD. Clinicopathologic correlations of surgically excised type 1 and type 2 submacular choroidal neovascular membranes. Am J Ophthalmol 1998;126:59–69.

37. Sarks SH. Ageing and degeneration in the macular region: a clinico-pathological study. Br J Ophthalmol 1976;60:324–341.

38. Gass JD. Pathogenesis of disciform detachment of the neuroepithelium. Am J Ophthalmol 1967; 63(Suppl):1–139.

39. Green WR, Gass JD. Senile disciform degeneration of the macula. Retinal arterialization of the fibrous plaque demonstrated clinically and histopathologically. Arch Ophthalmol 1971;86:487–494.

40. Lafaut BA, Aisenbrey S, Vanden Broecke C, et al. Clinicopathological correlation of deep retinal vascular anomalous complex in age related macular degeneration. Br J Ophthalmol 2000;84:1269–1274.

41. Shimada H, Kawamura A, Mori R, et al. Clinicopathological findings of retinal angiomatous proliferation. Graefes Arch Clin Exp Ophthalmol 2007;245:295–300.

42. MacCumber MW, Dastgheib K, Bressler NM, et al. Clinicopathologic correlation of the multiple recurrent serosanguineous retinal pigment epithelial detachments syndrome. Retina 1994;14:143–152.

43. Uyama M, Matsubara T, Fukushima I, et al. Idiopathic polypoidal choroidal vasculopathy in Japanese patients. Arch Ophthalmol 1999;117:1035–1042.

44. Yannuzzi LA, Nogueira FB, Spaide RF, et al. Idiopathic polypoidal choroidal vasculopathy: a peripheral lesion. Arch Ophthalmol 1998;116:382–383.

45. Yannuzzi LA, Wong DW, Sforzolini BS, et al. Polypoidal choroidal vasculopathy and neovascularized age-related macular degeneration. Arch Ophthalmol 1999;117:1503–1510.

46. Watzke RC, Klein ML, Hiner CJ, et al. A comparison of stereoscopic fluorescein angiography with indocyanine green videoangiography in age-related macular degeneration. Ophthalmology 2000;107:1601–1606.

47. Kaiser PK, Blodi BA, Shapiro H, et al. Angiographic and optical coherence tomographic results of the MARINA study of ranibizumab in neovascular age-related macular degeneration. Ophthalmology 2007; 114:1868–1875.

48. Vujosevic S, Vaclavik V, Bird AC, et al. Combined grading for choroidal neovascularisation: colour, fluorescein angiography and autofluorescence images. Graefes Arch Clin Exp Ophthalmol 2007;245:1453–1460.
49. Holz FG, Jorzik J, Schutt F, et al. Agreement among ophthalmologists in evaluating fluorescein angiograms in patients with neovascular age-related macular degeneration for photodynamic therapy eligibility (FLAP Study). Ophthalmology 2003;110:400–405.
50. Kwiterovich KA, Maguire MG, Murphy RP, et al. Frequency of adverse systemic reactions after fluorescein angiography. Results of a prospective study. Ophthalmology 1991;98:1139–1142.
51. Sallet G, Lafaut BA, De Laey JJ. Indocyanine green angiography and age-related serous pigment epithelial detachment. Graefes Arch Clin Exp Ophthalmol 1996;234:25–33.
52. Guyer DR, Yannuzzi LA, Slakter JS, et al. Classification of choroidal neovascularization by digital indocyanine green videoangiography. Ophthalmology 1996;103:2054–2060.
53. Guyer DR, Yannuzzi LA, Slakter JS, et al. Digital indocyanine-green videoangiography of occult choroidal neovascularization. Ophthalmology 1994;101:1727–1735; discussion 1735–1737.
54. Fernandes LH, Freund KB, Yannuzzi LA, et al. The nature of focal areas of hyperfluorescence or hot spots imaged with indocyanine green angiography. Retina 2002;22:557–568.
55. Eandi CM, Ober MD, Freund KB, et al. Selective photodynamic therapy for neovascular age-related macular degeneration with polypoidal choroidal neovascularization. Retina 2007;27:825–831.
56. Spaide RF, Yannuzzi LA, Slakter JS, et al. Indocyanine green videoangiography of idiopathic polypoidal choroidal vasculopathy. Retina 1995;15:100–110.
57. Da Pozzo S, Parodi MB, Ravalico G. A pilot study of ICG-guided laser photocoagulation for occult choroidal neovascularization presenting as a focal spot in age-related macular degeneration. Int Ophthalmol 2001;24:187–194.
58. Yannuzzi LA, Negrao S, Iida T, et al. Retinal angiomatous proliferation in age-related macular degeneration. Retina 2001;21:416–434.
59. Slakter JS, Yannuzzi LA, Schneider U, et al. Retinal choroidal anastomoses and occult choroidal neovascularization in age-related macular degeneration. Ophthalmology 2000;107:742–753; discussion 753–754.
60. Sandhu SS, Talks SJ. Correlation of optical coherence tomography, with or without additional colour fundus photography, with stereo fundus fluorescein angiography in diagnosing choroidal neovascular membranes. Br J Ophthalmol 2005;89:967–9670.
61. Coscas F, Coscas G, Souied E, et al. Optical coherence tomography identification of occult choroidal neovascularization in age-related macular degeneration. Am J Ophthalmol 2007;144:592–599.
62. Salinas-Alaman A, Garcia-Layana A, Maldonado MJ, et al. Using optical coherence tomography to monitor photodynamic therapy in age related macular degeneration. Am J Ophthalmol 2005;140:23–28.
63. Liakopoulos S, Ongchin SC, Bansal A, et al. Quantitative optical coherence tomography findings in various subtypes of neovascular age-related macular degeneration. Invest Ophthalmol Vis Sci 2008;49:5048–5054.
64. Hughes EH, Khan J, Patel N, et al. In vivo demonstration of the anatomic differences between classic and occult choroidal neovascularization using optical coherence tomography. Am J Ophthalmol 2005;139:344–346.
65. Truong SN, Alam S, Zawadzki RJ, et al. High resolution Fourier-domain optical coherence tomography of retinal angiomatous proliferation. Retina 2007;27:915–925.
66. Brancato R, Introini U, Pierro L, et al. Optical coherence tomography (OCT) angiomatous prolifieration (RAP) in retinal. Eur J Ophthalmol 2002;12:467–472.
67. Rogers AH, Martidis A, Greenberg PB, et al. Optical coherence tomography findings following photodynamic therapy of choroidal neovascularization. Am J Ophthalmol 2002;134:566–576.
68. Fung AE, Lalwani GA, Rosenfeld PJ, et al. An optical coherence tomography-guided, variable dosing regimen with intravitreal ranibizumab (Lucentis) for neovascular age-related macular degeneration. Am J Ophthalmol 2007;143:566–583.
69. Krebs I, Binder S, Stolba U, et al. Optical coherence tomography guided retreatment of photodynamic therapy. Br J Ophthalmol 2005;89:1184–1187.
70. Keane PA, Liakopoulos S, Ongchin SC, et al. Quantitative subanalysis of optical coherence tomography after treatment with ranibizumab for neovascular age-related macular degeneration. Invest Ophthalmol Vis Sci 2008;49:3115–120.
71. Bolz M, Ritter M, Polak K, et al. [The role of Stratus OCT in anti-VEGF therapy: qualitative and quantitative assessment of neovascular AMD.] Ophthalmolog 2008;105:650–655.
72. Emerson GG, Flaxel CJ, Lauer AK, et al. Optical coherence tomography findings during pegaptanib therapy for neovascular age-related macular degeneration. Retina 2007;27:724–729.
73. Framme C, Bunse A, Sofroni R, et al. Fundus autofluorescence before and after photodynamic therapy for choroidal neovascularization secondary to age-related macular degeneration. Ophthalmic Surg Lasers Imaging 2006;37:406–414.
74. McBain VA, Townend J, Lois N. Fundus autofluorescence in exudative age-related macular degeneration. Br J Ophthalmol 2007;91:491–496.
75. Vaclavik V, Vujosevic S, Dandekar SS, et al. Autofluorescence imaging in age-related macular degeneration complicated by choroidal neovascularization: a prospective study. Ophthalmology 2008;115:342–346.
76. Bindewald A, Bird AC, Dandekar SS, et al. Classification of fundus autofluorescence patterns in early age-related macular disease. Invest Ophthalmol Vis Sci 2005;46:3309–3314.

77. Dandekar SS, Jenkins SA, Peto T, et al. Autofluorescence imaging of choroidal neovascularization due to age-related macular degeneration. Arch Ophthalmol 2005;123:1507–1513.

78. von Ruckmann A, Fitzke FW, Bird AC. Fundus autofluorescence in age-related macular disease imaged with a laser scanning ophthalmoscope. Invest Ophthalmol Vis Sci 1997;38:478–486.

79. Lois N, Halfyard AS, Bird AC, et al. Quantitative evaluation of fundus autofluorescence imaged "in vivo" in eyes with retinal disease. Br J Ophthalmol 2000;84:741–745.

80. Stanga PE, Kychenthal A, Fitzke FW, et al. Functional assessment of the native retinal pigment epithelium after the surgical excision of subfoveal choroidal neovascular membranes type II: preliminary results. Int Ophthalmol 2001;23:309–316.

81. Lois N, Owens SL, Coco R, et al. Fundus autofluorescence in patients with age-related macular degeneration and high risk of visual loss. Am J Ophthalmol 2002;133:341–349.

82. Spaide RF. Fundus autofluorescence and age-related macular degeneration. Ophthalmology 2003;110: 392–399.

83. Keilhauer CN, Delori FC. Near-infrared autofluorescence imaging of the fundus: visualization of ocular melanin. Invest Ophthalmol Vis Sci 2006;47:3556–3564.

84. Weinberger AW, Lappas A, Kirschkamp T, et al. Fundus near infrared fluorescence correlates with fundus near infrared reflectance. Invest Ophthalmol Vis Sci 2006;47:3098–3108.

85. Sarna T. Properties and function of the ocular melanin—a photobiophysical view. J Photochem Photobiol B 1992;12:215–258.

86. Wang Z, Dillon J, Gaillard ER. Antioxidant properties of melanin in retinal pigment epithelial cells. Photochem Photobiol 2006;82:474–479.

87. Sarna T, Burke JM, Korytowski W, et al. Loss of melanin from human RPE with aging: possible role of melanin photooxidation. Exp Eye Res 2003;76:89–98.

88. Weiter JJ, Delori FC, Wing GL, et al. Retinal pigment epithelial lipofuscin and melanin and choroidal melanin in human eyes. Invest Ophthalmol Vis Sci 1986;27:145–152.

89. Boulton M, Dayhaw-Barker P. The role of the retinal pigment epithelium: topographical variation and ageing changes. Eye 2001;15:384–389.

90. Rozanowski B, Cuenco J, Davies S, et al. The phototoxicity of aged human retinal melanosomes. Photochem Photobiol 2008;84:650–657.

91. Bynoe LA, Chang TS, Funata M, et al. Histopathologic examination of vascular patterns in subfoveal neovascular membranes. Ophthalmology 1994;101:1112–1117.

92. Gass J. Sterioscopic atlas of macular diseases: diagnosis and treatment, 4th ed. St. Louis: Mosby, 1996:554.

93. Kozak I, Mojana F, Morrison VL, et al. Autofluorescence imaging in exudative age-related macular degeneration after anti-VEGF treatment. ARVO 2008;264.

94. Perumal B, Lee JJ, Bearely S, et al. Correlation of RPE atrophy measured with fundus autofluorescence with visual acuity outcomes in patients with NVAMD responsive to anti-VEGF therapy. ARVO 2008;2238.

10C

Steffen Schmitz-Valckenberg   Hendrik P.N. Scholl

Monika Fleckenstein   Frank G. Holz

Almut Bindewald-Wittich

Fundus Autofluorescence in Atrophic Age-Related Macular Degeneration

Atrophic age-related macular degeneration (AMD) represents the late stage of "dry" AMD. It is characterized by the development of atrophic patches, which may initially occur in the parafoveal area (1–4). These atrophic areas appear funduscopically as sharply demarcated areas of depigmentation through which deep choroidal vessels can be seen. During the natural course of the disease, the areas of atrophy slowly enlarge over time. In atrophic AMD, characteristically, the fovea remains uninvolved until the advanced stages of the disease, a phenomenon referred to as "foveal sparing." A widely established term used to refer to this advanced form of dry AMD is "geographic atrophy" (GA). By contrast, the term "areolar choroidal atrophy" is usually used to refer to findings that are similar but caused by monogenetic retinal macular dystrophies, which may manifest earlier in life.

Severe visual loss secondary to GA occurs in about 20% of all patients with AMD (5–8). Hence, GA is, after choroidal neovascularization (CNV), the second most common cause of legal blindness due to AMD. Patients with primary GA tend to be older than those with neovascular forms of AMD at the time of initial presentation, and it has been speculated that GA occurs in eyes in which a neovascular angiogenic event has not developed. As opposed to the recent breakthrough with anti-VEGF (vascular endothelial growth factor) therapy for active neovascular AMD, there is to date no treatment available for patients with GA, other than visual aids and visual rehabilitation. Therefore, a better understanding of the pathogenesis of GA appears to be mandatory. Sensitive diagnostic tools and prognostic markers to evaluate disease stage and future progression in the individual patient are needed.

It is clinically well established that GA atrophy can affect one or both eyes (9,10). The fellow eye can be affected by any other AMD manifestation and development, including CNV or disciform scarring. It has been reported that eyes demonstrating typical early features of GA can also develop CNV; in these patients, severe and sudden visual loss occurs (11). When CNV develops in an eye with previously diagnosed pure GA, it usually has an evanescent appearance and it is often difficult to outline its borders and differentiate between hyperfluorescence resulting from the CNV and that caused by atrophic areas. In this context, careful slit-lamp biomicroscopy may allow the identification of subretinal fluid or hemorrhage, which would indicate the presence of a CNV. Optical coherence tomography (OCT) may also be helpful in identifying a CNV in these cases.

PATHOPHYSIOLOGY

Areas of GA in AMD occur at sites where macular changes at the level of the retinal pigment epithelium (RPE) and Bruch's membrane, such as pigmentary alterations and drusen, are present (9,10,12,13). Regression of confluent, large, soft drusen may lead to atrophy (1). Similarly, calcified deposits seem to correlate well with the development of atrophy (14). In some cases, GA occurs following the collapse and flattening of RPE detachments (1).

The pathophysiological mechanisms underlying the atrophic process are not completely understood. It is believed that lipofuscin, a by-product of incompletely digested photoreceptor outer segments that accumulates in RPE cells in atrophic AMD, plays a key role in the disease process (see also Chapters 1 and 2) (15). Histopathological studies have shown that clinical visible areas of atrophy are confined to areas of RPE and photoreceptor cell loss, and choriocapillaris closure (13,16,17). Furthermore, lipofuscin and melanolipofuscin-engorged RPE cells have been observed in the junctional zone between the atrophic and the relatively normal retina, whereas in areas of atrophy there is loss of RPE and thus of lipofuscin granules (17).

These postmortem observations suggest that lipofuscin may play a direct pathogenetic role in atrophic AMD by causing RPE cell death, with subsequent deleterious effects on photoreceptors and choriocapillaries. Alternatively, it is possible that the excessive accumulation of lipofuscin is an expression of RPE cell dysfunction and is thus the result, not the cause, of it.

IMAGING TECHNIQUES

Fundus Photography

The discrete areas of loss of RPE associated with loss of overlying photoreceptors in GA appear as areas of depigmentation on slit-lamp biomicroscopy in comparison with surrounding normal retina. The decreased retinal thickness at such sites is usually not visible on nonstereo images. Deep, large choroidal vessels may be apparent and more distinctly visible through areas of atrophic retina. Due to the low contrast, particularly in the red spectrum, the distinction of GA on fundus photographs is challenging and other imaging modalities are required to accurately identify atrophic patches.

Fluorescein Angiography

On fluorescein angiography (FA), atrophic areas are much better delineable. These appear as areas of discrete hyperfluorescence, representing a transmission defect with mild late staining. It may be difficult to differentiate between areas of atrophy and areas with fibrosis, regressed CNV, or hyperfluorescence from other causes.

Indocyanine Green Angiography

Due to atrophy of the choriocapillaris, GA appears as areas of discrete hypofluorescence with loss of the normal background signal on indocyanine green (ICG) angiography. Larger, deeper choroidal vessels are clearly visible. Compared to FA, it appears to be more difficult to distinguish between atrophic and nonatrophic retina using ICG.

Optical Coherence Tomography

Retinal thinning with loss of outer retina is observed over GA on OCT scans. Spectral-domain OCT with simultaneous confocal scanning laser ophthalmoscopy (cSLO) allows for better 3D assessment of retinal abnormalities. Recent data suggest that OCT can reveal highly variable morphological alterations in the atrophic area and in the surrounding retina in eyes with funduscopically uniform-appearing GA (18).

Fundus Autofluorescence

Findings on Fundus Autofluorescence in Geographic Atrophy

Fundus AF findings in patients with GA are in accordance with histopathologic findings (19,20). Thus, because of the lack of RPE lipofuscin, which contains the dominant fluorophores involved in the AF signal (see Chapter 3), AF imaging shows a markedly reduced AF signal at the site of atrophic areas (Fig. 10C.1). Compared with drusen, which may also exhibit a decreased AF signal, atrophic areas typically show an even stronger reduction of AF (21). The high-contrast difference between atrophic and nonatrophic retina allows for much better delineation of atrophic areas with AF

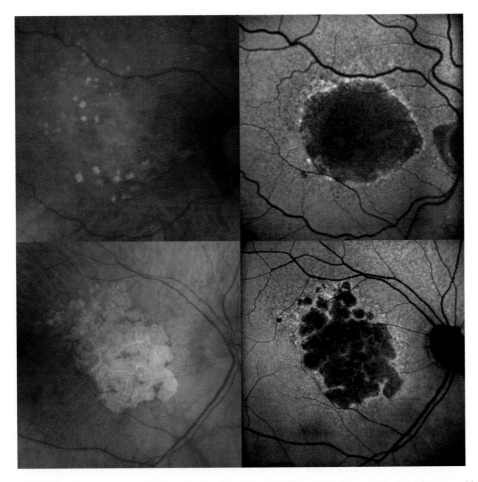

FIGURE 10C.1.   Fundus photographs and autofluorescence (AF) images of two patients with geographic atrophy (GA) secondary to age-related macular degeneration (AMD). In one of these patients an ill-defined area of hypopigmentation is observed, as well as calcified drusen (*top left*). A fundus AF image obtained from the same patient (*top right*) better delineates the area of atrophy. Furthermore, surrounding areas of atrophy, at the junctional zone between atrophic and relatively preserved retina, markedly increased AF signal is detected (*top right*); this does not correlate clinically with any obvious changes. Similar findings are observed in another patient (*bottom left* and *right*) with atrophic AMD.

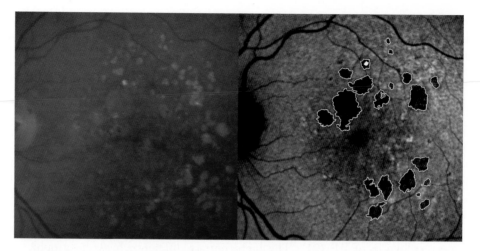

FIGURE 10C.2. Fundus photograph of the left eye of a patient with atrophic AMD (*left*). Single atrophic patches are clearly detected and quantified by customized image analysis software (detected areas are marked by a *white circle*) on the fundus AF image (*right*). Note that drusen and pigment abnormalities seen on the fundus photograph can be easily differentiated from atrophic areas with fundus AF imaging.

imaging compared to conventional fundus photographs (22,23). In contrast to FA, AF imaging is a noninvasive and less time-consuming method.

AF imaging has been applied to detect and precisely quantify atrophic areas in combination with customized image analysis software (Fig. 10C.2) (22,23). This software enables automated segmentation of atrophic areas by a region algorithm. Interfering retinal blood vessels, which have similar AF intensities, are recognized by the software and can be excluded from the measurements. Further developments include the alignment of AF images at different examinations using retinal landmarks to correct for different scan angles and magnifications. This allows the progression of the atrophic process to be accurately assessed over time, and can be used in longitudinal observations, including interventional trials.

An even more striking finding of AF imaging in GA patients, which does not usually correlate with obvious changes on fundus photography or FA, is the frequent visualization of high-intensity levels of AF surrounding the atrophic patches at the junctional zone of atrophy (Fig. 10C.1) (24). This observation is in accordance with histopathological data showing lipofuscin-engorged RPE cells surrounding areas of atrophy (see above).

Clinical Significance of Fundus Autofluorescence Findings in Geographic Atrophy

Studies of photoreceptor function have underscored the importance of abnormal AF intensities around atrophy and the pathophysiological role of increased RPE lipofuscin accumulation in patients with GA due to AMD. Scholl and coworkers (25) demonstrated that rod photoreceptor function is more severely affected than cone function over areas with increased AF using fine-matrix mapping. With a combination of SLO-based microperimetry and AF imaging, impaired photopic sensitivity has been observed in areas of abnormal AF in the junctional zone (26). Because normal photoreceptor function is dependent on normal RPE function, particularly with regard to the constant phagocytosis of shed distal outer segment discs for photoreceptor cell renewal, a negative feedback mechanism has been proposed whereby cells with lipofuscin-loaded secondary lysosomes would phagocytose fewer shed photoreceptor outer segments, subsequently leading to impaired retinal sensitivity in areas with increased AF intensity. This would also be in accordance with experimental data showing that compounds of lipofuscin, such as A2-E (N-retinylidene-N-retinylethanolamin), possess toxic properties and may interfere with normal RPE cell function (see also Chapter 2) (27,28). The higher susceptibility of the rod system relative to the cone system may be explained by the relative retinoid deficiency in cones.

The Fundus Autofluorescence in Age-related Macular Degeneration (FAM) Study Group introduced a classification system for distinct patterns of abnormal elevated AF in the junctional zone of GA (29). This morphological classification is based on information that is solely detectable by AF imaging and consists of five main patterns: none, focal, banded, diffuse, and patchy. The "diffuse" pattern is further subdivided into five subtypes. These distinct AF phenotypes may reflect heterogeneity of the underlying disease process. The concomitant observation of a high degree of symmetry of AF patterns in patients with bilateral GA in the presence of a high degree of interindividual variability also suggests that genetic determinants rather than nonspecific aging changes may be involved (30).

Impact of Fundus Autofluorescence Findings on Geographic Atrophy Progression

While the presence of atrophy represents a nonspecific end-stage manifestation of various retinal degenerations, the identification of elevated levels of AF at the junctional zone of atrophy is of particular interest. The distinct patterns of AF observed surrounding areas of GA, as described in a cross-sectional study undertaken by the FAM Study Group (see above), seem to be of prognostic value for predicting the speed of atrophy progression. This may be even more important when one considers the high variability of atrophy progression over time among patients with GA, which has been independently demonstrated by several natural history studies (2,31,32). Current data on the spread of atrophy suggest that atrophy expands linearly over time, and that the best predictor for this expansion appears to be the growth rate observed in the previous year (33). Atrophy enlargement of very small areas (less than one disc area or ca. 2.5 mm^2) has been shown to be less rapid than that of larger areas; however, the overall difference of atrophy progression between eyes (0–13.8 mm^2/per year) could not be explained by baseline atrophy or by any other tested demographic factors (34).

Early pilot studies with AF imaging for atrophy progression in GA patients demonstrated the occurrence of new atrophic patches and the spread of preexisting atrophy solely in areas with abnormally high levels of AF at baseline, suggesting that levels of increased AF precede cell death and, therefore, absolute scotoma (24). With larger groups of patients and longer follow-up, it was shown that the extension of the total area of increased AF surrounding areas of atrophy at baseline had a strong positive correlation with the rate of progression of atrophy over time (35). A recent analysis of atrophy progression rates over time and AF patterns at baseline revealed that variation in GA growth rates is dependent on the specific phenotype of abnormal AF at baseline (31). The progression rates in eyes with banded (median 1.81 mm^2/year, $n = 24$ eyes) and diffuse (1.77 mm^2/year, $n = 112$) AF patterns were significantly higher compared to those in eyes without AF abnormalities (0.38 mm^2/year, $n = 17$) and focal FAF patterns (0.81 mm^2/year, $n = 14$, $p < 0.0001$; Figs. 10C.3 and 10C.4). Within the group of the diffuse pattern, eyes with the diffuse-trickling pattern exhibited an even higher spread rate (median 3.02 mm^2/year, $n = 9$) compared to the other diffuse types (1.67 mm^2/year, $p = 0.001$; Fig. 10C.4). This study represents the largest longitudinal study of AF findings in GA patients so far (median follow-up 1.80 years, range 0.52–7.14; $n = 195$ eyes of 129 patients). Overall, phenotypic features of AF abnormalities had a much stronger impact on atrophy progression than any other risk factor (including size

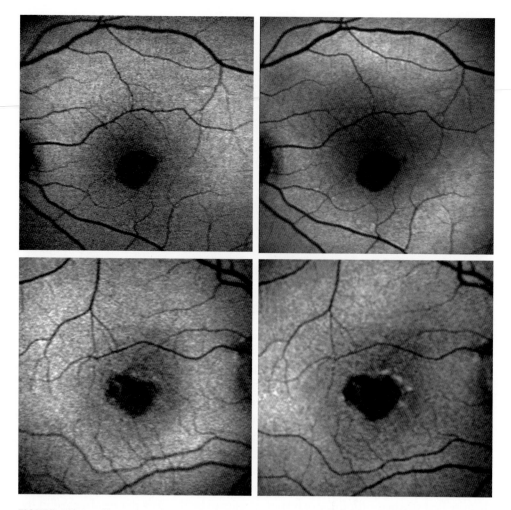

FIGURE 10C.3.   Illustration of the relationship between specific fundus AF phenotypes and atrophy progression in patients with GA due to AMD (Part I: slow progressors) showing the baseline AF image (*left*) and the follow-up AF image (*right*) for each eye, respectively. Eyes with no abnormal AF changes (*top row*: atrophy progression 0.02 mm²/year, follow-up 12 months) and with only small areas of focally increased AF at the margin of the atrophic patch (*bottom row*: 0.36 mm²/year, follow-up 15 months) usually have very slow progression over time. (Adapted from Holz FG, Bindewald-Wittich A, Fleckenstein M, et al. Progression of geographic atrophy and impact of fundus autofluorescence patterns in age-related macular degeneration. Am J Ophthalmol 2007;143:463–472.)

of baseline atrophy, history of smoking, hypertension, diabetes, age >80 years, hyperlipidemia, and family history) that has been addressed in previous studies on progression of GA due to AMD. These findings also suggest that AF phenotypes may be used to explain the great heterogeneity of atrophy progression rates among different patients (36).

Fundus Autofluorescence to Evaluate the Response to Future Therapeutic Strategies

Currently, there is no treatment available to halt or slow the progression of atrophic AMD. With the noninvasive visualization of prognostic determinants, the metabolic mapping of functional changes and the ability to accurately monitor the disease over time, AF imaging may not only contribute to the understanding of atrophic AMD, it may also be used to develop and assess new emerging therapeutic strategies for this disease.

Visual cycle modulators, which aim to target the detrimental accumulation of toxic lipofuscin in the RPE, are pharmaceutical agents that may slow down the progression

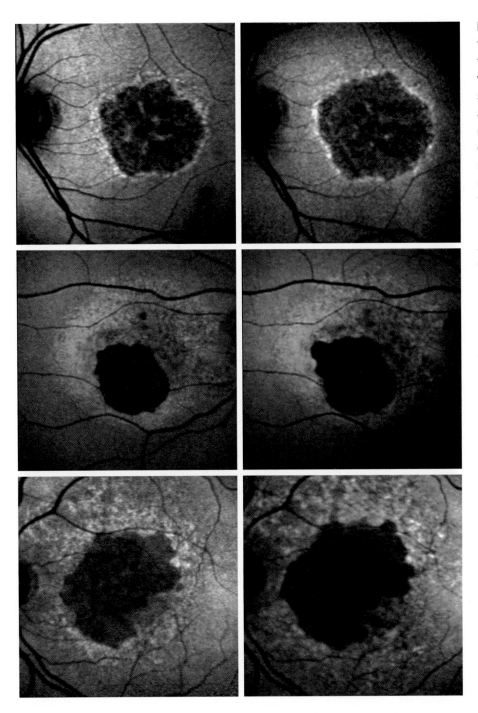

FIGURE 10C.4. Illustration of the relationship between specific fundus AF phenotypes and atrophy progression in patients with GA due to AMD (Part I: slow progressors) showing the baseline AF image (*left*) and the follow-up AF image (*right*) for each eye, respectively. Eyes with no abnormal AF changes (*top row*: atrophy progression 0.02 mm²/year, follow-up 12 months) and with only small areas of focally increased AF at the margin of the atrophic patch (*bottom row*: 0.36 mm²/year, follow-up 15 months) usually have very slow progression over time. (Adapted from Holz FG, Bindewald-Wittich A, Fleckenstein M, et al. Progression of geographic atrophy and impact of fundus autofluorescence patterns in age-related macular degeneration. Am J Ophthalmol 2007;143:463–472.)

of atrophy. One agent is Fenretinide (N-[4-hydroxyphenyl]retinamide), an oral compound that has been shown to lower the production of toxic fluorophores in the RPE in a dose-dependent manner in albino ABCA4$^{-/-}$ mice (37). This vitamin A derivative acts by competing with serum retinol for the binding sites of retinal-binding protein and promotes renal clearance of retinol. The bioavailability of retinol for the RPE and photoreceptors is consequently reduced and less toxic retinoid by-products, such as A2-E, are generated. A Phase II randomized, double-masked, placebo-controlled multicenter study that included over 200 GA patients was initiated in 2006 (Sirion Therapeutics, Tampa, FL; http://www.siriontherapeutics.com). The therapeutic concept of Fenretinide is underscored by growing evidence from experimental and clinical studies, including AF findings, on the pathophysiological role of deleterious accumulation of lipofuscin. To reduce the observational period in a slowly progressive disease, minimize the sample size, and better demonstrate possible treatment effects, patient recruitment in this study involves the identification of high-risk features according to the AF pattern classification described by the FAM Study Group, and only "rapid progressors" are included in this large interventional trial in patients with GA secondary to AMD.

DIFFERENTIAL DIAGNOSIS

The differential diagnosis of GA includes scar tissue or fibrosis following regression of CNV, trauma, postinflammation, or other causes. Notably, GA is a nonspecific disease manifestation and can be the result of retinal disorders other than AMD, such as retinal and macular dystrophies (e.g., Stargardt disease and Best disease), central areolar macular dystrophy, and cone dystrophy. To establish the diagnosis of GA, it might be helpful to evaluate retinal changes in the fellow eye and look for retinal abnormalities surrounding the area of atrophy. For example, hard and soft drusen might be very indicative of GA, while focal yellow flecks would suggest Stargardt disease. AF imaging may be helpful for evaluating retinal abnormalities surrounding areas of atrophy.

SUMMARY

Fundus AF imaging allows for accurate delineation of areas of atrophy. Precise quantification of these areas is possible with AF, which is also useful for monitoring the progression of the disease. Distinct phenotypic patterns of abnormal AF in the junctional zone of atrophy are associated with significant differences in rates of atrophy progression over time, and appear to have the strongest predictive value compared to other factors, including smoking, age, and size of the area of atrophy at baseline. Areas of increased AF in the junctional zone of atrophy are correlated with decreased retinal sensitivity, which may reflect the pathophysiologic role of increased lipofuscin accumulation. AF imaging has enhanced our understanding of the disease and may prove to be essential in monitoring the response to therapeutic interventions.

REFERENCES

1. Blair CJ. Geographic atrophy of the retinal pigment epithelium. A manifestation of senile macular degeneration. Arch Ophthalmol 1975;93:19–25.
2. Sunness JS. The natural history of geographic atrophy, the advanced atrophic form of age-related macular degeneration. Mol Vis 1999;5:25.
3. Maguire P, Vine AK. Geographic atrophy of the retinal pigment epithelium. Am J Ophthalmol 1986; 102:621–625.
4. Schatz H, McDonald HR. Atrophic macular degeneration. Rate of spread of geographic atrophy and visual loss. Ophthalmology 1989;96:1541–1551.
5. Klein R, Klein BE, Knudtson MD, et al. Fifteen-year cumulative incidence of age-related macular degeneration: the Beaver Dam Eye Study. Ophthalmology 2007;114:253–262.
6. Wang JJ, Rochtchina E, Lee AJ, et al. Ten-year incidence and progression of age-related maculopathy: the Blue Mountains Eye Study. Ophthalmology 2007;114:92–98.
7. Augood CA, Vingerling JR, de Jong PT, et al. Prevalence of age-related maculopathy in older Europeans: the European Eye Study (EUREYE). Arch Ophthalmol 2006;124:529–535.
8. Klaver CC, Wolfs RC, Vingerling JR, et al. Age-specific prevalence and causes of blindness and visual impairment in an older population: the Rotterdam Study. Arch Ophthalmol 1998;116:653–658.
9. Gass JD. Drusen and disciform macular detachment and degeneration. Arch Ophthalmol 1973;90:206–217.
10. Green WR, Key 3rd SN. Senile macular degeneration: a histopathologic study. Trans Am Ophthalmol Soc 1977;75:180–254.

11. Sunness JS, Gonzalez-Baron J, Bressler NM, et al. The development of choroidal neovascularization in eyes with the geographic atrophy form of age-related macular degeneration. Ophthalmology 1999;106:910–919.

12. Sarks SH. Drusen patterns predisposing to geographic atrophy of the retinal pigment epithelium. Aust J Ophthalmol 1982;10:91–97.

13. Sarks JP, Sarks SH, Killingsworth MC. Evolution of geographic atrophy of the retinal pigment epithelium. Eye 1988;2:552–577.

14. AREDS. A randomized, placebo-controlled, clinical trial of high-dose supplementation with vitamins C and E, beta carotene, and zinc for age-related macular degeneration and vision loss: AREDS report no. 8. Arch Ophthalmol 2001;119:1417–1436.

15. Sparrow JR, Boulton M. RPE lipofuscin and its role in retinal pathobiology. Exp Eye Res 2005;80:595–606.

16. Green WR, Engel C. Age-related macular degeneration: histopathologic studies: the 1992 Lorenz E. Zimmermann Lecture. Ophthalmology 1992;100:1519–1535.

17. Sarks SH. Ageing and degeneration in the macular region: a clinico-pathological study. Br J Ophthalmol 1976;60:324–341.

18. Fleckenstein M, Charbel Issa P, Helb HM, et al. High resolution spectral domain-OCT imaging in geographic atrophy associated with age-related macular degeneration. Invest Ophthalmol 2008;49:4137–4144.

19. von Ruckmann A, Fitzke FW, Bird AC. Distribution of fundus autofluorescence with a scanning laser ophthalmoscope. Br J Ophthalmol 1995;79:407–412.

20. Holz FG, Bellmann C, Margaritidis M, et al. Patterns of increased in vivo fundus autofluorescence in the junctional zone of geographic atrophy of the retinal pigment epithelium associated with age-related macular degeneration. Graefes Arch Clin Exp Ophthalmol 1999;237:145–152.

21. Delori FC, Fleckner MR, Goger DG, et al. Autofluorescence distribution associated with drusen in age-related macular degeneration. Invest Ophthalmol Vis Sci 2000;41:496–504.

22. Schmitz-Valckenberg S, Jorzik J, Unnebrink K, et al. Analysis of digital scanning laser ophthalmoscopy fundus autofluorescence images of geographic atrophy in advanced age-related macular degeneration. Graefes Arch Clin Exp Ophthalmol 2002;240:73–78.

23. Deckert A, Schmitz-Valckenberg S, Jorzik J, et al. Automated analysis of digital fundus autofluorescence images of geographic atrophy in advanced age-related macular degeneration using confocal scanning laser ophthalmoscopy (cSLO). BMC Ophthalmol 2005;5:8.

24. Holz FG, Bellman C, Staudt S, et al. Fundus autofluorescence and development of geographic atrophy in age-related macular degeneration. Invest Ophthalmol Vis Sci 2001;42:1051–1056.

25. Scholl HP, Bellmann C, Dandekar SS, et al. Photopic and scotopic fine matrix mapping of retinal areas of increased fundus autofluorescence in patients with age-related maculopathy. Invest Ophthalmol Vis Sci 2004;45:574–583.

26. Schmitz-Valckenberg S, Bultmann S, Dreyhaupt J, et al. Fundus autofluorescence and fundus perimetry in the junctional zone of geographic atrophy in patients with age-related macular degeneration. Invest Ophthalmol Vis Sci 2004;45:4470–4476.

27. Zhou J, Jang YP, Kim SR, et al. Complement activation by photooxidation products of A2E, a lipofuscin constituent of the retinal pigment epithelium. Proc Natl Acad Sci USA 2006;103:16182–16187.

28. Bergmann M, Schutt F, Holz FG, et al. Inhibition of the ATP-driven proton pump in RPE lysosomes by the major lipofuscin fluorophore A2-E may contribute to the pathogenesis of age-related macular degeneration. FASEB J 2004;18:562–564.

29. Bindewald A, Schmitz-Valckenberg S, Jorzik JJ, et al. Classification of abnormal fundus autofluorescence patterns in the junctional zone of geographic atrophy in patients with age related macular degeneration. Br J Ophthalmol 2005;89:874–878.

30. Bellmann C, Jorzik J, Spital G, et al. Symmetry of bilateral lesions in geographic atrophy in patients with age-related macular degeneration. Arch Ophthalmol 2002;120:579–584.

31. Holz FG, Bindewald-Wittich A, Fleckenstein M, et al. Progression of geographic atrophy and impact of fundus autofluorescence patterns in age-related macular degeneration. Am J Ophthalmol 2007;143:463–472.

32. Sunness J, Margalit E, Srikurnaran D, et al. The long-term natural history of geographic atrophy from age-related macular degeneration. Ophthalmology 2007;114:271–277.

33. Dreyhaupt J, Mansmann U, Pritsch M, et al. Modelling the natural history of geographic atrophy in patients with age-related macular degeneration. Ophthalmic Epidemiol 2005;12:353–362.

34. Sunness JS, Gonzalez-Baron J, Applegate CA, et al. Enlargement of atrophy and visual acuity loss in the geographic atrophy form of age-related macular degeneration. Ophthalmology 1999;106:1768–1779.

35. Schmitz-Valckenberg S, Bindewald-Wittich A, Dolar-Szczasny J, et al. Correlation between the area of increased autofluorescence surrounding geographic atrophy and disease progression in patients with AMD. Invest Ophthalmol Vis Sci 2006;47:2648–2654.

36. Schmitz-Valckenberg S, Fleckenstein M, Scholl HP, et al. Fundus autofluorescence and progression of age-related macular degeneration. Surv Ophthalmol 2009;54(1):96–117.

37. Radu RA, Han Y, Bui TV, et al. Reductions in serum vitamin A arrest accumulation of toxic retinal fluorophores: a potential therapy for treatment of lipofuscin-based retinal diseases. Invest Ophthalmol Vis Sci 2005;46:4393–4401.

11A

Anthony G. Robson
Isabelle Audo
Phil Hykin
Andrew R. Webster

Fundus Autofluorescence in Retinitis Pigmentosa

R etinitis pigmentosa (RP) is a heterogeneous group of disorders characterized by progressive retinal dysfunction affecting mainly rods with secondary cone involvement. Patients with RP classically present with impaired night vision and progressive visual field constriction with ultimate loss of central vision. Typically, as photoreceptors die, intraretinal pigment migration ("bone-spicules") is observed along the midperipheral retina. Retinal blood vessel attenuation and disc pallor are seen in advanced stages. Fundus examination can be normal, especially early in the course of the disease. Full-field electroretinogram (ERG) demonstrates rod-cone dysfunction and may be essential in establishing the diagnosis and severity of the condition.

Autosomal dominant (AD), recessive (AR), and X-linked forms of inheritance can be observed in families affected with RP, with rare cases of mitochondrial and digenic forms. In general, AD RP has a better prognosis for retention of central vision than recessive or X-linked disease, although there is wide mutation-specific variability. In addition, RP can be isolated or be part of a syndrome. More than 180 genes implicated in retinal dystrophies have been mapped and more 120 genes have been cloned, highlighting the complexity of the disease (for a recent summary, see the Retinal Information Network, http://www.sph.uth.tmc.edu/Retnet/). However, more than half of all cases are due to unidentified genetic defects. Thus, precise phenotyping is critical to better understand the disorder, identify candidate genes, and to develop novel therapies.

MOLECULAR BASIS AND PATHOLOGY

The majority of cases of RP are nonsyndromic (isolated); about 25% occur as part of a syndrome, the most common being Usher syndrome (RP and neurosensory hearing loss), which represents 14% of all RP cases (1). Other syndromic forms include Bardet-Biedl syndrome (RP, polydactyly, obesity, renal abnormality, and mental retardation), Refsum disease, and other disorders associated with renal, metabolic, skeletal, or neurological disease (2,3). The prevalence of isolated RP varies according to the inheritance pattern; recent estimates suggest that AD RP forms account for approximately 30%, AR RP for 20%, and X-linked for 15% of cases (4). A further 5% have been classified as early-onset forms of RP (Leber congenital amaurosis). The other 30% represent sporadic cases, which are most likely to be AR, but X-linked or de novo dominant forms might also be included in this group (4). To add to the complexity, different genes have been implicated in similar patterns of inheritance. Since the identification of the *RHODOPSIN* (*RHO*) gene as the first gene implicated in AD RP (5), more than 180 genes have been linked to the physiopathology of retinal dystrophies. The products of these genes are implicated in very diverse cellular functions, including the phototransduction cascade, retinoid cycle, photoreceptor structures, transcription factors, outer segment renewal, splicing factors, and intracellular trafficking (3). For most of these genes, expression is restricted to the photoreceptors, especially rods, and/or the retinal pigment epithelium (RPE), but others, such as splicing factors, are more ubiquitously expressed. The mechanism by which a ubiquitously expressed gene is responsible for a restricted photoreceptor disease is not well understood, but it may relate to the uniquely high metabolic demand of the photoreceptors.

In addition, in AD RP, nonpenetrance has been described associated with certain genotypes (e.g., *PRPF31* mutations [6]), which may complicate genetic counseling. Some genes are implicated in different phenotypes; for instance, *RHO* is the gene most commonly implicated in AD RP (20%–30% of AD RP [7]), but it can also be involved (less commonly) in AR RP and AD congenital stationary night blindness (8,9). Similarly, *NR2E3*, which is responsible for Enhanced S Cone syndrome (10), a recessive disorder, can be found in 1%–3% of cases of AD RP (11,12).

Because of the genetic heterogeneity of RP, the precise molecular mechanisms leading to photoreceptor cell death are still not fully understood. It is thought that photoreceptors degenerate through a common final pathway by apoptosis (13,14), which may involve calpains (15,16). Causes of apoptosis include ionic imbalance, protein aggregates, or default in photoreceptor structure (3). Explanations have also been given to the secondary cone cell death in the case of mutation in genes expressed only in rods, and evidence suggests that cones rely on rods to survive (17,18).

FINDINGS ON FUNDUS EXAMINATION

Fundus examination can be normal (RP *sine pigmento*), especially in the early stages of the disease. In the course of RP, RPE changes will appear in the midperiphery with pigment migration into the inner retinal layers as photoreceptors die. Blood vessel attenuation and pallor of the optic disc are hallmarks of advanced stages and are thought to result from the decreased metabolic demand with photoreceptor degeneration. The posterior pole is usually preserved until late in the course of the disorder. However, in about 63% of all cases of RP, foveal lesions are present, including atrophic changes (43%) and cystic changes (20%), mainly oedematous, that can be documented with fluorescein angiography (FA) or optical coherence tomography (OCT) (19–21) (see below). These macular changes will cause early loss of central vision. Premature posterior subcapsular cataract may also occur, resulting in impaired visual acuity.

ELECTRODIAGNOSTIC FINDINGS

ERG is essential for establishing the diagnosis of RP when there are no or only subtle abnormalities on fundus examination. In RP, the dark-adapted bright flash ERG a-wave, which predominantly reflects rod photoreceptor hyperpolarization, is abnormal with milder photopic ERG abnormalities, indicating milder cone-system involvement. The degree of macular cone system involvement varies among patients and may be assessed by pattern ERG (PERG) (22) and multifocal ERG (mfERG) (23). The PERG P50 component is a response to an alternating checkerboard stimulus that depends on the integrity of macular cones and has been used extensively as an objective index of macular function (24,25). Multifocal ERG is typically performed using a stimulus array comprised of 61 or 103 hexagonal stimulus elements centered at the fovea and usually extending over the central 55–60 degrees. The mfERG responses are mathematically derived using a cross-correlation algorithm and allow assessment of localized cone-system function at multiple retinal locations across the posterior pole (26). Both PERG (27–31) and mfERG (32–35) recordings have been used to objectively assess macular function in RP. The extent of macular involvement is not always related to the severity of generalized or peripheral dysfunction, and serial testing with either technique may prove to be of prognostic value for predicting functional sparing of the macula or the rate of disease progression.

IMAGING TECHNIQUES

Fluorescein Angiography

Historically, fluorescein angiography (FA) has played a major role in assessing morphological abnormalities in RP, but it has been replaced by noninvasive techniques such as fundus autofluorescence (AF) and OCT. FA classically shows a variable mottled increased fluorescence in affected areas due to window defects (transmission defects though atrophic changes in the RPE). Pigment clumping/bone spicules block fluorescence transmission from blood in the retinal vessels or from the choroid. Narrowing of blood vessels with no filling delay is also a classical sign. Vascular leakage is not unusual in the course of the disease; cystoid macular oedema (CMO) may also occur and can be documented by FA (36).

Indocyanine-Green Angiography

Because of the physical properties of its dye, indocyanin green (ICG) angiography is mainly used to assess the choroidal vasculature and its involvement in retinal disease. This imaging technique has little value in the management of primarily photoreceptor diseases and is currently not performed for the diagnosis or management of patients with RP.

Optical Coherence Tomography

OCT is increasingly being used in the evaluation of patients with RP. This noninvasive and noncontact imaging technique is at least as sensitive as FA in the detection of CMO, and is valuable for the accurate diagnosis and management of patients with nonleaking CMO (37–39). OCT can also document atrophic changes. Ultra-high-resolution OCT allows a more precise assessment of changes in the neurosensory retina (40) and may be used in combination with scanning laser ophthalmoscopy (SLO; for review see Podoleanu and Rosen [41]). These new and complementary techniques will allow a better evaluation of macular photoreceptor changes during the course of RP and will be especially useful for monitoring future treatments.

Fundus Autofluorescence

Fundus AF imaging can reveal otherwise invisible manifestations of disrupted RPE metabolism, and the technique has an increasingly important role in the assessment and management of RP. Early detection of macular involvement may have prognostic implications for retention of central vision, and attempts to establish functional correlates of abnormal AF have outlined its value in monitoring disease progression.

Early reports documented a close spatial correspondence between absent AF and outer retinal atrophy in RP (42). Almost all adult patients with RP have a decreased AF signal in the midperiphery (43). More recently, OCT has demonstrated a spatial correspondence between the lateral extension of the outer retinal high-reflectance band and preserved macular AF (44), suggesting preservation of outer retinal structure within this area. At the central macula, abnormal patterns of increased fundus AF may be present (43–45) and are usually associated with impaired visual acuity. In patients with CMO, round or oval areas of increased AF can be detected at the fovea. In chronic CMO, RPE atrophy may ensue and a reduced AF signal may be observed.

An abnormal parafoveal ring of increased AF, not visible on slit-lamp biomicroscopy (Fig. 11A.1), is commonly observed and has been reported in AD, AR, sporadic cases (28,30,31,44,46), and X-linked RP (47). The ring has been described in patients as young as 2 years old (48), but is not always present in affected children. A cross-sectional analysis of dominant pedigrees suggested that the ring can be a relatively late manifestation of RP, manifesting only in adolescence or adulthood (28). Few surveys have quantified the incidence of this abnormality, but estimates range from about 50% in a heterogeneous group of RP patients (31) to 95% in a cohort with Usher syndrome type 2 (45). Fundus AF is usually preserved in areas internal and external to this ring of abnormal AF, but in adults there is often a patchy or reduced AF signal in more eccentric regions that usually encroach upon the vascular arcades (Fig. 11A.1D). The diameter of the ring has been reported to vary between approximately 3–20 degrees and usually exhibits a high degree of interocular symmetry.

Parafoveal rings of increased AF are not specific to RP. Similar annular AF abnormalities have been documented in other retinal dystrophies, including Leber congenital

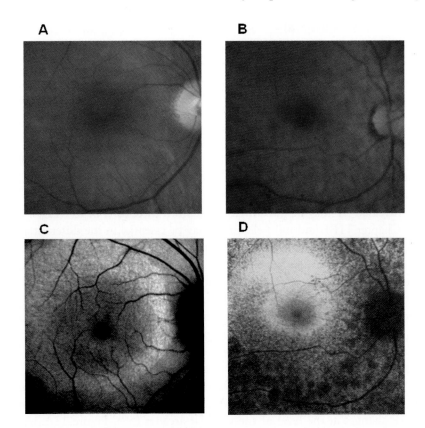

FIGURE 11A.1.   Fundus photographs **(A,B)** and typical examples of abnormal AF in two unrelated individuals with RP, showing a parafoveal ring of increased AF **(C,D)**.

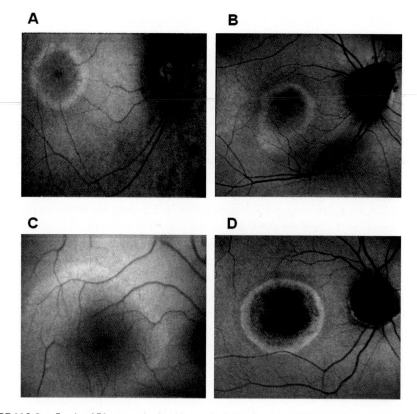

FIGURE 11A.2. Fundus AF images obtained in two individuals with AD RP (mutation in *PRPF3*-RP18) and good visual acuity **(A,C)** compared with two individuals with X-linked cone-rod dystrophy (mutation in exon ORF15 of *RPGR*-RP3 **[B,D]**). **(A)** from the maternal aunt (35 years old) of **(C)** (17 years old); **(B)** from the maternal nephew (40 years old) of **(D)** (74 years old).

amaurosis (see also Chapter 11D) (49), cone-rod dystrophy (Fig. 11A.2B,D) (50–54) and "cone dystrophy with supernormal rod ERG" (see also Chapter 11B) (55,56), Best disease (see also Chapter 11F) (57), X-linked retinoschisis (see also Chapter 11C) (58), and other forms of maculopathy (59,60). The incidence of parafoveal rings of increased AF in non-RP cases was recently reviewed (30). In cone-rod dystrophy, the annular areas of increased AF may be indistinguishable from those seen in RP (Fig. 11A.2A,B) (see also Chapter 11B), and full-field ERG may be essential in the differential diagnosis. However, once the cone-rod dystrophy progresses, atrophic macular RPE changes usually ensue, demonstrating a reduced AF signal within the ring (Fig. 11A.2D). An important caveat is that dense macular pigment may resemble early atrophic changes at the fovea, and two-wavelength AF (61) utilizing wavelengths that are differently absorbed by luteal pigment may help to identify subtle abnormalities. Unlike in RP, the ring of increased AF in cone-rod dystrophy evolves differently as the maculopathy worsens (see later).

In sector RP, fundus AF can be decreased within the inferior vascular arcades, showing approximate correspondence with areas of superior visual field loss (62). A semicircular parafoveal arc of increased AF may be present inferior to the fovea with patchy AF changes at the level of the vascular arcades (59). Figure 11A.3A shows a typical example from a patient with sector RP who had full-field ERGs consistent with restricted photoreceptor disease; multifocal ERG reduction and superior visual field loss were concordant with the localized inferior retinal area of abnormal AF.

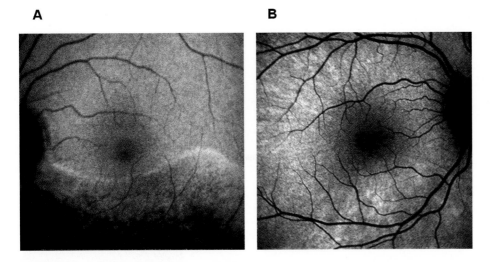

FIGURE 11A.3.   **(A)** Fundus AF in a patient with sector RP, showing an arc of high density and an inferior area of abnormally reduced AF that corresponds with a superior visual field defect. **(B)** Radial pattern of increased AF corresponding to a typical "tapetal reflex" in an obligate carrier for X-linked RP.

Functional Significance of Annular Autofluorescence Abnormalities in Retinitis Pigmentosa

Several electrophysiological and psychophysical studies have sought to determine the functional significance of the ring of increased AF. In a heterogeneous group of RP patients with normal visual acuity, ring size was not directly related to the severity of generalized retinal dysfunction, as determined by full-field ERG (28). This, however, was expected since full-field ERG does not provide information regarding macular function.

In a heterogeneous group of patients with RP and normal visual acuity, a high positive correlation between the radius of the ring and the pattern ERG P50 component was found (28,30,31), suggesting that only areas within the ring contribute to the generation of the pattern ERG. This hypothesis was first substantiated by recording pattern ERGs to checkerboards of different diameters. Pattern ERGs to small stimulus fields were comparable to those recorded in normal subjects, but there was a cutoff in the expected enlargement when the checkerboard stimulus diameter exceeded that of the ring (28,29). Multifocal ERGs corroborated the pattern ERG findings, showing widespread response attenuation over parafoveal areas with sparing or relative sparing over the central macula (31,35). The lateral extent of mfERG response preservation varied between patients and was related to both the ring size and the approximate area of central visual field preservation ascertained using automated Humphrey (35) or Goldman perimetry (36). Figure 11A.4 illustrates typical AF abnormalities (Fig. 11A.4A), small-field pattern ERGs (Fig. 11A.4B), visual field constriction (Fig. 11A.4D), and corresponding mfERGs (Fig. 11A.4C) in a representative patient with RP and normal visual acuity.

Fine matrix mapping involves psychophysical measurement of photopic and scotopic thresholds, typically at more than 100 retinal locations within a 9 × 9 degree macular area. The technique has been used to measure cone and rod system sensitivity in numerous retinal disorders (29,63–65). Photopic fine matrix mapping in individuals with RP and good visual acuity revealed preserved cone sensitivity within the ring of increased AF (Fig. 11A.5). There was a steep gradient of threshold elevation across the ring and severe sensitivity loss over more eccentric areas (Fig. 11A.5C) (29,35,66),

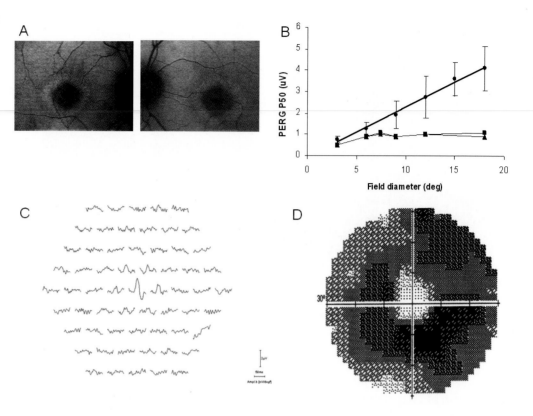

consistent with the PERG and mfERG data. The ring corresponded with the internal edge of photopic visual field constriction. Perhaps not surprisingly, given that patients had predominantly rod photoreceptor disease, scotopic sensitivity losses were more severe than photopic sensitivity losses and encroached upon central macular areas encircled by the ring (Fig. 11A.5D). These observations suggest that rod macular dysfunction precedes significant lipofuscin accumulation and increased AF (see below). The significance of a similar ring in patients with impaired visual acuity is not known.

The above-mentioned studies show that retinal function may be severely impaired outside the ring of increased AF, despite normal or near-normal levels of AF (Figs. 11A.5 and 11A.6). There is evidence that lipofuscin, and specifically A2E, rapidly fragments when exposed to light, and this could be a triggering factor for the complement system that would predispose the macula to disease (67). If the time course of lipofuscin degradation were similar in vivo, then its presence in the RPE would suggest continuing outer segment turnover and metabolic demand (42). Preservation of AF may occur in the presence of dysfunctional but intact photoreceptors, and it has been suggested that these cells may be amenable to functional rescue. Identification of viable retinal areas has become increasingly important given recent advances in gene therapy (68,69). It is also possible that clinicians will use AF as an outcome measure when assessing the efficacy of future treatments. However, recent OCT evidence has indicated disruption of the presumed photoreceptor layer in regions of preserved AF external to the ring (44). An implication is that maintenance of normal lipofuscin levels may not be dependent on normal photoreceptor structure. Further studies are required to examine this possibility.

Serial Imaging of Fundus Autofluorescence Abnormalities in Retinitis Pigmentosa

In some RP pedigrees, ring size may be related to the age of the patient or the duration of the disease (Fig. 11A.2A,C) (28). It was anticipated that the ring would

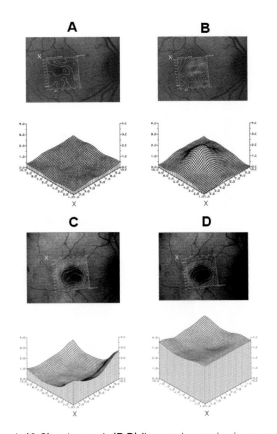

FIGURE 11A.5. Photopic **(A,C)** and scotopic **(B,D)** fine matrix mapping in one normal subject **(A,B)** and in one individual with a clinical diagnosis of RP and normal visual acuity **(C,D)**. Contour plots (rows 1 and 3) show sensitivity gradients over tested retinal areas; corresponding 3D plots (rows 2 and 4) show retinal location (abscissa, degrees) and thresholds (ordinate, log units). Labeling (x) shows correspondence between the orientation of contour and threshold plots. Pattern ERG, mfERG, and visual field from the same individual are shown in Fig. 11A.4. In the patient with RP, photopic thresholds at the fovea are normal, in keeping with preserved cone system function, but show marked elevation over areas external to the ring of increased AF. The ring aproximates to the internal edge of visual field constriction. Under dark-adapted conditions, threshold elevation is seen internal and external to the ring **(D)**, in keeping with rod system dysfunction over both the central macula and more eccentric areas.

constrict as the severity of the disease and macular involvement progressed; however, to date, only one longitudinal study has documented serial changes in RP. In 9 of 12 patients monitored over periods of up to 5 years, ring size and pattern ERG P50 amplitude were stable. In the remaining three individuals there was progressive constriction and narrowing of the ring of increased AF (35). Progressive ring constriction resulted in proportionate attenuation of the pattern ERGs to large but not small stimulus fields (Fig. 11A.6) and, as in previous studies, fine matrix mapping showed that the internal edge of visual field constriction was spatially concordant with the ring of increased AF (35). It was concluded that the visual field loss in RP mirrors the constriction of the AF ring, and follows progressive rod photoreceptor dysfunction over concentric macular areas within the ring.

The ring of increased AF may be of prognostic value in patients with normal visual acuity, but longitudinal imaging studies may be necessary to establish the stability or rate of ring constriction. Small rings of increased AF are sometimes associated

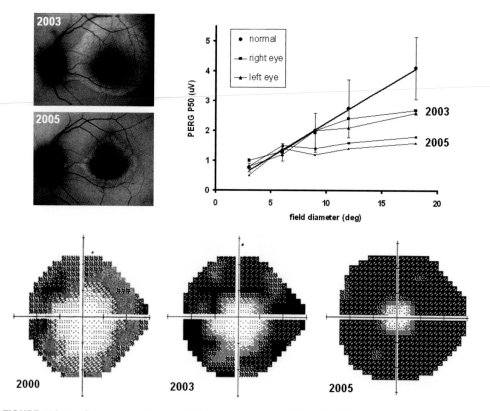

FIGURE 11A.6.   Comparison of fundus AF images and pattern ERGs with different sizes of checkerboards and Humphrey visual fields in a patient with Usher syndrome type 2 (mutation of USH2A) and normal visual acuity. Testing was repeated after 24 months. The ring of increased AF shows progressive constriction over the 2-year period, consistent with pattern ERG reduction and progressive visual field constriction. Filled circles and error bars in the graph show mean values and standard deviations for eight normal subjects; triangles and squares show patient data from right and left eyes. (From Robson AG, Saihan Z, Jenkins SA, et al. Functional characterisation and serial imaging of abnormal fundus autofluorescence in patients with retinitis pigmentosa and normal visual acuity. Br J Ophthalmol 2006;90:472–479, reproduced with permission from the BMJ Publishing Group.)

with mild foveal photopic sensitivity loss (29). Snellen visual acuity may be preserved, but such cases may have a poorer prognosis for retention of central vision.

Unlike cases of RP, some individuals with cone-rod dystrophy manifest rings that show progressive enlargement with time (54), suggesting an expanding centrifugal front of macular photoreceptor dysfunction. This was also suggested by a cross-sectional analysis within families (54): older individuals tended to have larger AF rings (Fig. 11A.2B,D) that surrounded areas of central RPE atrophy (Fig. 11A.2D). It is possible that rings associated with other causes of maculopathy (other than RP) may also expand with time as lesions become larger with age.

Fundus Autofluorescence in X-Linked Retinitis Pigmentosa

X-linked RP accounts for approximately 5% to 20% of RP cases (4,70–72); it generally has a severe phenotype with early onset and often leads to complete blindness by the fourth or fifth decade of life. Most cases are consequent upon mutation in *RPGR* or *RP2*. Typical fundus features of RP are present, which are usually severe in adults (73,74). Perhaps not surprisingly, given the severity of the phenotype, there is a paucity of data specifically describing AF in male patients with XLRP. One report described a ring of increased AF at an eccentricity of 3.5–15 degrees in a young affected male (47).

The detection of carrier status is important for genetic counseling purposes. Heterozygous carriers of XLRP can manifest a wide range of fundus and/or full-field ERG abnormalities that may be asymmetrical, resulting from random inactivation of the X-chromosome during embryogenesis. Carriers may have a normal fundus and a normal ERG when young, but often manifest a typical radially orientated "tapetal sheen" that has been considered pathognomonic of the disorder (75). The prevalence of either abnormal fundus or abnormal ERG increases with age (76). In one study of female carriers of XLRP (*RPGR*), abnormal AF was found in 9 of 11 individuals (47). Most of these showed a distinctive patchy, radially distributed pattern of increased AF in the parafovea that was not seen in other forms of RP (Fig. 11A.3B). The radial pattern of increased AF could be asymmetrical and occurred over parafoveal areas associated with the most pronounced sensitivity losses. Such changes can occur in the absence of severe fundus abnormalities and may prove useful in identifying carriers, and patient management.

DIFFERENTIAL DIAGNOSIS

RP must be distinguished from other causes of inherited or acquired pigmentary retinopathies and from other causes of night blindness that may occur with or without fundus changes. The differential diagnoses include the following:

1. Genetically determined causes of inherited retinal degenerations other than typical RP, including choroideremia, gyrate atrophy, enhanced S-cone syndrome/Goldman-Favre, inherited vitreoretinopathies such as familial exudative vitreo retinopathy (FEVR) and Wagner-Stickler syndrome, cone-rod dystrophies, Stargardt disease, and Sorsby fundus dystrophy.
2. Abnormal retinal pigmentation, including X-linked choroideremia carriers, X-linked ocular albinism carriers, and congenital hypertrophy of the RPE. Unilateral pigmentary retinopathy usually results from an acquired disease caused by retinal inflammation (toxoplasmosis and diffuse subacute unilateral neuroretinitis) or trauma (contusion, intraocular foreign body, and secondary siderosis).
3. RP *sine pigmento* must be differentiated from other causes of night vision impairment with normal fundus, including various forms of congenital stationary night blindness, vitamin A deficiency, carcinoma associated retinopathy, or autoimmune retinopathy.
4. Inflammatory conditions (syphilis, rubella, or other causes of posterior uveitis or chorioretinitis).
5. Drug toxicity (thioridazine, clofazimine, and chloroquine).
6. Resolved rhegmatogenous or exudative retinal detachments.

Family history, clinical context, and ancillary studies such as electrophysiology and fundus AF will be critical for accurate diagnosis.

SUMMARY

Fundus AF imaging is a useful tool in the diagnosis and evaluation of patients with RP and allows a precise characterization of the disease in conjunction with electrophysiology and OCT. An abnormal AF pattern may be observed in some patients with no other fundus abnormalities, indicating the presence of the disease. Functional correlation studies in cases of abnormal AF with preserved visual acuity have outlined its potential prognostic value in terms of predicting central macular involvement (i.e., stability on the ring of increased AF at the macula is likely to indicate a better prognosis in terms of retention of central vision). Distinctive radial patterns of increased AF may help identify carriers of X-linked RP and thus facilitate genetic counseling and patient management, and enable targeted mutational screening. With the development of new treatments, identification of viable retinal areas has become increasingly important, and this can be accomplished noninvasively by AF. In this context, AF will be important both for the selection of suitable candidates for future therapeutic interventions and as an outcome measurement in the evaluation of future treatments aimed at photoreceptor neuroprotection and/or restoration of function.

ACKNOWLEDGMENTS

The Foundation Fighting Blindness (AGR, IA), EVI-GENORET FP6 Integrated Project LSHG-CT-2005-512036 (ARW, IA), Steffen Suchert Foundation (IA).

REFERENCES

1. Williams DS. Usher syndrome: animal models, retinal function of Usher proteins, and prospects for gene therapy. Vision Res 2008;48:433–441.
2. Adams NA, Awadein A, Toma HS. The retinal ciliopathies. Ophthalmic Genet 2007;28:113–125.
3. Hartong DT, Berson EL, Dryja TP. Retinitis pigmentosa. Lancet 2006;368: 1795–1809.
4. Daiger SP, Bowne SJ, Sullivan LS. Perspective on genes and mutations causing retinitis pigmentosa. Arch Ophthalmol 2007;125:151–158.
5. Dryja TP, McGee TL, Reichel E, et al. A point mutation of the rhodopsin gene in one form of retinitis pigmentosa. Nature 1990;343:364–366.
6. Al-Maghtheh M, Vithana E, Tarttelin E, et al. Evidence for a major retinitis pigmentosa locus on 19q13.4 (RP11) and association with a unique bimodal expressivity phenotype. Am J Hum Genet 1996;59:864–871.
7. Sullivan LS, Bowne SJ, Birch DG, et al. Prevalence of disease-causing mutations in families with autosomal dominant retinitis pigmentosa: a screen of known genes in 200 families. Invest Ophthalmol Vis Sci 2006;47:3052–3064.
8. Dryja TP. Molecular genetics of Oguchi disease, fundus albipunctatus, and other forms of stationary night blindness: LVII Edward Jackson Memorial Lecture. Am J Ophthalmol 2000;130:547–563.
9. Zeitz C, Gross AK, Leifert D, et al. A novel constitutively active rhodopsin mutation (p.Ala295Val) causes autosomal dominant CSNB. Invest Ophthalmol Vis Sci 2008;49:4105–4114.
10. Audo I, Michaelides M, Robson AG, et al. Phenotypic variation in enhanced S-cone syndrome. Invest Ophthalmol Vis Sci 2008;49:2082–2093.
11. Coppieters F, Leroy BP, Beysen D, et al. Recurrent mutation in the first zinc finger of the orphan nuclear receptor NR2E3 causes autosomal dominant retinitis pigmentosa. Am J Hum Genet 2007;81:147–157.
12. Gire AI, Sullivan LS, Bowne SJ, et al. The Gly56Arg mutation in NR2E3 accounts for 1–2% of autosomal dominant retinitis pigmentosa. Mol Vis 2007;13:1970–1975.
13. Chang GQ, Hao Y, Wong F. Apoptosis: final common pathway of photoreceptor death in rd, rds, and rhodopsin mutant mice. Neuron 1993;11:595–605.
14. Portera-Cailliau C, Sung CH, Nathans J, et al. Apoptotic photoreceptor cell death in mouse models of retinitis pigmentosa. Proc Natl Acad Sci USA 1994;91:974–878.
15. Paquet-Durand F, Azadi S, Hauck SM, et al. Calpain is activated in degenerating photoreceptors in the rd1 mouse. J Neurochem 2006;96:802–814.
16. Paquet-Durand F, Johnson L, Ekström P. Calpain activity in retinal degeneration. J Neurosci Res 2007; 85:693–702.
17. Léveillard T, Mohand-Saïd S, Lorentz O, et al. Identification and characterization of rod-derived cone viability factor. Nat Genet 2004;36:755–759.
18. Sahel JA. Saving cone cells in hereditary rod diseases: a possible role for rod-derived cone viability factor (RdCVF) therapy. Retina 2005;25:S38–S39.
19. Fishman GA, Fishman M, Maggiano J. Macular lesions associated with retinitis pigmentosa. Arch Ophthalmol 1977;95:798–803.
20. Fishman GA, Maggiano JM, Fishman M. Foveal lesions seen in retinitis pigmentosa. Arch Ophthalmol 1977;95:1993–1996.

21. Hajali M, Fishman GA. The prevalence of cystoid macular oedema on optical coherence tomography in retinitis pigmentosa patients without cystic changes on fundus examination. Eye 2008;92:1065–1068.

22. Holder GE, Brigell MG, Hawlina M, et al. ISCEV standard for clinical pattern electroretinography—2007 update. Doc Ophthalmol 2007;114:111–116.

23. Hood DC, Bach M, Brigell M, et al. ISCEV guidelines for clinical multifocal electroretinography (2007 edition). Doc Ophthalmol 2008;116:1–11.

24. Berninger TA, Arden GB. The pattern electroretinogram. Eye 1988;2: S257–S283.

25. Holder GE, Robson AG, Hogg CR, et al. Pattern ERG: clinical overview, and some observations on associated fundus autofluorescence imaging in inherited maculopathy. Doc Ophthalmol 2003;106:17–23.

26. Hood DC. Assessing retinal function with the multifocal technique. Prog Retin Eye Res 2000;19:607–646.

27. Holder GE, Robson AG. Paediatric electrophysiology: a practical approach. In: Lorenz B, ed. Essentials in Ophthalmology. Berlin: Springer-Verlag, 2006, 133–155.

28. Robson AG, El-Amir A, Bailey C, et al. Pattern ERG correlates of abnormal fundus autofluorescence in patients with retinitis pigmentosa and normal visual acuity. Invest Ophthalmol Vis Sci 2003;44:3544–3550.

29. Robson AG, Egan CA, Luong VA, et al. Comparison of fundus autofluorescence with photopic and scotopic fine-matrix mapping in patients with retinitis pigmentosa and normal visual acuity. Invest Ophthalmol Vis Sci 2004;45: 4119–4125.

30. Robson AG, Michaelides M, Saihan Z, et al. Functional characteristics of patients with retinal dystrophy that manifest abnormal parafoveal annuli of high density fundus autofluorescence; a review and update. Doc Ophthalmol 2008;116:79–89.

31. Popovic P, Jarc-Vidmar M, Hawlina M. Abnormal fundus autofluorescence in relation to retinal function in patients with retinitis pigmentosa. Graefes Arch Clin Exp Ophthalmol 2005;243:1018–1027.

32. Kondo M, Miyake Y, Horiguchi M, et al. Clinical evaluation of multifocal electroretinogram. Invest Ophthalmol Vis Sci 1995;36:2146–2150.

33. Hood DC, Holopigian K, Greenstein V, et al. Assessment of local retinal function in patients with retinitis pigmentosa using the multi-focal ERG technique. Vision Res 1998;38:163–179.

34. Granse L, Ponjavic V, Andreasson S. Full-field ERG, multifocal ERG and multifocal VEP in patients with retinitis pigmentosa and residual central visual fields. Acta Ophthalmol Scand 2004;82:701–706.

35. Robson AG, Saihan Z, Jenkins SA, et al. Functional characterisation and serial imaging of abnormal fundus autofluorescence in patients with retinitis pigmentosa and normal visual acuity. Br J Ophthalmol 2006;90:472–479.

36. Newsome DA. Retinal fluorescein leakage in retinitis pigmentosa. Am J Ophthalmol 1986;101:354–360.

37. Hirakawa H, Iijima H, Gohdo T, et al. Optical coherence tomography of cystoid macular edema associated with retinitis pigmentosa. Am J Ophthalmol 1999;128:185–191.

38. Apushkin MA, Fishman GA, Janowicz MJ. Monitoring cystoid macular edema by optical coherence tomography in patients with retinitis pigmentosa. Ophthalmology 2004;111:1899–1904.

39. Chung H, Hwang JU, Kim JG, et al. Optical coherence tomography in the diagnosis and monitoring of cystoid macular edema in patients with retinitis pigmentosa. Retina 2006;26:922–927.

40. Witkin AJ, Ko TH, Fujimoto JG, et al. Ultra-high resolution optical coherence tomography assessment of photoreceptors in retinitis pigmentosa and related diseases. Am J Ophthalmol 2006;142:945–952.

41. Podoleanu AG, Rosen RB. Combinations of techniques in imaging the retina with high resolution. Prog Retin Eye Res 2008;27:464–499.

42. von Rückmann A, Fitzke FW, Bird AC. Distribution of fundus autofluorescence with a scanning laser ophthalmoscope. Br J Ophthalmol 1995;79:407–412.

43. von Rückmann A, Fitzke FW, Bird AC. Distribution of pigment epithelium autofluorescence in retinal disease state recorded in vivo and its change over time. Graefes Arch Clin Exp Ophthalmol 1999;237: 1–9.

44. Murakami T, Akimoto M, Ooto S, et al. Association between abnormal autofluorescence and photoreceptor disorganization in retinitis pigmentosa. Am J Ophthalmol 2008;145:87–94.

45. Saihan Z, Robson AG, Haralambous E, et al. Analysis of fundal autofluorescence images in a cohort of individuals with mutations in USH2A. Invest Ophthalmol Vis Sci 2007;48: ARVO E-abstract 3686.

46. Audo I, Robson AG, Hykin P, et al. FAF imaging of retinal diseases. Rev Ophthalmol 2005;12.

47. Wegscheider E, Preising MN, Lorenz B. Fundus autofluorescence in carriers of X-linked recessive retinitis pigmentosa associated with mutations in RPGR, and correlation with electrophysiological and psychophysical data. Graefes Arch Clin Exp Ophthalmol 2004;242:501–511.

48. Wabbels B, Demmler A, Paunescu K, et al. Fundus autofluorescence in children and teenagers with hereditary retinal diseases. Graefes Arch Clin Exp Ophthalmol 2006;244:36–45.

49. Scholl HP, Chong NH, Robson AG, et al. Fundus autofluorescence in patients with leber congenital amaurosis. Invest Ophthalmol Vis Sci 2004;45: 2747–2752.

50. Downes SM, Holder GE, Fitzke FW, et al. Autosomal dominant cone and cone-rod dystrophy with mutations in the guanylate cyclase activator 1A gene-encoding guanylate cyclase activating protein-1. Arch Ophthalmol 2001;119: 96–105.

51. Downes SM, Payne AM, Kelsell RE, et al. Autosomal dominant cone-rod dystrophy with mutations in the guanylate cyclase 2D gene encoding retinal guanylate cyclase-1. Arch Ophthalmol 2001;119:1667–1673.

52. Michaelides M, Holder GE, Hunt DM, et al. A detailed study of the phenotype of an autosomal dominant cone-rod dystrophy (CORD7) associated with mutation in the gene for RIM1. Br J Ophthalmol 2005;89:198–206.

53. Ebenezer ND, Michaelides M, Jenkins SA, et al. Identification of novel RPGR ORF15 mutations in X-linked progressive cone-rod dystrophy (XLCORD) families. Invest Ophthalmol Vis Sci 2005;46: 1891–1898.
54. Robson AG, Michaelides M, Luong VA, et al. Functional correlates of fundus autofluorescence abnormalities in patients with RPGR or RIMS1 mutations causing cone or cone-rod dystrophy. Br J Ophthalmol 2008;92:95–102.
55. Michaelides M, Holder GE, Webster AR, et al. A detailed phenotypic study of "cone dystrophy with supernormal rod ERG." Br J Ophthalmol 2005;89: 332–339.
56. Robson AG, Michaelides M, Wu H, et al. Fundus autofluorescence and intensity-response functions in "cone dystrophy with supernormal rod electroretinogram" consequent upon mutation in KCNV2. Invest Ophthalmol Vis Sci 2008;49:ARVO E-abstract 2167.
57. Jarc-Vidmar M, Kraut A, Hawlina M. Fundus autofluorescence imaging in Best's vitelliform dystrophy. Klin Monatsbl Augenheilkd 2003;220:861–867.
58. Tsang SH, Vaclavik V, Bird AC, et al. Novel phenotypic and genotypic findings in X-linked retinoschisis. Arch Ophthalmol 2007;125:259–267.
59. Fleckenstein M, Charbel Issa P, Fuchs HA, et al. Discrete arcs of increased fundus autofluorescence in retinal dystrophies and functional correlate on microperimetry. Eye 2008; March 14 [Epub ahead of print].
60. Poloschek CM, Hansen LL, Bach M. Annular fundus autofluorescence abnormality in a case of macular dystrophy. Doc Ophthalmol 2008;116:91–95.
61. Wüstemeyer H, Jahn C, Nestler A, et al. A new instrument for the quantification of macular pigment density: first results in patients with AMD and healthy subjects. Graefes Arch Clin Exp Ophthalmol 2002;240:666–671.
62. Meyerle CB, Fisher YL, Spaide RF. Autofluorescence and visual field loss in sector retinitis pigmentosa. Retina 2006;26:248–250.
63. Chen JC, Fitzke FW, Pauleikhoff D, et al. Functional loss in age-related Bruch's membrane change with choroidal perfusion defect. Invest Ophthalmol Vis Sci 1992;33:334–340.
64. Westcott MC, Garway-Heath DF, Fitzke FW, et al. Use of high spatial resolution perimetry to identify scotomata not apparent with conventional perimetry in the nasal field of glaucomatous subjects. Br J Ophthalmol 2002;86:761–766.
65. Scholl HP, Bellmann C, Dandekar SS, et al. Photopic and scotopic fine matrix mapping of retinal areas of increased fundus autofluorescence in patients with age-related maculopathy. Invest Ophthalmol Vis Sci 2004;45:574–583.
66. Robson AG, Moreland JD, Pauleikhoff D, et al. Macular pigment density and distribution: comparison of fundus autofluorescence with minimum motion photometry. Vision Res 2003;43:1765–1775.
67. Zhou J, Jang YP, Kim SR, et al. Complement activation by photooxidation products of A2E, a lipofuscin constituent of the retinal pigment epithelium. Proc Natl Acad Sci USA 2006;103:16182–16187.
68. Bainbridge JW, Smith AJ, Barker SS, et al. Effect of gene therapy on visual function in Leber's congenital amaurosis. N Engl J Med 2008;358:2231–2239.
69. Maguire AM, Simonelli F, Pierce EA, et al. Safety and efficacy of gene transfer for Leber's congenital amaurosis. N Engl J Med 2008;358:2240–2248.
70. Jay M. On the heredity of retinitis pigmentosa. Br J Ophthalmol 1982;66: 405–416.
71. Bird AC, Heckenlively JR. X-linked recessive retinitis pigmentosa (X-linked pigmentary retinopathies). In: Heckenlively JR, ed. Retinitis Pigmentosa. Philadelphia: JB Lippincott, 1988:162–176.
72. Prokisch H, Hartig M, Hellinger R, et al. A population-based epidemiological and genetic study of X-linked retinitis pigmentosa. Invest Ophthalmol Vis Sci 2007;48:4012–4018.
73. Flaxel CJ, Jay M, Thiselton DL, et al. Difference between RP2 and RP3 phenotypes in X linked retinitis pigmentosa. Br J Ophthalmol 1999;83:1144–1148.
74. Lorenz B, Andrassi M, Kretschmann U. Phenotype in two families with RP3 associated with RPGR mutations. Ophthalmic Genet 2003;24:89–101.
75. Heckenlively JR, Weleber RG. X-linked recessive cone dystrophy with tapetal-like sheen. A newly recognized entity with Mizuo-Nakamura phenomenon. Arch Ophthalmol 1986;104:1322–1328.
76. Jenkins SA, Bird AC, Moore AT, et al. What is the reduced risk of carrier status in females of X-linked retinal dystrophy families when the fundus and ERG are normal? ARVO 2006;E-abstract 1021.

Fundus Autofluorescence in Cone and Cone-Rod Dystrophies

INTRODUCTION

The cone dystrophies (COD) and cone-rod dystrophies (CORD) are a heterogeneous group of disorders in terms of both clinical features and underlying genetic basis. They are characterized by reduced central vision, color vision abnormalities, visual field loss, and a variable degree of nystagmus and photophobia. There is absent or severely impaired cone function on electroretinography (ERG) and psychophysical testing. Patients with CORD develop additional rod system abnormalities that lead to night-blindness later in the disease process.

Disorders of cone function can be usefully divided into stationary (cone dysfunction syndromes) and progressive (COD and CORD) disorders (1,2). The stationary cone dysfunction syndromes often present shortly after birth or in infancy. Progressive cone dystrophies usually present in childhood or early adulthood, with many patients developing rod photoreceptor involvement later in life, thereby leading to considerable overlap between progressive COD and CORD. In this chapter the term CORD is used to describe those disorders in which subjects have significant secondary involvement of the rod system at an early stage, in contrast to progressive COD, in which rod involvement, if present, occurs late in the disease process.

COD and CORD can be inherited as autosomal dominant (AD), autosomal recessive (AR), or X-linked (XL) recessive traits. When an inheritance pattern can be reliably established, it is most commonly AD (3,4). Mutations in 14 genes have been described to date, with mutations in *peripherin/RDS*, *ABCA4*, and *RPGR* being the most common causes of AD, AR, and XL COD and CORD, respectively (2,5).

This chapter will concentrate only on progressive disorders, including COD and CORD, since data on fundus autofluorescence (AF) imaging in the various stationary cone dysfunction syndromes are, to date, very limited (6).

MOLECULAR BASIS

The molecular basis of COD and CORD is complex because of their genetic heterogeneity. The molecular basis of some of the most common forms of COD and CORD is discussed below (see Fundus Autofluorescence subsection).

CLINICAL FEATURES

Patients with COD are not usually symptomatic until late childhood or early adulthood. The age of onset of visual loss and the rate and degree of progression is variable; however, visual acuity usually deteriorates over time to the level of 20/200-counting

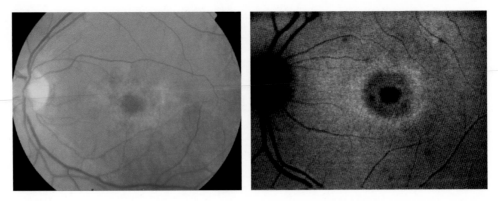

FIGURE 11B.1. Color fundus photograph (*left*) and AF image (*right*) in a patient with cone dystrophy and bull's-eye maculopathy.

fingers. Photophobia is often a prominent early symptom. Individuals with CORD will, in addition, complain of night-blindness. The retinal dystrophy is usually isolated but may be associated with systemic abnormalities (2).

In COD, fundus examination may show a typical bull's-eye appearance (Fig. 11B.1). However, in some cases there may only be minor macular retinal pigment epithelium (RPE) disturbance. The optic discs show a variable degree of temporal pallor. The retinal periphery is usually normal. In CORD, fundus examination may show a bull's-eye appearance in the early stages, with macular atrophy developing over time. Peripheral RPE atrophy, retinal pigmentation, arteriolar attenuation, and optic disc pallor can be seen in the late stages of the disease, similarly to the rod-cone dystrophies (see Chapter 11A). The sign of the "dark choroid" may be seen on fluorescein angiography (7). A tapetal-like sheen, which may change in appearance on dark adaptation (the Mizuo-Nakamura phenomenon), has been described in association with XL-CORD (8).

DIAGNOSTIC TESTS

Electrophysiology

In COD or in the early stages of CORD, ERG shows normal rod responses but significantly abnormal cone responses. The 30Hz flicker ERG is usually of increased implicit time, but rarely the implicit time is normal and amplitude reduction is the only abnormality (Table 11B.1) (9,10). In CORD, both rod and cone thresholds are elevated on psychophysical testing and the ERG shows reduced rod and cone amplitudes, with the cone ERGs being more abnormal than the rod ERGs. A negative ERG can be also observed in some patients (Table 11B.1). An unusual form of CORD with abnormal cone function and supernormal rod responses has been also described (11,12). Obligate carriers of XL COD and CORD may show evidence of cone dysfunction on electrophysiological or psychophysical testing (13–15).

Imaging Studies

Fluorescein angiography, indocyanine green angiography, and optical coherence tomography do not, to date, have a significant role in the evaluation of patients with COD and CORD.

TABLE 11B.1   **Genetics, Age of Onset, Fundus Features, Autofluorescence, and Electrophysiological Abnormalities in Cone and Cone-Rod Dystrophies**

Gene Defect (inheritance)	Age of Onset	Phenotype	Fundus Changes	AF	PERG	ERG
GUCA1A (AD)	3rd–5th decade	COD, CORD	ranges from mild macular RPE disturbance to RPE atrophy, with normal peripheral retina	focal increased AF at the macula; perifoveal rings of increased AF; reduced AF in areas of atrophy	severely reduced or undetectable	severely reduced amplitude of single flash and flicker with minimal or no 30Hz flicker implicit time shift; in CORD, additional reduction in rod responses
GUCY2D (AD)	1st, 2nd decade	CORD	macular and peripheral atrophy	increased foveal in areas of atrophy AF; reduced AF in areas of atrophy	severely reduced or undetectable	reduced cone and rod responses;* "negative ERG"
Peripherin (AD)	2nd, 3rd decade	CORD	macular RPE mottling, macular atrophy, peripheral retinal atrophy and areas of peripheral RPE hyperpigmentation	"speckled" AF	reduced responses	reduced cone and rod responses
CRX (AD)	1st decade	CORD	macular and later peripheral retinal degeneration	reduced AF in areas of atrophy, "speckled" AF in the midperipheral retina	reduced responses	reduced cone and rod responses; "negative ERG"
RIMS 1 (AD)	2nd–5th decade	CORD	ranges from mild macular RPE disturbance to atrophy and pigmentation•	reduced AF at the center of the macula surrounded by a ring of increased AF	absent or severely reduced	reduced cone and rod responses, often normal 30Hz flicker implicit time
ABCA4 (AR)	1st–3rd decade	COD, CORD	macular atrophy, bull's eye appearance, peripheral pigmentary changes in advanced disease	reduced AF at the center of the macula surrounded by a ring of increased AF; reduced AF only	absent or severely reduced	severely reduced cone responses; in CORD, additional reduction in rod responses
KCNV2 (AR)	1st, 2nd decade	COD	RPE disturbance at the macula	most commonly reduced AF at the center of the macula surrounded by a ring of increased AF	absent or severely reduced	reduced rod b-wave amplitude with low intensity stimulus; often higher than normal with high flash energies, cone responses severely reduced
RPGR (X-linked)	5th decade	COD	macular atrophy	perifoveal ring of increased AF	absent or severely reduced	reduced cone responses
RPGR (X-linked)	2nd–4th decade	CORD	range from mild macular RPE disturbance to extensive atrophy and hyperpigmentation	reduced macular AF, reduced AF surrounded by a ring of increased AF	absent or severely reduced	reduced cone and rod responses

AF, autofluorescence; ERG, full-field electroretinogram; PERG, pattern electroretinogram; RPE, retinal pigment epithelium; *, ERG is usually nonrecordable by the fourth decade of life; •, attenuation of retinal blood vessels and peripheral retinal atrophy can occasionally be observed.
See text for detailed description of AF findings. In CORD, ERG reveals greater reductions in cone than in rod responses. AD, autosomal dominant; AR, autosomal recessive.

Fundus Autofluorescence

Fundus AF imaging has been used to assist in the diagnosis, to aid detailed description of the phenotype, and to provide insights into the natural history and underlying pathophysiology of COD and CORD.

COD and CORD are classified below based on their mode of inheritance and their causative genes (only those for which well-documented AF data are available will be discussed in this section). Fundus AF features will be described herein. The clinical, electrophysiological, and AF findings are summarized in Table 11B.1.

Fundus Autofluorescence Findings in Autosomal Dominant Disease

To date, seven genes have been associated with AD disease. AF data are available for COD and CORD caused by mutations in *GUCA1A, GUCY2D, Peripherin/RDS, CRX,* and *RIMS1,* as described below.

COD and CORD Associated with *GUCA1A*

Photophobia, reduced central vision, and generalized dyschromatopsia, with no evidence of nystagmus, are usually observed. In some subjects, RPE changes may be subtle, especially in the early stages of the disease. In these patients, AF imaging is helpful in confirming the macular abnormality by identifying localized area(s) of increased macular AF (Fig. 11B.2) (9,16). In some individuals, perifoveal rings of increased AF have been described that are similar to those observed in retinitis pigmentosa (see Chapter 11, Retinitis Pigmentosa subsection) (9); these rings are increasingly recognized as features of COD and CORD (17,18). In older subjects with macular atrophy, corresponding areas of decreased AF are seen (Fig. 11B.3).

The gene *GUCA1A* encodes the phototransduction protein guanylate cyclase activating protein-1 (GCAP1). Mutant GCAP1 protein activates retinal guanylate cyclase-1 (RetGC1) at low Ca^{2+} concentrations but fails to inactivate it at high Ca^{2+} concentrations, thereby leading to a constant activation of RetGC1 in photoreceptors, even at the high Ca^{2+} concentrations of the dark-adapted state (Fig. 11B.4). The consequent dysregulation of intracellular Ca^{2+} and cGMP levels is believed to lead to cell death.

CORD Associated with *GUCY2D*

Moderate myopia is common, with photophobia and pendular nystagmus seen in affected individuals, who experience the major visual reduction in the second or third decade of life (19–21). Initially there is only absent tritan color discrimination, but this progresses to complete loss of color vision over time.

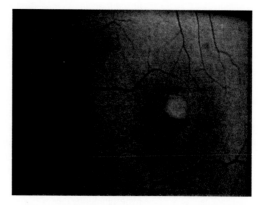

FIGURE 11B.2. AD-COD and CORD (*GUCA1A*). Fundus AF image showing localized increased macular AF.

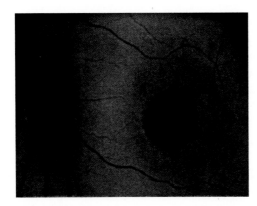

FIGURE 11B.3. AD-COD and CORD (*GUCA1A*). Fundus AF image showing decreased macular AF.

The earliest AF abnormality is increased AF at the fovea, suggesting that this is the site of initial dysfunction (21). A markedly reduced AF signal is detected at the site of macular atrophy, indicating loss of photoreceptor cells, or at least their outer segments. In the later stages, subjects have an annulus of increased AF surrounding areas of central atrophy (see below). Increased AF at the edge of atrophy is likely to indicate an area destined to become atrophic (17,18).

Families with AD-CORD associated with single *GUCY2D* missense mutations have a much milder phenotype (only mild rod involvement) than subjects with complex mutations (moderate to severe rod loss) (19–23).

The gene *GUCY2D* encodes retinal guanylate cyclase 1 (RetCG1) (Fig. 11B.4). Mutant RetGC1 has been shown to have a higher apparent affinity for GCAP1 than wild-type RetGC1, and an altered Ca^{2+} sensitivity of the GCAP1 activation, with marked residual activity at high Ca^{2+} concentrations (24). Therefore, as seen in GCAP1 mutations, RetGC1 mutations result in a failure to inactivate cyclase activity at high physiological Ca^{2+} concentrations in the photoreceptors, with a subsequent

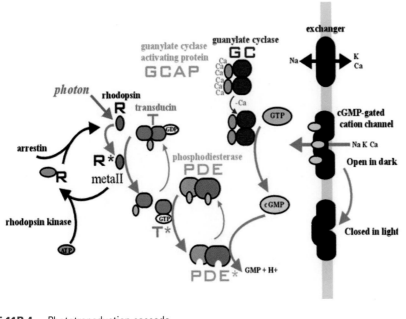

FIGURE 11B.4. Phototransduction cascade.

abnormal phototransduction recovery phase. This dysregulation of intracellular Ca^{2+} and cGMP levels may lead to cell death.

It is plausible that RetGC1, in addition to having a role in phototransduction, may have a function at the photoreceptor synaptic terminal, as suggested by the "negative ERG" often observed in patients carrying mutations in *GUCY2D* (25).

CORD Associated with *Peripherin/RDS*

To date, four mutations in *peripherin/RDS* have been reported in Japanese families and a large British family (26–29). Affected individuals in the Japanese families had typical symptoms, electrophysiological findings associated with CORD, and little intrafamilial variability. Ophthalmoscopy revealed macular RPE atrophy with peripheral retinal degeneration in the later stages. Although mutations in the Arg172Trp (R172W) *peripherin/RDS* were previously reported to cause a fully penetrant progressive macular dystrophy with high intra- and interfamilial consistency of phenotype (30,31), this mutation has now also been described in a large British family with marked intrafamilial phenotypic variation, including a CORD phenotype (29). The majority of affected individuals had reduced central vision starting in the second or third decade, and several individuals became aware of nyctalopia and slow dark adaptation at a later stage.

AF imaging in the majority of patients reveals a highly characteristic speckled macular appearance with areas of increased and decreased AF (Fig. 11B.5).

The peripherin/RDS protein is found in rod and cone photoreceptor outer segment discs in a complex with ROM1. It is believed to function as an adhesion molecule involved in the stabilization and maintenance of a compact arrangement of outer segment discs (32,33). To date, four mutations in *peripherin/RDS* have been associated with a CORD phenotype: Asn244His (26,27), Tyr184Ser (27), Val200Glu (28), and Arg172Trp (29). The amino acids Arg172, Tyr184, Val200, and Asn244 are all located in the second intradiscal loop (EC-2) of the peripherin/RDS protein, which contains seven conserved cysteine residues, six of which are important for protein folding (33). The seventh cysteine (C150) in the EC-2 domain forms an intermolecular disulfide bond with the C150 residue in another molecule of either peripherin/RDS or ROM1 to form higher-order oligomeric complexes that are necessary for outer segment disc generation and stabilization (33). This loop, within which the CORD-associated mutations are located, is therefore critical for the functioning of the protein.

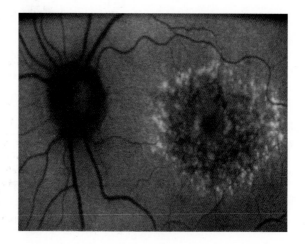

FIGURE 11B.5.   AD-CORD (*peripherin/RDS*). AF imaging showing florid typical abnormal speckled appearance, with areas of increased and decreased macular AF.

CORD Associated with *CRX*

A severe early-onset AD-CORD phenotype associated with *CRX* mutations (cone-rod homeobox-containing gene) has been reported in patients of diverse origin, with little or no visual function remaining after the age of 50 years (34–37).

AF imaging undertaken in a German CORD family with CRX mutations revealed that AF was severely reduced in areas of atrophy but otherwise well preserved at the posterior pole (37). A speckled appearance with areas of increased and decreased AF was noted in the mid-periphery in several but not all subjects. This feature may prove helpful in suggesting *CRX* as the underlying genetic cause (Fig. 11B.6) (37).

CRX is a photoreceptor-specific transcription factor and plays a crucial role in the differentiation and maintenance of photoreceptor cells (38,39). The electronegative ERG changes seen in patients with *CRX* mutations suggest that inner retinal function is primarily impaired. Since retinal expression of *CRX* is limited to photoreceptors (38,39), this dysfunction may be the result of abnormal photoreceptor communication with second-order retinal neurones. This is supported by the finding that photoreceptors in *CRX* knockout mice have severely abnormal synaptic endings in the outer plexiform layer (40).

In addition to directly regulating the expression of several photoreceptor-specific genes (including the opsins and arrestin), *CRX* also interacts with the transcription factors *NRL* (neural retina leucine zipper) and *NR2E3* to affect expression of genes critical to photoreceptor morphogenesis and function (41,42).

CORD Associated with *RIMS1*

A CORD phenotype associated with a point mutation in *RIMS1* (formerly known as *RIM1*), a gene encoding a photoreceptor synaptic protein, was reported in a four-generation British family (43,44). Most of these individuals had experienced

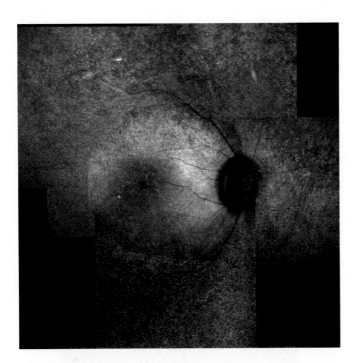

FIGURE 11B.6.   AD-CORD (*CRX*). AF image showing reduced AF in areas of atrophy, but otherwise good preservation at the posterior pole. A speckled appearance with areas of increased and decreased AF is seen in the mid-periphery.

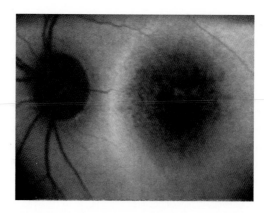

FIGURE 11B.7.   AD-CORD (*RIMS1*). Fundus AF image showing decreased AF centrally with a surrounding ring of increased AF.

progressive deterioration in central vision, night vision, and peripheral visual field constriction, especially during the third and fourth decades. They had mild photophobia and no nystagmus. Mild to moderate generalized dyschromatopsia was detected in the majority of the individuals.

AF imaging revealed decreased macular AF centrally surrounded by a ring of increased AF in the majority of patients (Figs. 11B.7 and 11B.8) (17,18,43). A perifoveal ring of increased AF was also detected in the youngest individual (18 years old), who had very mild RPE disturbance at the macula and was asymptomatic (Fig. 11B.8). The presence of a perifoveal ring of increased AF may be very helpful in establishing an early diagnosis in such cases. The size of the AF ring correlated with the age of the patient and enlarged over time (17). Photopic and scotopic fine matrix mapping and multifocal ERG (mfERG) demonstrated that the rings of increased AF were associated with a gradient of scotopic and photopic sensitivity loss when comparing to retinal locations internal and external to the ring of increased AF (see also Chapter 11A). Pattern ERG P50 amplitude, when detectable, was inversely related to the size of the AF ring (see also Chapter 11A). Increased AF was therefore associated with reduced rod and cone sensitivity, rather than photoreceptor cell death. Bull's-eye lesions, present in two individuals, consisted of a ring of decreased perifoveal AF bordered peripherally and centrally by increased AF (Fig. 11B.9). The normal ERG recorded in these patients suggests that there is no widespread dysfunction of the RPE.

RIMS1 is expressed in brain and retinal photoreceptors, where it is localized to the presynaptic ribbons in ribbon synapses. The protein product is believed to play an

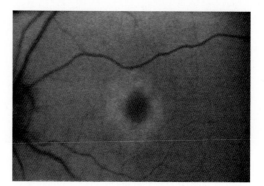

FIGURE 11B.8.   AD-CORD (*RIMS1*). AF image showing a perifoveal ring of relative increased AF.

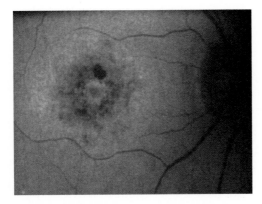

FIGURE 11B.9.   AD-CORD (*RIMS1*). Fundus AF image showing concentric rings of increased and decreased AF in a bull's-eye maculopathy-like pattern.

important role in synaptic transmission and plasticity (45). Mutations in *RIMS1* may alter the rate of synaptic vesicle docking and fusion in response to a Ca^{2+} signal (44).

Fundus Autofluorescence in Autosomal Recessive Disease

To date, six genes have been associated with AR disease. Data are available for COD and CORD caused by mutations in *ABCA4* and *KCNV2*, as described below.

COD and CORD Associated with *ABCA4*

Mutations in *ABCA4* are the most common cause of AR-CORD (46–48). All patients experience visual loss early in life, impaired color vision, and a central scotoma (47).

Subjects with COD may have a ring of increased AF surrounding decreased foveal AF (Fig. 11B.10). Although some patients with CORD have the same pattern of AF, the majority have decreased foveal AF only (Fig. 11B.11) (49,50). In a recent study involving patients with disease-causing variants in *ABCA4* and either Stargardt disease (STGD) or CORD, a peripapillary ring of normal-appearing AF was visible at all stages of disease (51). This finding is highly suggestive of *ABCA4*-related retinopathy.

ABCA4 encodes a transmembrane rim protein (an outwardly directed flippase of all-*trans* retinal) that is located in the discs of rod and cone outer segments and is involved in ATP-dependent transport of retinoids from photoreceptor to RPE during

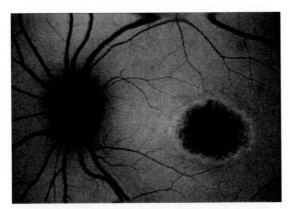

FIGURE 11B.10.   AR-COD (*ABCA4*). AF image showing a ring of increased AF surrounding decreased foveal AF.

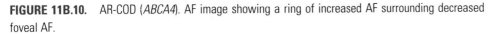

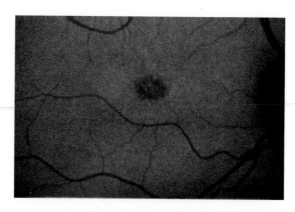

FIGURE 11B.11.   AR-CORD (*ABCA4*) AF image showing decreased foveal AF.

the visual cycle. Failure of this transport results in deposition of A2E (N-retinylidene-N-retinylethanolamine) in the RPE, with RPE cell dysfunction and subsequent loss of photoreceptors (see also Chapter 11, Stargardt-Fundus flavimaculatus subsection).

COD Associated with *KCNV2* (COD/SuperROD)

An unusual AR-CORD has been described with abnormal photopic responses associated with supernormal and delayed rod ERG b-waves (11,12,52). Subjects present with reduced central vision and marked photophobia, are usually myopic, and have reduced color discrimination predominantly along the red-green axes. Patients with more advanced disease complain of nyctalopia.

In most patients, AF imaging reveals a perifoveal ring of increased AF. In some patients (generally older), however, an area of increased AF may be seen at the central macula (Fig. 11B.12), suggesting that accumulation of AF material at the center of the macula may occur over time. In the oldest subject studied, central atrophy was present surrounded by an annulus of relatively increased AF (Fig. 11B.13), indicating that the accumulated autofluorescent material may lead to cell death (18,52). The electrophysiological data (see Table 11B.1) are consistent with the site of dysfunction being post-phototransduction but pre-inner nuclear layer, most probably at the first synapse (52,53).

KCNV2 encodes a voltage-gated K$^+$ channel subunit expressed in rods and cones (54). The effects of these mutations suggest that *KCNV2* is involved in setting the resting potential and voltage response of photoreceptors.

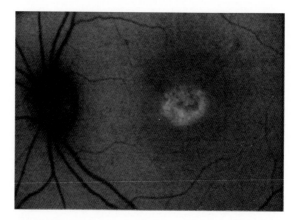

FIGURE 11B.12.   Cone dystrophy with supernormal rod ERG (*KCNV2*). Fundus AF image showing markedly increased macular AF surrounded by a ring of relative decreased AF.

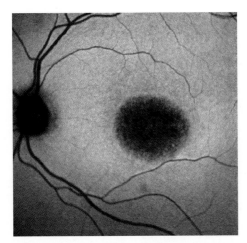

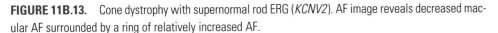

FIGURE 11B.13.   Cone dystrophy with supernormal rod ERG (*KCNV2*). AF image reveals decreased macular AF surrounded by a ring of relatively increased AF.

Fundus Autofluorescence in X-Linked Disease

Mutations in *RPGR* are a common cause of XL-CORD (14,55) and have also been identified in patients with XL-COD (14,56).

COD and CORD Associated with *RPGR*

Only two families with XL-COD have been reported, with patients having typical COD findings (Table 11B.1) (56). However, they were unusual in having a late onset of reduced vision in the fifth decade. In XL-CORD, affected males experience progressive deterioration in central vision and subsequently night vision, mild photophobia, and moderate to high myopia (14).

AF imaging in COD patients may reveal a perifoveal ring of increased AF (14). Detailed AF imaging has been assessed in two unrelated XL-CORD families (14). A ring of increased AF around the fovea is often observed; older affected subjects may also have decreased AF corresponding to areas of atrophy seen ophthalmoscopically (Fig. 11B.14). The ring of increased AF can be the sole abnormality detected in otherwise asymptomatic patients (Fig. 11B.15) (14), underlining the importance of AF imaging in establishing an early diagnosis. Unlike female carriers of rod-cone

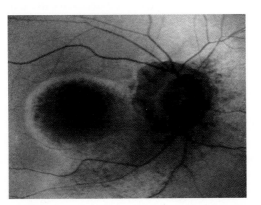

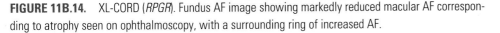

FIGURE 11B.14.   XL-CORD (*RPGR*). Fundus AF image showing markedly reduced macular AF corresponding to atrophy seen on ophthalmoscopy, with a surrounding ring of increased AF.

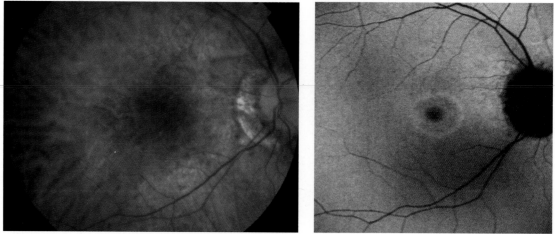

FIGURE 11B.15. XL-CORD (*RPGR*). Color fundus photograph **(A)** shows no abnormalities in an asymptomatic patient in whom AF imaging **(B)** revealed a ring of increased AF.

dystrophy associated with *RPGR* mutations (57), CORD carrier females have normal AF reported to date (14).

Mutations in the retinitis pigmentosa GTPase regulator (*RPGR*) gene are also a major cause of XL RP. RPGR has been shown to interact with RPGRIP1. Both proteins colocalize to the outer segments of rod and cone photoreceptors, principally in connecting cilia of rods and cones, and thus are thought to have an important role in intracellular transport.

SUMMARY

COD and CORD represent an important cause of blindness in children and young adults for which there is currently no treatment available. It is important, however, to establish a correct diagnosis to provide patients with an accurate prognosis and informed genetic counseling.

Fundus AF imaging plays an important role in the evaluation of patients with COD and CORD. As shown in this chapter, in many instances, AF imaging may aid in establishing an early diagnosis before the onset of symptoms and before any ophthalmoscopic abnormalities are detected. Furthermore, the pattern of AF may be so characteristic and recognizable (e.g., the speckled AF appearance associated with mutations in *peripherin/RDS*) that it may help the clinician to not identify the disorder on clinical grounds alone, but also to target genetic testing. The distribution of AF has been helpful also in shedding light on the natural history and pathogenesis of these disorders. For example, in CORD associated with *GUCY2D*, the earliest abnormality of increased AF at the fovea implies that this is the site of initial dysfunction, in contrast to bull's-eye dystrophies, in which there is central sparing in the early stages of the disease. Moreover, the high correlation found between AF and PERG, and mfERG and photopic and scotopic fine matrix mapping in patients with perifoveal rings of increased AF demonstrates that AF abnormalities have functional significance. Therefore, AF imaging may help in identifying suitable patients and viable areas of retina amenable to future therapies, and may also have a role in assessing the response to these treatments.

REFERENCES

1. Michaelides M, Hunt DM, Moore AT. The cone dysfunction syndromes. Br J Ophthalmol 2004;88: 291–297.

2. Michaelides M, Hardcastle AJ, Hunt DM, et al. Progressive cone and cone-rod dystrophies: phenotypes and underlying molecular genetic basis. Surv Ophthalmol 2006;51:232–258.

3. Krill AE, Deutman AF, Fishman M. The cone degenerations. Doc Ophthalmol 1973;35:1–80.

4. Moore AT. Cone and cone-rod dystrophies. J Med Genet 1992;29:289–290.

5. Maugeri A, Klevering BJ, Rohrschneider K, et al. Mutations in the *ABCA4* (*ABCR*) gene are the major cause of autosomal recessive cone-rod dystrophy. Am J Hum Genet 2000;67:960–966.

6. Michaelides M, Aligianis IA, Holder GE, et al. Cone dystrophy phenotype associated with a frameshift mutation (M280fsX291) in the α-subunit of cone-specific transducin (*GNAT2*). Br J Ophthalmol 2003;87:1317–1320.

7. Uliss A, Moore AT, Bird AC. The dark choroid in posterior retinal dystrophies. Ophthalmology 1987;94: 1423–1428.

8. Jacobson DM, Thompson S, Bartley JA. X-linked progressive cone dystrophy. Clinical characteristics of affected males and female carriers. Ophthalmology 1989;96:885–895.

9. Downes SM, Holder GE, Fitzke FW, et al. Autosomal dominant cone and cone-rod dystrophy with mutations in the guanylate cyclase activator 1A gene-encoding guanylate cyclase activating protein-1. Arch Ophthalmol 2001;119: 96–105.

10. Payne AM, Downes SM, Bessant DA, et al. A mutation in guanylate cyclase activator 1A (*GUCA1A*) in autosomal dominant cone dystrophy mapping to a new locus on chromosome 6p21.1. Hum Mol Genet 1998;7:273–277.

11. Gouras P, Eggers HM, MacKay CJ. Cone dystrophy, nyctalopia, and supernormal rod responses. A new retinal degeneration. Arch Ophthalmol. 1983;101:718–724.

12. Alexander KR, Fishman GA. Supernormal scotopic ERG in cone dystrophy. Br J Ophthalmol 1984;68:69–78.

13. Reichel E, Bruce AM, Sandberg MA, et al. An electroretinographic and molecular genetic study of X-linked cone degeneration. Am J Ophthalmol 1989; 108:540–547.

14. Ebenezer ND, Michaelides M, Jenkins SA, et al. Identification of novel *RPGR* ORF15 mutations in X-linked progressive cone-rod dystrophy (XLCORD) families. Invest Ophthalmol Vis Sci 2005;46: 1891–1898.

15. Jacobson DM, Thompson S, Bartley JA. X-linked progressive cone dystrophy. Clinical characteristics of affected males and female carriers. Ophthalmology 1989;96:885–895.

16. Michaelides M, Wilkie SE, Jenkins S, et al. Mutation in the gene *GUCA1A*, encoding guanylate cyclase activating protein-1 (GCAP1) causes cone, cone-rod and macular dystrophy. Ophthalmology 2005; 112:1442–1447.

17. Robson AG, Michaelides M, Luong VA, et al. Functional correlates of fundus autofluorescence abnormalities in patients with RPGR or RIMS1 mutations causing cone or cone rod dystrophy. Br J Ophthalmol 2008;92:95–102.

18. Robson AG, Michaelides M, Saihan Z, et al. Functional characteristics of patients with retinal dystrophy that manifest abnormal parafoveal annuli of high density fundus autofluorescence; a review and update. Doc Ophthalmol 2008;116:79–89.

19. Gregory-Evans K, Kelsell RE, Gregory-Evans CY, et al. Autosomal dominant cone-rod retinal dystrophy (CORD6) from heterozygous mutation of *GUCY2D*, which encodes retinal guanylate cyclase. Ophthalmology 2000; 107:55–61.

20. Ito S, Nakamura M, Nuno Y, et al. Novel complex GUCY2D mutation in Japanese family with cone-rod dystrophy. Invest Ophthalmol Vis Sci 2004;45:1480–1485.

21. Downes SM, Payne AM, Kelsell RE, et al. Autosomal dominant cone-rod dystrophy with mutations in the guanylate cyclase 2D gene encoding retinal guanylate cyclase-1. Arch Ophthalmol 2001;119:1667–1673.

22. Payne AM, Morris AG, Downes SM, et al. Clustering and frequency of mutations in the retinal guanylate cyclase (*GUCY2D*) gene in patients with dominant cone-rod dystrophies. J Med Genet 2001;38:611–614.

23. Perrault I, Rozet JM, Gerber S, et al. A retGC-1 mutation in autosomal dominant cone-rod dystrophy. Am J Hum Genet 1998;63:651–654.

24. Wilkie SE, Newbold RJ, Deery E, et al. Functional characterization of missense mutations at codon 838 in retinal guanylate cyclase correlates with disease severity in patients with autosomal dominant cone-rod dystrophy. Hum Mol Genet 2000;9:3065–3073.

25. Liu X, Seno K, Nishizawa Y, et al. Ultrastructural localization of retinal guanylate cyclase in human and monkey retinas. Exp Eye Res 1994;59:761–768.

26. Nakazawa M, Kikawa E, Chida Y, et al. Asn244His mutation of the *peripherin/RDS* gene causing autosomal dominant cone-rod degeneration. Hum Mol Genet 1994;3:1195–1196.

27. Nakazawa M, Kikawa E, Chida Y, et al. Autosomal dominant cone-rod dystrophy associated with mutations in codon 244 (Asn244His) and codon 184 (Tyr184Ser) of the *peripherin/RDS* gene. Arch Ophthalmol 1996;114: 72–78.

28. Nakazawa M, Naoi N, Wada Y, et al. Autosomal dominant cone-rod dystrophy associated with a Val200Glu mutation of the *peripherin/RDS* gene. Retina 1996;16:405–410.

29. Michaelides M, Holder GE, Bradshaw K, et al. Cone-rod dystrophy, intra-familial variability and incomplete penetrance associated with the R172W mutation in the *peripherin/RDS* gene. Ophthalmology 2005;112:1592–1598.

30. Downes SM, Fitzke FW, Holder GE, et al. Clinical features of codon 172 RDS macular dystrophy: similar phenotype in 12 families. Arch Ophthalmol 1999;117:1373–1383.

31. Nakazawa M, Wada Y, Tamai M. Macular dystrophy associated with monogenic Arg172Trp mutation of the peripherin/RDS gene in a Japanese family. Retina 1995;15:518–523.

32. Arikawa K, Molday LL, Molday RS, et al. Localization of peripherin/RDS in the disk membranes of cone and rod photoreceptors: relationship to disk membrane morphogenesis and retinal degeneration. J Cell Biol 1992;116: 659–667.

33. Loewen CJ, Molday RS. Disulfide-mediated oligomerization of peripherin/RDS and Rom-1 in photoreceptor disk membranes. Implications for photoreceptor outer segment morphogenesis and degeneration. J Biol Chem 2000;275:5370–5378.

34. Evans K, Duvall-Young J, Fitzke FW, et al. Chromosome 19q cone-rod retinal dystrophy: ocular phenotype. Arch Ophthalmol 1995;113:195–201.

35. Itabashi T, Wada Y, Sato H, et al. Novel 615delC mutation in the CRX gene in a Japanese family with cone-rod dystrophy. Am J Ophthalmol 2004;138: 876–877.

36. Papaioannou M, Bessant D, Payne A, et al. A new family of Greek origin maps to the CRD locus for autosomal dominant cone-rod dystrophy on 19q. J Med Genet 1998;35:429–431.

37. Paunescu K, Preising MN, Janke B, et al. Genotype-phenotype correlation in a German family with a novel complex CRX mutation extending the open reading frame. Ophthalmology 2007;114:1348–1357.

38. Freund CL, Gregory-Evans CY, Furukawa T, et al. Cone-rod dystrophy due to mutations in a novel photoreceptor-specific homeobox gene (*CRX*) essential for maintenance of the photoreceptor. Cell 1997; 91:543–553.

39. Furukawa T, Morrow EM, Cepko CL, et al. Crx, a novel otx-like homeobox gene, shows photoreceptor-specific expression and regulates photoreceptor differentiation. Cell 1997;91:531–541.

40. Morrow EM, Furukawa T, Raviola E, et al. Synaptogenesis and outer segment formation are perturbed in the neural retina of Crx mutant mice. BMC Neurosci 2005;6:5.

41. Peng GH, Ahmad O, Ahmad F, et al. The photoreceptor-specific nuclear receptor Nr2e3 interacts with Crx and exerts opposing effects on the transcription of rod versus cone genes. Hum Mol Genet. 2005;14:747–764.

42. Pittler SJ, Zhang Y, Chen S, et al. Functional analysis of the rod photoreceptor cGMP phosphodiesterase alpha-subunit gene promoter: Nrl and Crx are required for full transcriptional activity. J Biol Chem 2004;279:19800–19807.

43. Michaelides M, Holder GE, Hunt DM, et al. A detailed study of the phenotype of an autosomal dominant cone-rod dystrophy (CORD7) associated with mutation in the gene for RIM1. Br J Ophthalmol 2005;89:198–206.

44. Johnson S, Halford S, Morris AG, et al. Genomic organisation and alternative splicing of human *RIM1*, a gene implicated in autosomal dominant cone-rod dystrophy (CORD7). Genomics 2003;81:304–314.

45. Sun L, Bittner MA, Holz RW. RIM, a component of the presynaptic active zone and modulator of exocytosis, binds 14-3-3 through its N-terminus. J Biol Chem 2003;278:38301–38309.

46. Fishman GA, Stone EM, Eliason DA, et al. *ABCA4* gene sequence variations in patients with autosomal recessive cone-rod dystrophy. Arch Ophthalmol 2003;121:851–855.

47. Klevering BJ, Blankenagel A, Maugeri A, et al. Phenotypic spectrum of autosomal recessive cone-rod dystrophies caused by mutations in the ABCA4 (ABCR) gene. Invest Ophthalmol Vis Sci 2002;43:1980–1985.

48. Maugeri A, Klevering BJ, Rohrschneider K, et al. Mutations in the *ABCA4* (ABCR) gene are the major cause of autosomal recessive cone-rod dystrophy. Am J Hum Genet 2000;67:960–966.

49. Michaelides M, Chen LL, Brantley Jr MA, et al. ABCA4 mutations and discordant ABCA4 alleles in patients and siblings with bull's-eye maculopathy. Br J Ophthalmol 2007;91:1650–1655.

50. Kurz-Levin MM, Halfyard AS, Bunce C, et al. Clinical variations in assessment of bull's-eye maculopathy. Arch Ophthalmol 2002;120:567–575.

51. Cideciyan AV, Swider M, Aleman TS, et al. ABCA4-associated retinal degenerations spare structure and function of the human parapapillary retina. Invest Ophthalmol Vis Sci 2005;46:4739–4746.

52. Michaelides M, Holder GE, Webster AR, et al. A detailed phenotypic study of "cone dystrophy with supernormal rod ERG." Br J Ophthalmol 2005;89:332–339.

53. Hood DC, Cideciyan AV, Halevy DA, Jacobson SG. Sites of disease action in a retinal dystrophy with supernormal and delayed rod electroretinogram b-waves. Vision Res 1996;36:889–901.

54. Wu H, Cowing JA, Michaelides M, et al. Mutations in the gene KCNV2 encoding a voltage-gated potassium channel subunit cause "cone dystrophy with supernormal rod electroretinogram" in humans. Am J Hum Genet 2006;79:574–579.

55. Demirci FY, Rigatti BW, Wen G, et al. X-linked cone-rod dystrophy (locus COD1): identification of mutations in *RPGR* exon ORF15. Am J Hum Genet 2002;70:1049–1053.

56. Yang Z, Peachey NS, Moshfeghi DM, et al. Mutations in the *RPGR* gene cause X-linked cone dystrophy. Hum Mol Genet 2002;11:605–611.

57. Wegscheider E, Preising MN, Lorenz B. Fundus autofluorescence in carriers of X-linked recessive retinitis pigmentosa associated with mutations in RPGR, and correlation with electrophysiological and psychophysical data. Graefes Arch Clin Exp Ophthalmol 2004;242:501–511.

Irena Tsui
Stephen H. Tsang

Fundus Autofluorescence in X-Linked Retinoschisis

X-linked retinoschisis (XLRS), also known as juvenile retinoschisis, is the most common cause of macular degeneration in young men (1,2), with an incidence between 1:5000 and 1:25,000 (3). Rarely, a homozygous female from a consanguineous marriage can be affected. The disease occurs in all races, with the highest prevalence in Finland (4).

Patients with XLRS have a highly variable clinical course. Patients present most commonly as school-aged boys who fail vision-screening examinations (60%) because of strabismus (30%) or vitreous hemorrhage (1,2,5). The classic "spoke wheel" appearance may be present in the fovea (3), but eventually nonspecific macular atrophy occurs in adulthood (6). Therefore, the diagnosis can be missed when patients present late or atypically.

RS1, the gene responsible for XLRS, is located on chromosome Xp22 and encodes the protein retinoschisin. It is not known to be expressed anywhere else in the body besides the retina and there are no systemic associations with XLRS. To date, there are 132 different pathogenic mutations known to cause XLRS (7). *RS1* gene defects have complete penetrance, but the phenotypic expression of the disease is variable (8) and there is no known genotype-phenotype correlation (9,10).

In children and young adults with XLRS, the differential diagnosis includes uveitic macular edema, myopic foveal schisis, and other inherited retinal diseases such as enhanced S-cone syndrome (ESCS)/Goldmann-Favre, congenital stationary night blindness, Stargardt disease, and familial exudative vitreoretinopathy. Adults with XLRS usually progress to macular atrophy, and the major differential diagnosis is age-related macular degeneration (AMD).

MOLECULAR BASIS AND PATHOLOGY OF XLRS

The cellular location of retinoschisin in the retina is a controversial issue. It was initially thought that retinoschisin is secreted by photoreceptors and ganglion cells. Specifically, it was first found in the photoreceptor inner segment microsomal and synaptic compartments (11–13).

In a more recent study using an epitope unmasking protocol, retinoschisin immunoreactivity was also found in the plasma membrane of inner retinal cells in addition to photoreceptors and ganglion cells (14). Since retinoschisin has not been conclusively detected in Müller cells (14,15), the long-standing hypothesis that Müller cells contribute to the pathogenesis of XLRS has yet to be verified experimentally.

In a mouse model of XLRS, loss of retinoschisin led to disrupted synaptic interactions between photoreceptors and bipolar neurons in the outer plexiform layer (OPL) (15,16). During development of XLRS mice, failure of centrifugal displacement of dendrites and synapses, as well as other inner retinal neurons and synapses, was thought to be responsible for the splitting of the putative fibers of Henle (14).

Improvement of the electronegative electroretinography (ERG) b-wave was found in adult *RS1*-deficient mice treated with adeno-associated virus (AAV) carrying the wild-type gene (16). A single injection of AAV-RS1 resulted in sustained RS1 expression and functional rescue. This demonstrated that even when loss of retinoschisin was long-standing, function could be recovered (16).

There is only one human pathology specimen of a patient with XLRS. In this 19-year-old man's enucleated eye, reduced levels of retinoschisin immunoactivity were observed in both the macula and the peripheral retina compared to a normal eye of an age-matched control (17). Clinically, about 50% of XLRS patients manifest peripheral retinoschisis, and some also have bridging vessels from the inner to the outer layer. Traction on these bridging vessels causes vitreous hemorrhage.

IMAGING AND DIAGNOSTIC TECHNIQUES

The classic foveal schisis seen in XLRS is best visualized at the slit lamp using red-free illumination. Similarly, red-free photos demonstrate the cavities better than color fundus photography (Fig. 11C.1A).

In XLRS, optical coherence topography (OCT) shows cystic spaces in the macula at the level of the retinal nerve fiber layer and inner nuclear layer, corresponding to the schisis cavities (Fig. 11C.1B). However, similar findings are observed in cystoid macular edema. As in other diseases with macular thickening, there is no correlation between foveal thickness and visual acuity in XLRS. Macular atrophy, which is often observed in late stages of XLRS, is another nonspecific finding on OCT. In the presence of vitreous hemorrhage, OCT is of limited value because the signal cannot penetrate dense vitreous opacities.

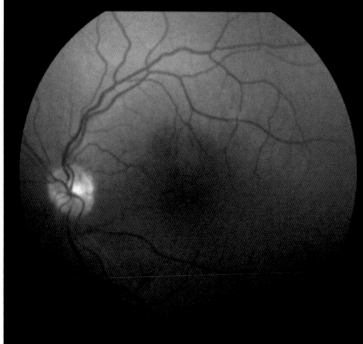

FIGURE 11C.1. A 34-year-old patient with XLRS. **(A)** Red-free fundus photograph shows stellate cystoid structures radiating from the fovea. **(B)** OCT with splitting of outer plexiform layer or Henle's fiber layer.

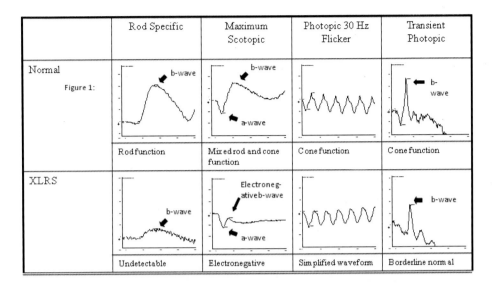

FIGURE 11C.2. Standardized full-field ERG in accordance with the International Society for Clinical Electrophysiology of Vision (ISCEV). Rod-specific, maximum scotopic, photopic flicker, and transient photopic responses in normal subjects (*above*) and electronegative XLRS patients (*below*) are shown.

On fluorescein angiography (FA), the cystic changes observed in XLRS do not fill or stain with fluorescein. Thus, FA is useful clinically to rule out leaking cystoid macular edema when the diagnosis of foveal cysts is uncertain. As in XLRS, patients with ESCS/Goldmann-Favre may also have nonleaking cystic spaces on FA. However, ESCS/Goldmann-Favre often can be distinguished from XLRS based on fundus appearance and the ERG findings.

Electrodiagnostic testing is essential in the work-up of XLRS and is important in establishing the diagnosis. Full-field ERG shows a reduced b-wave with a preserved a-wave (Fig. 11C.2). This finding, known as an electronegative ERG, is seen in a limited number of other inherited diseases, such as congenital stationary night blindness, Duchenne muscular dystrophy, Batten disease, and some forms of cone-rod dystrophy (CORD; see also Chapter 11B). Late in the course of the disease, both a- and b-waves may be reduced, but full-field ERG usually remains electronegative. Multifocal ERG may show reduced macular function, which is not specific to XLRS (8). There is no specific visual field defect associated with XLRS.

PHENOTYPES AND AUTOFLUORESCENCE FINDINGS

Defects in *RS1* have great allelic heterogeneity, with different mutations causing a wide spectrum of phenotypes. There are four distinct autofluorescence (AF) patterns found in XLRS. Three of them—early cystoid changes, intermediate hyperfluorescent rings, and eventual macular atrophy—are likely to represent different stages in the progression of the disease. The fourth AF pattern of XLRS is a rarer presentation of white dots on fundus examination, as recently described in the literature (18).

In young patients with foveal schisis, AF discloses a stellate pattern of round-oval areas with signal similar to that of the background. At this site, and in normal circumstances, a reduced AF signal is observed mainly related to blockage by luteal pigment. This AF pattern in XLRS seems to be the result of macular pigment displacement at the site of the cystic cavities (Fig. 11C.3); however, it is not specific for XLRS and can

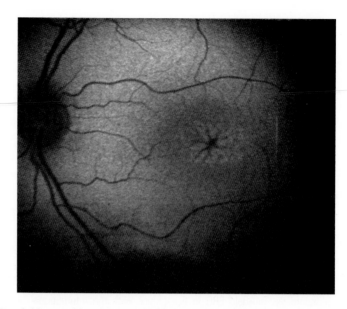

FIGURE 11C.3.   A 29-year-old patient with XLRS. AF shows pigment displacement of the macular pigment between cysts.

be seen also in ESCS/Goldmann-Favre, cystoid macular edema of any cause, and myopic foveal schisis (19).

In the intermediate state of XLRS, a high-density ring is seen in the macula on AF, indicating RPE involvement earlier than first realized (Fig. 11C.4). This ring is also seen in patients with retinitis pigmentosa, CORD, and bull's-eye macular dystrophy (20–22). High-density AF lesions suggest increased RPE accumulation of lipofuscin from increased or abnormal photoreceptor outer segment shedding. This disruption of RPE metabolism eventually leads to RPE atrophy.

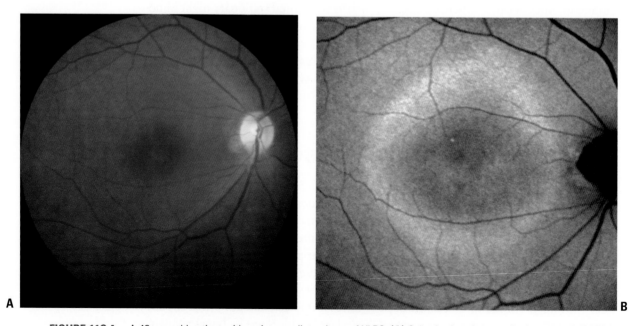

FIGURE 11C.4.   A 49-year-old patient with an intermediate phase of XLRS. **(A)** Color fundus photograph shows mottled RPE in the macula. **(B)** AF reveals a hyperfluorescent ring in the macula with early RPE atrophy in the center.

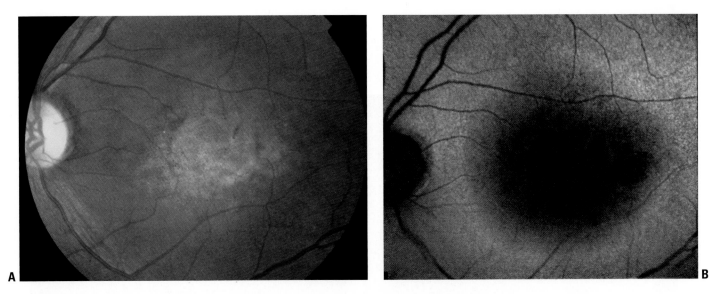

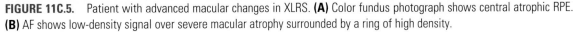

FIGURE 11C.5.   Patient with advanced macular changes in XLRS. **(A)** Color fundus photograph shows central atrophic RPE. **(B)** AF shows low-density signal over severe macular atrophy surrounded by a ring of high density.

In older patients, the schisis cavities often collapse, leaving nonspecific RPE atrophy, which is observed as an area of low AF signal (Fig. 11C.5). At this late stage, the diagnosis can be confused with AMD. XLRS can still be suspected, with clues such as decreased vision in childhood and a family history of similar problems in males. Even when the diagnosis is unclear in late stages of disease, the ERG remains electronegative. However, similar findings (atrophic macular changes and electronegative ERG) can be also found in some patients with CORD (see Chapter 11B).

Another unusual form of XLRS presents as atrophic changes associated with drusen-like multiple white dots (Fig. 11C.6). These dots differ from drusen associated with age-related maculopathy by their punctate appearance in individuals under age 50. Other conditions associated with foveal or parafoveal white dots and flecks include Stargardt-fundus flavimaculatus, retinitis punctata albescens, ESCS/Goldmann-Favre, Wagner vitreoretinal dystrophy, yellow dot dystrophy, and other forms of macular dystrophy (23). However, these other conditions have different funduscopic appearances and do not manifest an electronegative ERG (24,25).

Besides foveal cysts, another common presentation in childhood is vitreous hemorrhage from vitreous veils that have torn retinal vessels (4). The differential diagnosis of vitreous hemorrhage in childhood includes Norrie disease, familial exudative vitreoretinopathy, retinopathy of prematurity, persistent hyperplastic primary vitreous, and Coats disease. Ultrasonography is useful in such cases to rule out retinal detachment. AF is not as useful in this situation, but it would show a blocking defect from vitreous veils or hemorrhage (Fig. 11C.7).

RECENT INSIGHTS INTO THE PATHOGENESIS OF XLRS

The defective protein, retinoschisin, is expressed mainly in photoreceptors and then quickly taken up by Müller cells and transported to the inner retina (14). This may explain the electronegativity of the ERG b-wave that is typically seen in XLRS

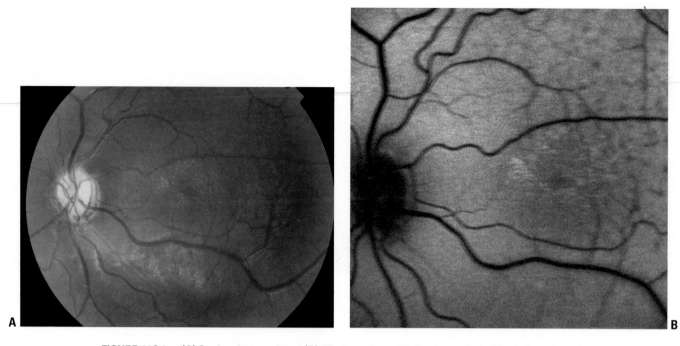

FIGURE 11C.6. **(A)** Fundus photograph and **(B)** AF of a patient with fine intraretinal white lesions along the venules and arterioles of the perifoveolar vascular network. Note that the AF images reveal increased AF signal corresponding to the white dots.

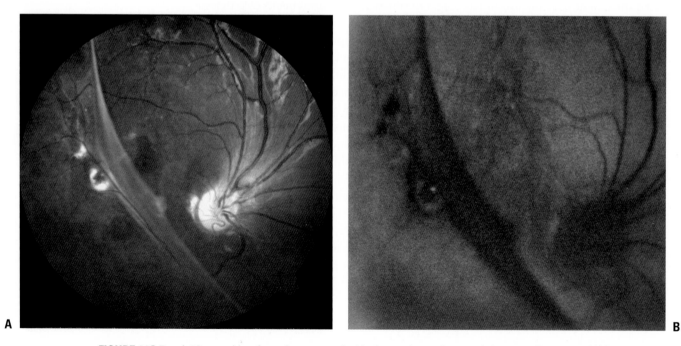

FIGURE 11C.7. A 12-year-old patient who presented with vitreous hemorrhage and vitreous veils at birth. **(A)** Red-free fundus photography. **(B)** AF showing a blocking defect caused by vitreous veils.

patients, which suggests that the disease causes post-phototransduction or inner-retinal pathology. The exact pathogenesis of the disease is still not completely understood, as retinal splitting occurs along all layers of the retina, most often superficially.

Fundus AF has provided new insights into the pathogenesis of XLRS. Although XLRS was previously thought to be primarily a disease of the retina, high-intensity signals on AF suggest that there is increased RPE metabolism early in the course of the disease. As seen in other conditions, such as retinitis pigmentosa, a ring of malfunctioning RPE may be due to improper photoreceptor outer segment shedding and subsequent accumulation of lipofuscin. This accumulation of lipofuscin eventually may lead to RPE dysfunction and atrophy. The exact role of RPE dysfunction in XLRS has only been recently realized and is not well understood.

SUMMARY

AF findings are useful in patients with suspected XLRS based on previous ocular or family history. Thus, if small round-oval areas of increased AF signal at the fovea are observed in a young male, the diagnosis of XLRS should be suspected. FA can confirm that these are truly schisis cavities if they are not hyperfluorescent, narrowing the diagnostic possibilities. In a patient with a central area of reduced AF signal in the macula, with or without a surrounding ring of increased AF, the diagnosis of XLRS should be added to the differential diagnosis.

Unlike FA, AF and OCT are noninvasive and take seconds to obtain. This is of great advantage when evaluating children and the elderly. However, AF, like OCT, is of limited value in the presence of vitreous hemorrhage or media opacities.

Fundus AF, in isolation, is of limited value for establishing with certainty the diagnosis of retinoschisis; it should be used with other imaging techniques and electrophysiology testing (see above). *RS1* gene testing is available to confirm a diagnosis of XLRS (http://www.nei.nih.gov/resources/eyegene.asp, http://www.ngrl.org.uk/Manchester/). Genetic testing also identifies female carriers of *RS1* (26,27). Early and accurate diagnosis may be important in genetic counseling of RS families. By age 60, the visual acuity of most XLRS individuals declines steadily to approximately 20/200.

Future *RS1* gene therapy will be of benefit for individuals with molecularly diagnosed XLRS (16). Imaging techniques such as AF, OCT, and electrophysiology will help in determining which patients are eligible for treatment.

ACKNOWLEDGMENTS

We thank the staff of the Medical Imaging Division of the Edward S. Harkness Eye Institute for their excellent work, and Brian Song for contributing to Figure 11C.1. We thank the members of the Graham Holder and Andrew Webster laboratories for sharing their advice and ideas. S.H.T. is a Burroughs-Wellcome Program in Biomedical Sciences Fellow and is also supported by the Charles E. Culpeper Scholarship, Foundation Fighting Blindness, Hirschl Trust, Schneeweiss Stem Cell Fund, Crowley Research Fund, Joel Hoffmann Scholarship, Barbara and Donald Jonas Family Fund, Hartford/American Geriatrics Society, Eye Surgery Fund, Bernard Becker-Association of University Professors in Ophthalmology-Research to Prevent Blindness, and National Institutes of Health (EY004081).

REFERENCES

1. Deutman AF, Pickers AJL, Aan de Kerk AL. Dominantly inherited cystoid macular edema. Am J Ophthalmol 1976;82:540–548.
2. Traboulsi E, ed. Genetic Disease of the Eye, 1st ed. Oxford: Oxford University Press, 1998:899.
3. George ND, Yates JR, Moore AT. X linked retinoschisis. Br J Ophthalmol 1995;79:697–702.
4. Tantri A, Vrabec TR, Cu-Unjieng A, Frost A, Annesley Jr WH, Donoso LA. X-linked retinoschisis: a clinical and molecular genetic review. Surv Ophthalmol 2004;49:214–230.
5. Pimenides D, George ND, Yates JR, et al. X-linked retinoschisis: clinical phenotype and RS1 genotype in 86 UK patients. J Med Genet 2005;42:e35.
6. Kellner U, Brummer S, Foerster MH, et al. X-linked congenital retinoschisis. Graefes Arch Clin Exp Ophthalmol 1990;228:432–437.
7. Consortium R. Functional implications of the spectrum of mutations found in 234 cases with X-linked juvenile retinoschisis. The Retinoschisis Consortium. Hum Mol Genet 1998;7:1185–1192.
8. Eksandh L, Andreasson S, Abrahamson M. Juvenile X-linked retinoschisis with normal scotopic b-wave in the electroretinogram at an early stage of the disease. Ophthalmic Genet 2005;26:111–117.
9. Inoue Y, Yamamoto S, Okada M, et al. X-linked retinoschisis with point mutations in the XLRS1 gene. Arch Ophthalmol 2000;118:93–96.
10. Taketani R, Yokoyama T, Hotta Y, et al. A case of juvenile retinoschisis diagnosed by analysis of the XLRS 1 gene. Jpn J Ophthalmol 2000;44:319.
11. Grayson C, Reid SN, Ellis JA, et al. Retinoschisin, the X-linked retinoschisis protein, is a secreted photoreceptor protein, and is expressed and released by Weri-Rb1 cells. Hum Mol Genet 2000;9:1873–1879.
12. Reid SN, Yamashita C, Farber DB. Retinoschisin, a photoreceptor-secreted protein, and its interaction with bipolar and Müller cells. J Neurosci 2003;23:6030–6040.
13. Molday LL, Hicks D, Sauer CG, et al. Expression of X-linked retinoschisis protein RS1 in photoreceptor and bipolar cells. Invest Ophthalmol Vis Sci 2001;42:816–825.
14. Takada Y, Fariss RN, Tanikawa A, et al. A retinal neuronal developmental wave of retinoschisin expression begins in ganglion cells during layer formation. Invest Ophthalmol Vis Sci 2004;45:3302–3312.
15. Weber BH, Schrewe H, Molday LL, et al. Inactivation of the murine X-linked juvenile retinoschisis gene, Rs1h, suggests a role of retinoschisin in retinal cell layer organization and synaptic structure. Proc Natl Acad Sci USA 2002;99:6222–6227.
16. Zeng Y, Takada Y, Kjellstrom S, et al. RS-1 gene delivery to an adult Rs1h knockout mouse model restores ERG b-wave with reversal of the electronegative waveform of X-linked retinoschisis. Invest Ophthalmol Vis Sci 2004;45:3279–285.
17. Mooy CM, Van Den Born LI, Baarsma S, et al. Hereditary X-linked juvenile retinoschisis: a review of the role of Müller cells. Arch Ophthalmol 2002;120:979–984.
18. Tsang SH, Vaclavik V, Bird AC, et al. Novel phenotypic and genotypic findings in X-linked retinoschisis. Arch Ophthalmol 2007;125:259–267.
19. Sayanagi K, Ikuno Y, Tano Y. Different fundus autofluorescence patterns of retinoschisis and macular hole retinal detachment in high myopia. Am J Ophthalmol 2007;144:299–301.
20. Robson AG, Saihan Z, Jenkins SA, et al. Functional characterisation and serial imaging of abnormal fundus autofluorescence in patients with retinitis pigmentosa and normal visual acuity. Br J Ophthalmol 2006;90:472–479.
21. Robson AG, Moreland JD, Pauleikhoff D, et al. Macular pigment density and distribution: comparison of fundus autofluorescence with minimum motion photometry. Vision Res 2003;43:1765–1775.
22. Robson A, Saihan Z, Jenkins S, et al. Macular function and serial imaging of abnormal fundus autofluorescence in patients with retinitis pigmentosa and good visual acuity. Invest Ophthalmol Vis Sci 2006;ARVO E-Abstract.
23. Audo I, Tsang SH, Fu AD, et al. Autofluorescence imaging in a case of benign familial fleck retina. Arch Ophthalmol 2007;125:714–715.
24. Tsui I, Song B, Lin C-S, et al. A practical approach to retinal dystrophies. Retin Physician 2007;4:18–26.
25. Robson AG, Richardson EC, Koh AH, et al. Unilateral electronegative ERG of non-vascular aetiology. Br J Ophthalmol 2005;89:1620–1626.
26. Sieving PA, Bingham EL, Kemp J, et al. Juvenile X-linked retinoschisis from XLRS1 Arg213Trp mutation with preservation of the electroretinogram scotopic b-wave. Am J Ophthalmol 1999;128:179–184.
27. Hewitt AW, FitzGerald LM, Scotter LW, et al. Genotypic and phenotypic spectrum of X-linked retinoschisis in Australia. Clin Exp Ophthalmol 2005;33:233–239.

Hendrik P.N. Scholl
Bettina Wabbels

Fundus Autofluorescence in Leber Congenital Amaurosis

INTRODUCTION

Leber congenital amaurosis (LCA) accounts for around 5% of all inherited retinal dystrophies and is the earliest and most severe form of inherited retinal disease (1–4). LCA is clinically and genetically heterogeneous, although most forms show autosomal recessive inheritance. Patients with nonsyndromic LCA typically have an onset of poor vision and nystagmus before 6 months of age, sluggish pupillary reactions, and undetectable electroretinogram (ERG) (5). Their vision, when they are old enough for formal assessment, is usually less than 20/400. Children with LCA are usually hyperopic and may demonstrate the oculodigital sign (repetitive pushing of the knuckle or finger into the eye). The appearance of the fundus is highly variable (6–8). A normal-appearing fundus may be encountered in infancy (6,8,9), although later in childhood a variety of fundus abnormalities may be present (6,7). These include typical retinitis pigmentosa (RP) (6,7,10), salt-and-pepper appearance of the fundus (10–15), increased granularity of the retinal pigment epithelium (RPE) (10,13,15), white spots or fundus flecks (6,10,16), macular coloboma (6–8,10,17), marbled fundus (6,7,10,18,19), peripheral nummular pigmentation (6,10,20), attenuation of the retinal vessels (14,15), and optic atrophy (11). Macular changes, peripapillary hypopigmentation, and lack of pigment migration into the retina (bone spicules) are common features observed in adult patients (15,21).

The clinical heterogeneity of the disease is reflected by the genetic heterogeneity. To date, 14 causative genes have been found to be mutated in patients with LCA and juvenile retinal degeneration, and explain approximately 70% of LCA cases (22). These genes are expressed preferentially in the retina or the RPE. Their putative functions are diverse and include vitamin A metabolism (*RPE65*) (23,24), phototransduction (*RetGC1/GUCY2D*) (25,26), retinal embryonic development (*CRX*) (27), protein trafficking (*AIPL1* and *RPGRIP1*) (28–30), photoreceptor cell structure (*CRB1*) (31), and G protein trafficking (*CEP290*) (32,33).

Compound heterozygous or homozygous mutations in RPE65 result in a number of different retinal degenerations, including LCA and early onset severe retinal dystrophy (EOSRD) (15,23,24,34–36). In various series, mutations in RPE65 accounted for 3% to 16% of cases of LCA/EOSRD (34,37–42). Very recently, *RPE65* has gained particular interest because of the initiation of small pilot studies in which patients with retinal dystrophies due to mutations in this gene received treatment with subretinal injections of recombinant adeno-associated virus vector expressing RPE65 complementary DNA (43–45). These studies represent the first attempt to use gene therapy to treat an eye disease. The results of similar treatments in animals have been very promising, and investigators were able to restore vision in a naturally occurring animal model (46–49). Patients with *RPE65* mutations have better visual function than is typically seen in LCA, especially in childhood (15,21,35). Although severe visual impairment is noted in infancy, with visual responses elicited only in bright surroundings, children with LCA and *RPE65* mutations generally have poor but useful vision in early life. Visual performance often improves during the first years of life, allowing the children to attend regular schools, but then gradually declines during the school-age years. A number of patients retain residual islands of peripheral vision, although it is considerably compromised in the third decade of life (39). In higher-age groups, progressive visual field loss and severe visual loss is the norm (50). Nystagmus is often present; however, the roving eye movements commonly seen in LCA are rarely seen in LCA caused by mutations in *RPE65* (5).

MOLECULAR BASIS AND PATHOLOGY

Clinical and genetic studies suggest that, although there is a relatively uniform loss of retinal function in LCA, the underlying pathophysiological mechanisms and retinal morphological changes may be extremely heterogeneous. As stated above, several genes have been found to be mutated in LCA; however, many others remain unknown (22). The complex disease mechanisms underlining LCA were recently reviewed by den Hollander and colleagues (22)

CEP290, *GUCY2D*, and *CRB1* are the genes most frequently involved in LCA (22). The protein codified by *CEP290* appears to have a role in intracellular protein trafficking in photoreceptor cells, specifically in ciliary transport processes (51). *GUCY2D* encodes a protein, RetGC-1, that is involved in the resynthesis of cGMP (see also Chapter 11B). cGMP is needed for the recovery of the dark state in photoreceptor cells following light exposure. Loss of function of RetGC-1 would mimic a situation in which the photoreceptors would be continuously exposed to light, which would lead to photoreceptor cell degeneration. CRB1 (RP12) appears to be essential in the morphogenesis and orientation of the photoreceptor outer segments (52).

Very few histopathology studies of genotyped patients with LCA have been published. In one such study (53), eyes obtained from a 33-week-old fetus with a mutation in the *RPE65* gene were examined. Compared with normal tissue, the *RPE65* mutated retina demonstrated cell loss and thinning in the photoreceptor cell layer (outer nuclear layer [ONL]), decreased immunoreactivity of phototransduction proteins, and aberrant synaptic and inner retinal organization. There was also thickening in Bruch's membrane and the choroid was abnormally vascularized.

Histopathology studies of the retinas obtained from an 11.5-year-old individual with LCA and a mutation in GUCY2D have also been presented (54). The affected patient had vision of only light perception, no measurable kinetic visual fields, and a flat ERG before death. Lack of photoreceptor outer segments was observed; however, there were reduced but present rods and cones in the macula and peripheral retina. The inner nuclear layer appeared normal in thickness and there were a reduced number of ganglion cells.

IMAGING AND DIAGNOSTIC TECHNIQUES

Imaging patients with LCA is often challenging because of their common inability to fixate and the presence of nystagmus. However, imaging techniques often provide very valuable information to the clinician, and will likely be essential in the evaluation of children and adults with this condition once treatments become available.

Fluorescein Angiography

Fluorescein angiography (FA) may be useful for determining RPE changes and atrophy that are not detected clinically. However, fundus autofluorescence (AF; see below), being noninvasive, has now replaced FA for this purpose.

Optical Coherence Tomography

Optical coherence tomography (OCT) studies in LCA are scarce, but they have provided important information regarding the retinal structure in patients with this disorder, including patients with mutations in *RPE65*, *RPGRIP1*, *CEP290*, *RDH12*, and *CRB1*.

In patients with LCA and mutations in *RPE65*, OCT demonstrated reduced ONL thickness at the fovea, even in the youngest patient studied (age 3 years) (55). Although reduced, measures of the foveal ONL thickness suggested preservation of some foveal cones even until later in life (55). RPE pigmentation (a measure of RPE integrity), as demonstrated by the sub-RPE backscattering index, was normal in LCA caused by mutations in *RPE65* (55).

OCT images obtained from a patient with LCA due to a mutation in the *RPGRIP1* gene demonstrated retained central retinal architecture with normal ONL thickness, which decreased to immeasurable levels outside the fovea (56). Similarly, OCT studies demonstrated that patients with mutations in *CEP290* retain photoreceptors and inner laminar architecture in the cone-rich central retina, independently of the severity of visual loss. Photoreceptor cell loss and distorted retina, suggesting neural-glial remodeling, were present elsewhere (57).

In contrast to patients with *RPE65*, *RPGRIP1*, and *CEP290*, patients with mutations in *RDH12* were found to have a lack of retinal lamination (distorted retinal structure) with variable retinal thickness (thin or thick) on OCT (58). Similarly, in those with mutations in *CRB1*, OCT demonstrated a very thick retina lacking on the normal retinal architecture and resembling immature retina (59).

On the basis of the above findings, patients with mutations in *RPE65*, *RPGRIP1*, and *CEP290* may be good potential candidates for gene replacement therapy. OCT appears to be an important tool to evaluate which patients might be eligible for potential treatments for this disease.

Fundus Autofluorescence

In vivo recording of RPE AF provides indirect information on the level of metabolic activity of the RPE, which is largely determined by the rate of turnover of photoreceptor outer segments. Progressive loss of lipofuscin occurs when there is reduced metabolic demand due to photoreceptor cell death. This is consistent with studies on patients with RP that showed a correspondence between areas of decreased AF and areas of photoreceptor cell loss (60). It suggests that decreased AF may be a good marker for the integrity of the RPE/photoreceptor cell complex, and that AF imaging may be useful to evaluate whether there is capacity to restore retinal function following treatment.

Patients with LCA and EOSRD may have a normal distribution of AF throughout the fundus (patient 1, Table 11D.1; Fig. 11D.1) (61,62). In some patients, a parafoveal ring of mildly increased AF can be detected (patients 2 and 3, Table 11D.1, Fig. 11D.1). A moderately decreased AF signal along the arcades and in the midperiphery can be detected. In contrast, patients with typical RP, who also often demon-

TABLE 11D.1	Summary of Clinical, Electrophysiological, and Funduscopic Findings				
	Patient 1	**Patient 2**	**Patient 3**	**Patient 4**	**Patient 5**
Diagnosis	LCA	LCA	LCA	EOSRD	EOSRD
Age at examination (years)	24	15	37	7	10
BCVA	Light perception	Light perception	Light perception	20/200–20/100 OU	20/400 RE, 20/500 LE (at 1 m)
Fundus features	Mild attenuation of the retinal vessels; otherwise normal	Mild pallor of the optic disc; mild attenuation of the retinal vessels; subtle salt-and-pepper appearance in the midperiphery	Pale optic discs, a normal macular appearance, attenuated retinal vessels, and both mild hypopigmentation at the level of the RPE and intraretinal pigment in the midperiphery	Pale optic disc, central RPE defect, pale fundus, clearly visible choroidal vessels	Pale optic disc, macula, and periphery, with spotty glittering reflexes
ERG (ISCEV standard)	Scotopic and photopic nondetectable	Scotopic and photopic nondetectable	Scotopic and photopic nondetectable	Scotopic: nonrecordable, maximal response amplitude 25% of mean; 30-Hz flicker: severely prolonged implicit times*	Scotopic and photopic nondetectable
Nystagmus	Yes	Yes	Yes	Yes after birth, none at present	Yes

BCVA, best-corrected visual acuity; EOSRD, early onset severe retinal dystrophy; ERG, electroretinogram; ISCEV, International Society for Clinical Electrophysiology of Vision; LE, left eye; OU, both eyes; RE, right eye; RPE, retinal pigment epithelium.
*Data from examination at the Department of Pathophysiology of Vision, University of Tübingen, Germany (Head Prof. Dr. E. Zrenner).

strate a ring of increased AF at the macula, have very reduced AF signal in the midperipheral retina (Fig 11D.1; see also Chapter 11A).

Preservation of the AF signal in LCA indicates the presence of structurally intact photoreceptors and the integrity of the photoreceptor/RPE complex (see below). The distinction between photoreceptor cell death and cell dysfunction is important and will be essential for distinguishing those patients who may benefit from future therapeutic interventions. If the photoreceptor cells are viable but dysfunctional, gene therapy might allow recovery of function; under such circumstances, cell transplantation would be inappropriate. In contrast, if loss of vision is due to photoreceptor cell death, gene therapy would serve to delay the progress of the disease by preventing cell death of compromised but surviving cells. Fundus AF and OCT findings (see above) suggest that the time course of progressive photoreceptor cell death may be slow in a subset of LCA families/patients; viable photoreceptors may still be present even until midlife in these patients. Thus, there should be a window of opportunity to treat some of the patients affected with this devastating disease.

As in patients with RP, a ring of increased AF can also be observed in patients with LCA (61,62). The significance of this ring of increased AF in patients with RP is explained in detail in Chapter 11A. However, the significance of this AF feature and its correlation to visual function in LCA is not known.

In contrast to the preserved AF signal in the above subset of LCA and EOSRD patients, patients with LCA/EOSRD associated with RPE65 mutations were found to

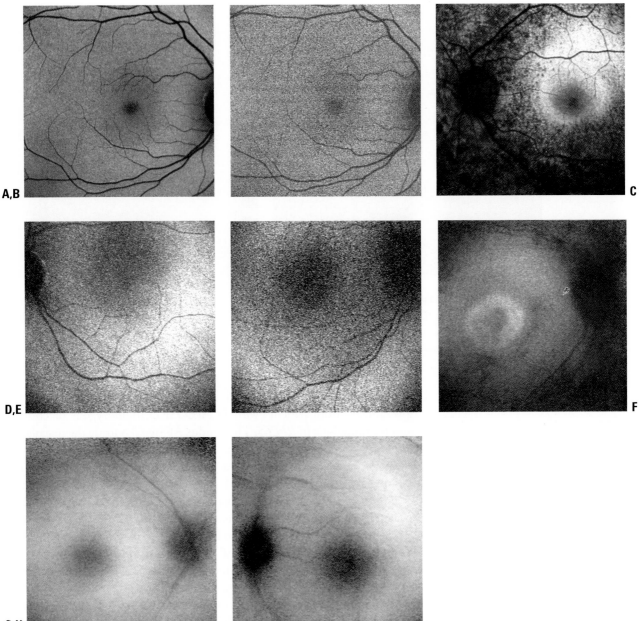

FIGURE 11D.1.   AF images of **(A,B)** a 32-year-old subject with no eye disease (**A**, image aligned from 16 single images; **B**, single frame of AF image), **(C)** a patient with RP, **(D–F)** three patients with LCA (patients 1–3, Table 11D.1), and **(G,H)** two patients with EOSRD (patients 4 and 5, Table 11D.1). Compared with the normal AF distribution **(A,B)**, the patient with RP **(C)** exhibits a parafoveal ring of moderately increased AF and severely decreased AF eccentric to the macula, including the periphery. **(D,E)** In two LCA patients (patients 1 and 2, Table 11D.1), a relatively normal distribution of AF is shown. **(F)** In one patient with LCA (patient 3, Table 11D.1), the AD distribution is normal at the fovea but there is a parafoveal ring of moderately increased AF. In the midperiphery, a moderately reduced AF signal with some topographic correspondence to areas of pigment migration into the retina is observed. **(G,H)** Patients with EOSRD (who were not associated with *RPE65* or *LRAT* mutations) demonstrated a clear AF signal.

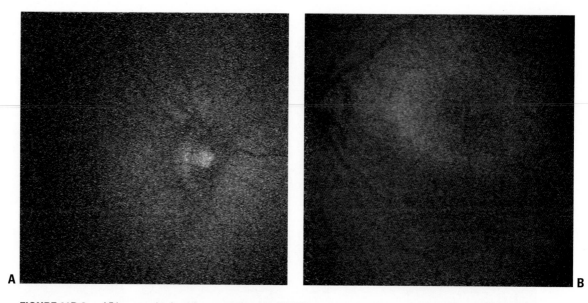

FIGURE 11D.2.   AF images obtained from patients with EOSRD associated with mutations in *RPE65*. **(A)** Nearly absent AF in a 10-year-old patient. **(B)** Very low AF signal is observed in a 14-year-old patient; some preservation of the AF signal is observed around the fovea.

have absent or very low AF signal beginning in the first decade of life (62). Figure 11D.2 shows images from patients with LCA/EOSRD, homozygous or compound heterozygous for mutations in *RPE65*. The fundus AF signal outside the macula is very low and very similar to that recorded at the optic nerve head and large retinal vessels. At the macula, the signal is low at the fovea, as seen also in individuals with no retinal disease, resulting from blockage of the AF signal by the macular pigment (see also Chapters 3 and 9), but is surrounded by an area where AF is present (Fig. 11D.2). The images are generally blurred and coarse-grained. With the detection sensitivity of commercially available instruments, such as the HRA2, it is difficult to detect any AF signal in most patients with LCA/EOSRD and *RPE65* mutations.

The finding of absent AF in patients with LCA/EOSRD and mutations in *RPE65* was not due to media opacities or a high refractive error. Because the AF signal was very low not only in the averaged images but also in the single-frame images, nystagmus can be ruled out as the underlying reason for the absent AF. In patients with nystagmus of other origins, although the averaged AF image may be sometimes dark due to eye movements, it is generally much brighter that those observed in LCA/EOSRD and mutations in *RPE65*, and single-frame images have a demonstrable AF signal (Fig 11D.1) (61–63). However, OCT findings in patients with LCA/EOSRD and mutations in *RPE65* indicated still-viable photoreceptors despite the absence of AF (see above) (55–59,62), suggesting that the lack of AF signal is not due to atrophy of the RPE.

The lack of AF observed in patients with LCA/EOSRD and mutations in *RPE65*, even from early on in the course of the disease, is characteristic and appears to be in accordance with the biochemical defect present in these patients and with findings in animal models of the disease. The *RPE65* gene encodes an RPE-specific 65 kD protein (RPE65) and is localized on chromosome 1p31 (24). RPE65 plays a key role in the metabolism of vitamin A in the retina because it controls the final isomerization step from all-*trans* retinyl ester to 11-*cis* retinal. $RPE65^{-/-}$ mice accumulate all-*trans* retinyl ester during illumination cycles (64). The absence of AF in

$RPE65^{-/-}$ mice was shown by Katz and Redmond (65) to result from a failure of lipofuscin fluorophore formation. Lipofuscin accumulates from lysosomal degradation end products of all-*trans* retinal from shed photoreceptor disks phagocytosed by the RPE (66). The absence of AF in patients with compound heterozygous or homozygous mutations in RPE65 indicates that in humans as well, the formation of lipofuscin fluorophores is dependent on the normal function of the visual cycle and a normal RPE65 gene product in the RPE. The absence of retinal, both all-*trans* and 11-*cis*, prevents the formation of lipofuscin fluorophores in both $RPE65^{-/-}$ mice and patients with *RPE65* mutations.

Recently, it was demonstrated that there may be some residual AF in some patients with *RPE65* mutations (42); to date, however, it remains unclear how this finding can be explained based on the biochemical data and findings in animal models (see above). Since these patients had the same mutation in *RPE65* as those in whom no AF signal was detected, it is possible that the residual AF signal observed was due to AF signal from the sclera. Further studies are needed to elucidate this discrepancy.

SUMMARY

It is important to evaluate the distribution of fundus AF in patients with LCA/EOSRD. Such an evaluation may serve as a guide for genetic testing (e.g., a lack of fundus AF signal, especially in young patients, would indicate the likely presence of a mutation in RPE65), and provide important information with regard to the potential for visual recovery in patients with this disease, once genetic treatments become clinically available. This imaging technique could be particularly helpful in young patients who are not capable of cooperating with procedures to obtain detailed measurements of visual function, ERG, or other imaging techniques, such as OCT. It may also guide the location where therapeutic subretinal injections should be performed.

REFERENCES

1. Perrault I, Rozet JM, Gerber S, et al. Leber congenital amaurosis. Mol Genet Metab 1999;68:200–208.
2. Kaplan J, Bonneau D, Frezal J, et al. Clinical and genetic heterogeneity in retinitis pigmentosa. Hum Genet 1990;85:635–642.
3. Foxman SG, Heckenlively JR, Bateman JB, et al. Classification of congenital and early onset retinitis pigmentosa. Arch Ophthalmol 1985;103:1502–1506.
4. Fazzi E, Signorini SG, Scelsa B, et al. Leber's congenital amaurosis: an update. Eur J Paediatr Neurol 2003;7:13–22.
5. Heckenlively JR. Retinitis Pigmentosa. Philadelphia: Lippincott, 1988.
6. De Laey JJ. Leber's congenital amaurosis. Bull Soc Belge Ophtalmol 1991;241:41–50.
7. Harris EW. Leber's congenital amaurosis and RPE65. Int Ophthalmol Clin 2001;41:73–82.
8. Margolis S, Scher BM, Carr RE. Macular colobomas in Leber's congenital amaurosis. Am J Ophthalmol 1977;83:27–31.
9. Lambert SR, Taylor D, Kriss A. The infant with nystagmus, normal appearing fundi, but an abnormal ERG. Surv Ophthalmol 1989;34:173–186.
10. Heher KL, Traboulsi EI, Maumenee IH. The natural history of Leber's congenital amaurosis. Age-related findings in 35 patients. Ophthalmology 1992;99:241–245.
11. Schappert-Kimmijser J, Henkes HE, Bosch J. Amaurosis congenita (Leber). Arch Ophthalmol 1959;61:211–218.
12. Francois J. Leber's congenital tapetoretinal degeneration. Int Ophthalmol Clin 1968;8:929–947.
13. Smith D, Oestreicher J, Musarella MA. Clinical spectrum of Leber's congenital amaurosis in the second to fourth decades of life. Ophthalmology 1990;97:1156–1161.
14. Perrault I, Rozet JM, Ghazi I, et al. Different functional outcome of RetGC1 and RPE65 gene mutations in Leber congenital amaurosis. Am J Hum Genet 1999;64:1225–1228.

15. Lorenz B, Gyurus P, Preising M, et al. Early-onset severe rod-cone dystrophy in young children with RPE65 mutations. Invest Ophthalmol Vis Sci 2000;41:2735–2742.

16. Edwards WC, Macdonald Jr R, Price WD. Congenital amaurosis of retinal origin (Leber). Am J Ophthalmol 1971;72:724–728.

17. Leighton DA, Harris R. Retinal aplasia in association with macular coloboma, keratoconus and cataract. Clin Genet 1973;4:270–274.

18. Franceschetti A, Forni S. Dégénérescence tapétorétinienne (type Leber) avec aspect marbré du fond de oeil périphérique. Ophthalmologica 1958;135:610–618.

19. Chew E, Deutman A, Pinckers A, et al. Yellowish flecks in Leber's congenital amaurosis. Br J Ophthalmol 1984;68:727–731.

20. Schroeder R, Mets MB, Maumenee IH. Leber's congenital amaurosis. Retrospective review of 43 cases and a new fundus finding in two cases. Arch Ophthalmol 1987;105:356–359.

21. Paunescu K, Wabbels B, Preising MN, et al. Longitudinal and cross-sectional study of patients with early-onset severe retinal dystrophy associated with RPE65 mutations. Graefes Arch Clin Exp Ophthalmol 2005;243:417–426.

22. den Hollander AI, Roepman R, Koenekoop RK, et al. Leber congenital amaurosis: genes, proteins and disease mechanisms. Prog Retin Eye Res 2008;27:391–419.

23. Marlhens F, Bareil C, Griffoin JM, et al. Mutations in RPE65 cause Leber's congenital amaurosis. Nat Genet 1997;17:139–141.

24. Gu SM, Thompson DA, Srikumari CR, et al. Mutations in RPE65 cause autosomal recessive childhood-onset severe retinal dystrophy. Nat Genet 1997;17:194–197.

25. Camuzat A, Dollfus H, Rozet JM, et al. A gene for Leber's congenital amaurosis maps to chromosome 17p. Hum Mol Genet 1995;4:1447–1452.

26. Perrault I, Rozet JM, Calvas P, et al. Retinal-specific guanylate cyclase gene mutations in Leber's congenital amaurosis. Nat Genet 1996;14:461–464.

27. Freund CL, Wang QL, Chen S, et al. De novo mutations in the CRX homeobox gene associated with Leber congenital amaurosis. Nat Genet 1998;18:311–312.

28. Sohocki MM, Bowne SJ, Sullivan LS, et al. Mutations in a new photoreceptor-pineal gene on 17p cause Leber congenital amaurosis. Nat Genet 2000;24:79–83.

29. den Hollander AI, Heckenlively JR, van den Born LI, et al. Leber congenital amaurosis and retinitis pigmentosa with Coats-like exudative vasculopathy are associated with mutations in the crumbs homologue 1 (CRB1) gene. Am J Hum Genet 2001;69:198–203.

30. Dryja TP, Adams SM, Grimsby JL, et al. Null RPGRIP1 alleles in patients with Leber congenital amaurosis. Am J Hum Genet 2001;68:1295–1298.

31. Lotery AJ, Jacobson SG, Fishman GA, et al. Mutations in the CRB1 gene cause Leber congenital amaurosis. Arch Ophthalmol 2001;119:415–420.

32. den Hollander AI, Koenekoop RK, Yzer S, et al. Mutations in the CEP290 (NPHP6) gene are a frequent cause of Leber congenital amaurosis. Am J Hum Genet 2006;79:556–561.

33. McEwen DP, Koenekoop RK, Khanna H, et al. Hypomorphic CEP290/NPHP6 mutations result in anosmia caused by the selective loss of G proteins in cilia of olfactory sensory neurons. Proc Natl Acad Sci USA 2007;104:15917–15922.

34. Morimura H, Fishman GA, Grover SA, et al. Mutations in the RPE65 gene in patients with autosomal recessive retinitis pigmentosa or Leber congenital amaurosis. Proc Natl Acad Sci USA 1998;95:3088–3093.

35. Hamel CP, Griffoin JM, Lasquellec L, et al. Retinal dystrophies caused by mutations in RPE65: assessment of visual functions. Br J Ophthalmol 2001;85:424–427.

36. Simovich MJ, Miller B, Ezzeldin H, et al. Four novel mutations in the RPE65 gene in patients with Leber congenital amaurosis. Hum Mutat 2001;18:164

37. Dharmaraj SR, Silva ER, Pina AL, et al. Mutational analysis and clinical correlation in Leber congenital amaurosis. Ophthalmic Genet 2000;21:135–150.

38. Lotery AJ, Namperumalsamy P, Jacobson SG, et al. Mutation analysis of 3 genes in patients with Leber congenital amaurosis. Arch Ophthalmol 2000;118:538–543.

39. Thompson DA, Gyurus P, Fleischer LL, et al. Genetics and phenotypes of RPE65 mutations in inherited retinal degeneration. Invest Ophthalmol Vis Sci 2000;41:4293–4299.

40. Gerber S, Perrault I, Hanein S, et al. Complete exon-intron structure of the RPGR-interacting protein (RP-GRIP1) gene allows the identification of mutations underlying Leber congenital amaurosis. Eur J Hum Genet 2001;9:561–571.

41. Hanein S, Perrault I, Gerber S, et al. Leber congenital amaurosis: comprehensive survey of the genetic heterogeneity, refinement of the clinical definition, and genotype-phenotype correlations as a strategy for molecular diagnosis. Hum Mutat 2004;23:306–317.

42. Simonelli F, Ziviello C, Testa F, et al. Clinical and molecular genetics of Leber's congenital amaurosis: a multicenter study of Italian patients. Invest Ophthalmol Vis Sci 2007;48:4284–4290.

43. Bainbridge JW, Smith AJ, Barker SS, et al. Effect of gene therapy on visual function in Leber's congenital amaurosis. N Engl J Med 2008;358:2231–2239.

44. Maguire AM, Simonelli F, Pierce EA, et al. Safety and efficacy of gene transfer for Leber's congenital amaurosis. N Engl J Med 2008;358:2240–2248.

45. Cideciyan AV, Aleman TS, Boye SL, et al. Human gene therapy for RPE65 isomerase deficiency activates the retinoid cycle of vision but with slow rod kinetics. Proc Natl Acad Sci USA 2008;105:15112–15117.

46. Narfstrom K, Wrigstad A, Nilsson SE. The Briard dog: a new animal model of congenital stationary night blindness. Br J Ophthalmol 1989;73:750–756.

47. Veske A, Nilsson SE, Narfstrom K, Gal A. Retinal dystrophy of Swedish Briard/Briard-beagle dogs is due to a 4-bp deletion in RPE65. Genomics 1999;57:57–61.

48. Acland GM, Aguirre GD, Ray J, et al. Gene therapy restores vision in a canine model of childhood blindness. Nat Genet 2001;28:92–95.

49. Narfstrom K, Katz ML, Bragadottir R, et al. Functional and structural recovery of the retina after gene therapy in the RPE65 null mutation dog. Invest Ophthalmol Vis Sci 2003;44:1663–1672.

50. Al-Khayer K, Hagstrom S, Pauer G, et al. Thirty-year follow-up of a patient with Leber congenital amaurosis and novel RPE65 mutations. Am J Ophthalmol 2004;137:375–377.

51. Chang B, Khanna H, Hawes N, et al. In-frame deletion in a novel centrosomal/ciliary protein CEP290/NPHP6 perturbs its interaction with RPGR and results in early-onset retinal degeneration in the rd16 mouse. Hum Mol Genet 2006;15:1847–1857.

52. Pellikka M, Tanentzapf G, Pinto M, et al. Crumbs, the *Drosophila* homologue of human CRB1/RP12, is essential for photoreceptor morphogenesis. Nature 2002;416:143–149.

53. Porto FB, Perrault I, Hicks D, et al. Prenatal human ocular degeneration occurs in Leber's congenital amaurosis (LCA2). J Gene Med 2002;4:390–396.

54. Milam AH, Barakat MR, Gupta N, et al. Clinicopathologic effects of mutant GUCY2D in Leber congenital amaurosis. Ophthalmology 2003;110:549–558.

55. Jacobson SG, Aleman TS, Cideciyan AV, et al. Human cone photoreceptor dependence on RPE65 isomerase. Proc Natl Acad Sci USA 2007;104:15123–15128.

56. Jacobson SG, Cideciyan AV, Aleman TS, et al. Leber congenital amaurosis caused by an RPGRIP1 mutation shows treatment potential. Ophthalmology 2007;114:895–898.

57. Cideciyan AV, Aleman TS, Jacobson SG, et al. Centrosomal-ciliary gene CEP290/NPHP6 mutations result in blindness with unexpected sparing of photoreceptors and visual brain: implications for therapy of Leber congenital amaurosis. Hum Mutat 2007;28:1074–1083.

58. Jacobson SG, Cideciyan AV, Aleman TS, et al. RDH12 and RPE65, visual cycle genes causing Leber congenital amaurosis, differ in disease expression. Invest Ophthalmol Vis Sci 2007;48:332–338.

59. Jacobson SG, Cideciyan AV, Aleman TS, et al. Crumbs homolog 1 (CRB1) mutations result in a thick human retina with abnormal lamination. Hum Mol Genet 2003;12:1073–1078.

60. von Rückmann A, Fitzke FW, Bird AC. Distribution of pigment epithelium autofluorescence in retinal disease state recorded in vivo and its change over time. Graefes Arch Clin Exp Ophthalmol 1999;237:1–9.

61. Scholl HPN, Chong NHV, Robson AG, et al. Fundus autofluorescence in patients with Leber congenital amaurosis. Invest Ophthalmol Vis Sci 2004;45:2747–2752.

62. Lorenz B, Wabbels B, Wegscheider E, et al. Lack of fundus autofluorescence to 488 nanometers from childhood on in patients with early-onset severe retinal dystrophy associated with mutations in RPE65. Ophthalmology 2004;111:1585–1594.

63. Wabbels B, Demmler A, Paunescu K, et al. Fundus autofluorescence in children and teenagers with hereditary retinal diseases. Graefes Arch Clin Exp Ophthalmol 2005;1–10.

64. Redmond TM, Yu S, Lee E, et al. Rpe65 is necessary for production of 11-cis-vitamin A in the retinal visual cycle. Nat Genet 1998;20:344–351.

65. Katz ML, Redmond TM. Effect of Rpe65 knockout on accumulation of lipofuscin fluorophores in the retinal pigment epithelium. Invest Ophthalmol Vis Sci 2001;42:3023–3030.

66. Holz FG, Schütt F, Kopitz J, et al. Inhibition of lysosomal degradative functions in RPE cells by a retinoid component of lipofuscin. Invest Ophthalmol Vis Sci 1999;40:737–743.

Susan M. Downes

Fundus Autofluorescence in Pattern Dystrophy

Pattern dystrophy (PD), a term coined by Marmor and Byers (1), refers to a group of inherited retinal dystrophies characterized by the deposition of a highly autofluorescent material at the level of the retinal pigment epithelium (RPE), with an onset late in life. The incidence and prevalence are not known; however, PD is considered to be rare. In most cases there is an autosomal dominant (AD) mode of inheritance, although penetrance is variable. However, some cases may be sporadic or inherited as an autosomal recessive (AR) trait (the latter in association with reticular dystrophy). Patients may be asymptomatic or present with blurred vision and/or metamorphopsia. In advanced stages of the disease, reduced central vision and reading difficulties may be noted as a result of the development of atrophy or, less frequently, choroidal neovascularization (CNV).

The most common form of PD, adult vitelliform macular dystrophy (AVMD), is characterized by a bilateral solitary yellow, round to oval subfoveal lesion with or without a central pigmented spot (2). The next most common forms are multifocal PD simulating Stargardt disease-fundus flavimaculatus (STGD-FFM) and butterfly-shaped PD (3,4). Rarer forms of PD include Sjogren reticular dystrophy, macroreticular dystrophy, and fundus pulverulentus. These various phenotypes can be seen in different individuals in the same family (5,6). Also, depending on the stage of the disease, the phenotype can change in appearance in the same individual over time (7,8).

PD may be present as an isolated condition or as part of a syndrome associated with other systemic disorders. PD has been found in a proportion of patients with maternally inherited diabetes and deafness (MIDDM) (9) (see Chapter 11H), myotonic dystrophy (10), pseudoxanthoma elasticum (PXE) (11), Friedreich ataxia (12), and Crohn disease (13).

HISTOPATHOLOGY AND MOLECULAR GENETICS

Clinicopathologic studies of patients with PD have shown similar findings (14–16). A histopathological study of the postmortem eyes of a 61-year-old female revealed focal atrophy of the RPE in the foveolar area bordered by hypertrophic RPE, with fusiform collagenous plaques of eosinophilic material located between the atrophic RPE and Bruch's membrane. The sensory retina over the abnormal RPE displayed significant atrophy of the outer nuclear layer with loss of photoreceptor inner layer and outer segments. Pigment-laden macrophages with periodic acid Schiff-positive material had migrated into the atrophic outer retina. Ultraviolet fluorescent microscopy demonstrated massive accumulation of lipofuscin within the macular RPE as well as within the macrophages in the atrophic outer retina. Scanning electron microscopy revealed a confluent area of flattened atrophic RPE cells surrounded by taller hypertrophic RPE cells. Transmission electron microscopy demonstrated that the RPE cells contained many lipofuscin granules (14,15). In three patients with AVMD, RPE and photoreceptor cell loss were observed in the central area. A moderate number of pigment-laden macrophages were present in the subretinal space and outer retina. The RPE was distended to both sides of the central lesion with abundant lipofuscin (16).

PD is genetically heterogeneous. To date, the most common genes known to harbor mutations that can cause nonsyndromic PD include *PRPH2* (Peripherin 2) (Stone, personal communication referred to in Grover et al. [17]) (18), *ELOVL4* (19), and *BEST1* (20) (previously known as *VMD2*; see also Chapter 11F). In addition, as noted above, gene mutations in DTM (myotonic dystrophy) and mtDNA 3243 may be associated with a "PD-like" phenotype.

PRPH2 encodes peripherin 2, a membrane-associated glycoprotein restricted to photoreceptor outer segment discs (21). Normal levels of this protein are required for the morphogenesis and maintenance of the photoreceptor outer segments (22). The *rds* mouse exhibiting the retinal degeneration slow phenotype was found to have a single spontaneous mutation (23). The phenotype in the *rds* mouse is characterized by abnormal development of photoreceptor outer segments in the retina followed by a slow degeneration of the rods and cones, resembling the phenotypes described in human retinal dystrophies associated with *PRPH2* mutations (24). A feature seen in both humans with *PRPH2* mutations and mice with the *rds* mutation is a loss of photoreceptor function. Ali et al. (25) demonstrated that a subretinal injection of recombinant adeno-associated virus (rAAV) encoding an rds transgene resulted in the stable generation of outer segment structures and formation of new stacks of discs, which were morphologically similar to normal outer segments, and electrophysiological tests confirmed function. rAAV-mediated gene replacement of peripherin 2 restored retinal ultrastructure and function for as long as 14 weeks in the *rds* mouse. In this model, however, AAV-mediated gene replacement was not sustained in the long term.

Although studies have described a common consistent phenotype caused by certain mutations in peripherin 2, such as the Arg172Tryp mutation associated with macular dystrophy (26), significant variation in phenotypic expressivity in the same family has also been described in PD associated with *PRPH2* mutations (5). For example, the same mutation can cause retinitis pigmentosa, PD, and fundus flavimaculatus in a single family (5). Yang et al. (4) described three separate families, each of which had a distinct PD phenotype that differed from those of the other families, although they all had the same mutation in *PRPH2* and an identical disease haplotype.

ELOVL4 is a photoreceptor-specific gene that is involved in the biosynthesis of very long chain fatty acids. It is expressed in retina and skin. Defective protein trafficking may underlie the molecular mechanism associated with degeneration of the macula (27). It is possible that some patients with multifocal PD simulating STGD-FFM have mutations in this gene, as mutations in *ELOVL4* have been found in patients with AD Stargardt-like disease (19,28).

CLINICAL FEATURES

The age of onset in PD is usually in late adulthood, but with a positive family history it may occur in early adulthood. The progression of visual loss is usually slow, and most patients maintain reading vision until later in life. The condition can be quite asymmetrical. Monitoring vision, especially in drivers, is important. Regular self-monitoring with an Amsler grid should be encouraged, and patients should be advised to seek ophthalmic review if sudden onset of blurring or distortion occurs, which could indicate the development of CNV. CNV was originally thought to be rare in PD (29), but is probably not uncommon (30,31). Macular atrophy has been observed both at presentation and over time in patients with PD (32).

Adult Vitelliform Macular Dystrophy

AVMD is most commonly dominantly inherited, with incomplete penetrance and highly variable expression, but there are a significant number of sporadic cases. In one study, 91% of patients with AVMD had no family history (8). Furthermore, lesions may be unilateral in a high proportion of patients (8). Typical findings include a yellow (Fig. 11E.1) or pigmented central deposit, around which a depigmented halo is often seen (Fig. 11E.2). There may be a central spot alone or there may be a few deposits near the lesion or in the peripheral retina (Fig. 11E.3). The electro-oculogram (EOG) light rise is usually normal or mildly affected. Color vision may be abnormal.

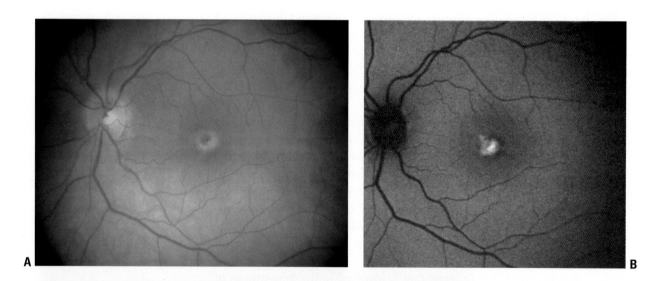

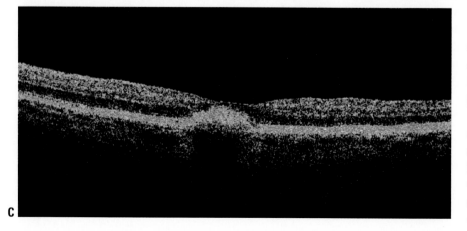

FIGURE 11E.1. Color fundus photograph **(A)**, AF image **(B)**, and OCT **(C)** obtained from a 64-year-old female with AVMD. Slit-lamp biomicroscopy disclosed a small yellow deposit at the left fovea **(A)**, with a highly increased signal on AF imaging **(B)**. OCT demonstrated a well-delineated, dome-shaped elevation of the anterior reflective band and increased reflectivity within the vitelliform lesion **(C)**. *PRPH2* testing demonstrated a mutation in the gene.

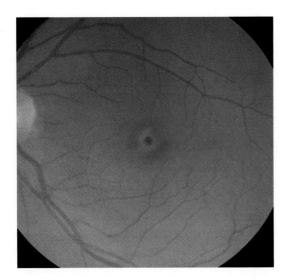

FIGURE 11E.2.   Color fundus photograph obtained from a 56-year-old male with central visual disturbance and AVMD. A central area of increased pigmentation surrounded by a halo of depigmentation is observed.

Butterfly-Shaped Pattern Dystrophy

Butterfly-shaped PD is characterized by an accumulation of yellow or brown pigment at the level of the RPE in a butterfly configuration (Fig. 11E.4). A subnormal EOG and normal or slightly diminished visual acuity have been described, as well as atrophic changes and an AD inheritance (3). Although Deutman proposed a relatively benign course for butterfly-shaped PD, it has now clear that butterfly-shaped PD, like other types of PD, is usually a progressive disorder with varying degrees of visual deterioration (3). Older individuals may have atrophic, depigmented lesions extending into the peripapillary region, with markedly reduced visual acuity (33).

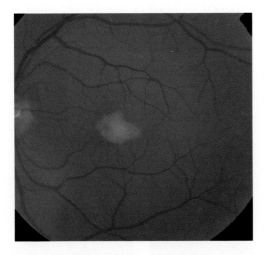

FIGURE 11E.3.   Color fundus photograph of a patient with AVMD demonstrating accumulation of yellow material at the fovea and additional deposits near this main lesion distributed throughout the macula and into the midperipheral retina.

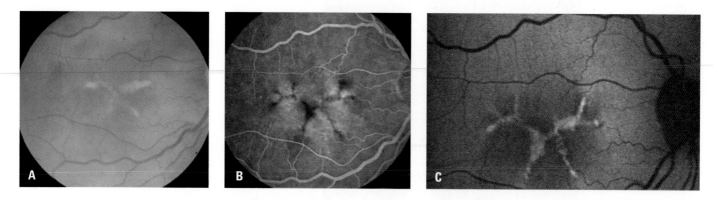

FIGURE 11E.4. Color fundus photograph (**A**), FFA image (**B**), and AF (**C**) obtained from an 82-year-old female with butterfly-shaped PD from a family with various PD phenotypes, AD inheritance, and a mutation in *PRPH2*. Deposition of yellow material in a "butterfly" distribution was observed on slit-lamp biomicroscopy (**A**), which demonstrated a high AF signal on AF imaging (**C**). FA demonstrated linear areas of hypofluorescence surrounded by ill-defined hyperfluorescence. (Courtesy of Professor Alan Bird, Moorfields Eye Hospital, London, England.)

Reticular and Macroreticular Pattern Dystrophy

Reticular dystrophy, first described by Sjogren (34) in 1950, is characterized by a pattern of pigment clumping that has been likened to a fishnet with knots (Fig. 11E.5A,B). Patients may have normal vision, normal electroretinogram (ERG) and EOG, and normal color vision and peripheral visual fields (34,35).

Macroreticular PD was described in 1970 (36). It is extremely rare. It is characterized by a larger meshwork of reticular changes in the fundus (Fig. 11E.5B). The ERG and EOG may be abnormal (37).

Fundus Pulverentulus

The term "fundus pulverentulus" has been used to describe a granular fundus appearance, and has been reported in families manifesting other PD phenotypes (Fig. 11E.6) (38,39).

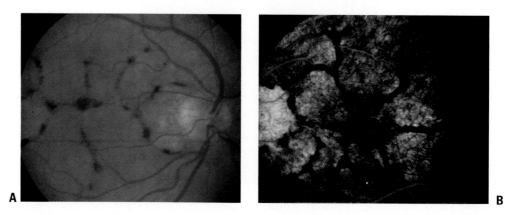

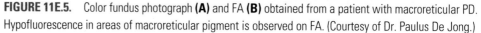

FIGURE 11E.5. Color fundus photograph (**A**) and FA (**B**) obtained from a patient with macroreticular PD. Hypofluorescence in areas of macroreticular pigment is observed on FA. (Courtesy of Dr. Paulus De Jong.)

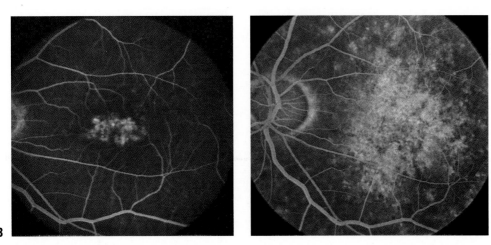

A,B

FIGURE 11E.6.   FA obtained from a 46-year-old patient with PD (a relative of the proband with butterfly dystrophy shown in Fig. 11E.4). In her left eye, at presentation, retinal pigment epithelial defects in a granular pulverentulus-like appearance at the central macula were seen (**A**). Twenty years later, these changes had become more diffuse (**B**). (Courtesy of Professor Alan Bird, Moorfields Eye Hospital, London, England.)

Multifocal Pattern Dystrophy Simulating Stargardt Disease-Fundus Flavimaculatus

The form of PD known as multifocal PD simulating STGD-FFM is characterized by the presence of fleck-like deposits and AD inheritance (Fig. 11E.7) (40). It may be indistinguishable from AD STGD-like fundus dystrophy associated with mutations in the *ELOVL4* gene, and molecular genetic testing may be necessary to differentiate between these two conditions.

IMAGING AND OTHER DIAGNOSTIC STUDIES IN PATTERN DYSTROPHY

Fluorescein and Indocyanine Green Angiography

With the advent of fundus autofluorescence (AF) imaging, fluorescein angiography (FA) and indocyanine green (ICG) angiography are probably better reserved for investigating complications of PD, such as CNV, rather than for diagnostic purposes.

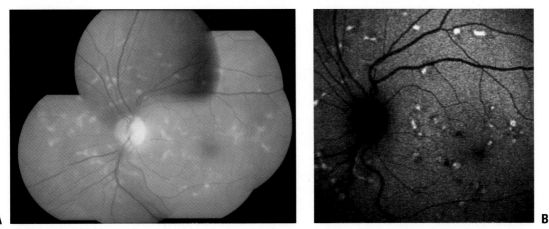

A   **B**

FIGURE 11E.7.   Color fundus photograph (**A**) and AF image (**B**) of a patient with Friedreich ataxia and multifocal PD simulating STGD-FFM (12). Visual acuity and retinal electrophysiology were normal until optic atrophy supervened as part of Friedreich ataxia.

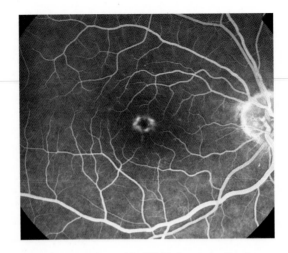

FIGURE 11E.8. FA obtained from a patient with AVMD demonstrating the corona sign, in which there is hyperfluorescence surrounding a central area of hypofluorescence. (Courtesy of Professor Alan Bird, Moorfields Eye Hospital, London, England.)

In the absence of AF imaging, FA is useful for highlighting changes in the RPE (31,39,41). FA can also demonstrate a "dark choroid" in some individuals with STGD-FFM (see Chapter 11G), which may help in the differentiation between PD and STGD-FFM (see later).

Typical features seen on FA in AVMD include a central hypofluorescent spot corresponding to the area of central increased pigmentation and a ring of hyperfluorescence around it (referred to as the "corona sign" [Fig. 11E.8]), which relates to a window defect in areas where atrophic changes have occurred (8,42). In a few patients, FA may be normal. On ICG angiography, a foveal nonfluorescent spot has been observed throughout the angiogram, with a hyperfluorescent area surrounding the central spot that is evident in early frames of the angiogram (43).

The ICG and FA findings from a 37-year-old female with reticular dystrophy complicated by CNV showed that in the areas of reticular changes there were significant abnormalities characterized by intense hyperfluorescence (31).

Da Pozzo et al. (44) suggested caution in interpreting ICG angiography, as vitelliform material present in PD may bind to the ICG molecule and cause hyperfluorescence simulating an occult CNV.

Optical Coherence Tomography (OCT)

OCT alone will not permit accurate diagnosis of AVMD or other types of PD. However, it can be a useful adjunct to fundus AF and color fundus imaging to exclude associated edema, as seen in cases complicated by CNV. In the latter, FA would be indicated.

Pierro et al. (45) carried out a retrospective review of 43 patients (72 eyes) with AVMD. In all eyes, OCT showed a well-defined central region of thickening in the reflective band representing the RPE. Similar findings have been reported by Hayami et el. (46). In patients with a thinner neurosensory retinal layer overlying the AVMD lesion, the visual acuity was reduced (45).

Benhamou et al. (47) described the OCT features in evolving lesions of AVMD as the disease progressed. In the vitelliform stage, a well-circumscribed dome-shaped elevation of the anterior reflective band, a moderate back scattering below the anterior reflective band, well-delineated posterior boundaries in the plane of the RPE, and an increase in the reflectivity within the vitelliform lesion as the lesion became smaller (atrophic stage) were observed. These authors pointed out that it was not possible to be certain about the exact location of the yellow material seen on histopathological studies because those observations were made in eyes with end-stage disease. According to Benhamou et al. (47), the posterior reflective band corresponds to the RPE, whereas the highly reflective anterior band represents the pseudo-vitelliform lesion (47). They stated that the lesion is located between the photoreceptor layer and the RPE, but it sometimes appears that the lesion is within the RPE.

Therefore, the common feature seen on OCT imaging in patients with PD is a thickened, well-circumscribed, central focal dome-shaped lesion that appears to lie in between the photoreceptors and RPE (Figs. 11E.1C and 11E.9). If a central lesion is observed in OCT images of patients with PD, as in AVMD, there does not seem to be any specific difference between the yellow deposit and the pigmented deposit. However, the discrete dome-shaped, smooth elevation on OCT seems to depend on the type of PD (i.e., the presence of AVMD) rather than, for instance, multifocal PD simulating STGD-FFM (personal observation). Findings from OCT alone, however, may not be specific enough to distinguish PD from a CNV. In cases of age-related macular degeneration (AMD)-associated CNV, OCT tends to show much more extensive changes throughout the retinal layers, in contrast to PD, in which changes are more focal and smooth in contour. However, in idiopathic, myopic, or inflammatory CNV, especially if it is inactive, OCT findings may be indistinguishable from those observed in PD. Under these circumstances, history and ancillary tests, such as AF, are very helpful. A very high AF signal is seen in PD and, most commonly, a reduced or mottled AF signal is seen at the site of a CNV.

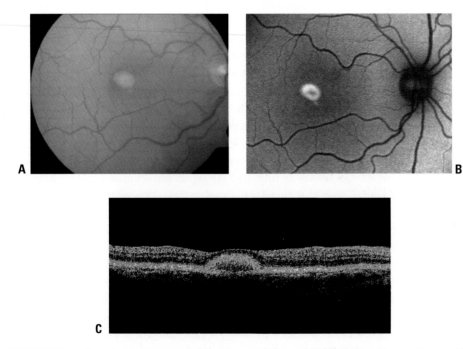

FIGURE 11E.9.   Color fundus photograph **(A)**, AF image **(B)**, and OCT **(C)** obtained from a 56-year-old female with AD PD with a mutation in *PRPH2*. Accumulation of yellow material at the fovea was observed on slit-lamp biomicroscopy **(A)**. The material demonstrated a very increased AF signal **(B)**. OCT disclosed a smooth, well-circumscribed, dome-shaped elevation in the area of the lesion, with a highly reflective band corresponding to the RPE **(C)**.

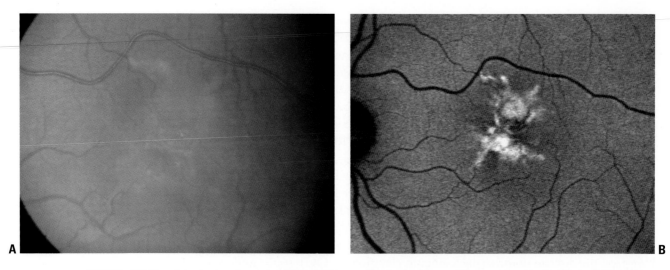

FIGURE 11E.10. Color fundus photograph **(A)** and AF image **(B)** obtained from a 63-year-old male with PD. A relatively large, ill-defined yellowish lesion at the macula was observed on slit-lamp biomicroscopy **(A)**. Fundus AF disclosed a significantly increased AF signal at the site of the lesion, suggesting accumulation of lipofuscin material as typically observed in PD **(B)**.

Fundus Autofluorescence

Fundus AF is very helpful in the diagnosis and evaluation of patients with PD. In AVMD a very characteristic well-circumscribed, very high AF signal is seen in the vitelliform stage (Figs. 11E.1B and 11E.9B). In patients with a central clump of pigment and a surrounding halo of depigmentation, AF images usually demonstrate a central area of significantly increased AF surrounded by a halo of reduced AF. The evolution of these appearances during the course of the disease has not been well documented, but with the disappearance of the vitelliform lesion a corresponding loss of AF signal is observed, indicating the occurrence of atrophy. AF imaging may allow the visualization of disease-specific distributions of lipofuscin in the RPE even when these changes are not yet visible on fundoscopy (48). Fundus AF can also be useful in the diagnosis of PD in cases with an amorphous deposit, allowing its differentiation from other lesions, such as a drusenoid pigment epithelial detachment (PED) (Fig. 11E.10).

In a study by Renner et al. (8) in which 13 patients (25 eyes) were imaged with fundus AF, a yellow lesion was present in 22 eyes, and central pigmentation was present in 6 eyes. In 19 of the 22 eyes (86%) an increased AF signal was seen, and in 8 of these there was an additional small spot of reduced AF signal at the center of the area of increased AF (8). Parodi et al. (49) evaluated 15 patients with AVMD by AF imaging and compared the findings with those observed in 10 healthy volunteers. AF imaging was performed with both short-wave conventional AF and near-infrared AF (NIA) (see also Chapter 6). The former technique revealed three different patterns of AF (normal, focal, and patchy), whereas only two patterns (focal and patchy) were seen with NIA. When AF patterns were correlated with functional tests (vision and microperimetry), it was found that patchy AF was associated with the worst functional outcome. Abnormal short-wave conventional AF was seen in 86% of patients with AVMD, and abnormal NIA was observed in 100%.

Saito et al. (50) evaluated six Japanese patients (12 eyes) with what they diagnosed as AVMD. Bilateral macular lesions were present in all patients and varied from the typical vitelliform (five eyes) to faded vitelliform changes with RPE atrophy (five eyes) or a normal fovea associated with small flecks around it (two eyes). AF imaging demonstrated small spots of increased AF throughout the posterior pole in all cases.

Multifocal ERGs (mFERGs) were significantly reduced not only in the macular area, but also in the outermost ring of the mFERGs (20–30 degrees). The authors suggested that morphological and functional abnormalities in AVMD may not be limited to the macula, but may be present throughout the posterior pole. This was supported by their electrophysiological findings (50). It is possible that these observations reflected previous reports describing the coexistence of fundus pulverentulus and AVMD. The images of the Japanese patients were not typical of AVMD; in one case, the lesions were larger than those typical of AVMD, and it is not clear from the EOG findings whether these patients might have had Best disease. Another case shown had a central lesion with multifocal vitelliform peripheral lesions, which could represent STGD-FFM or multifocal Best disease. The patients were not reported to be from the same family and had no family history. Thus, their findings on AF imaging do not appear to be typical of AVMD. However, it is still possible that these patients have an atypical phenotype of PD that has not been previously described, especially considering that most previously published cases of AVMD affected Caucasians.

AF imaging is expected to play a very important role in monitoring response to future therapies. It may also be useful for identifying individuals with no known genetic mutation, and those in whom the early signs are subtle on fundoscopy. Although AF imaging cannot identify all presymptomatic cases of PD, in many cases it can highlight deposits that are not clearly seen on slit-lamp biomicroscopy. AF imaging is very useful for distinguishing PD from other conditions, especially AMD (see later). AF imaging in PD has replaced FA and is much preferred by patients because it is noninvasive and less time-consuming. FA, however, is still indicated if a CNV is suspected.

Electrophysiology

In general, PD is not associated with gross electrophysiological abnormalities. The EOG may be normal or mildly abnormal; the ERG is most often normal (1,8,51). However, abnormal ERG values (b-wave amplitude of the maximum rod-cone response, single flash cone response, and 30-Hz flicker response) may be elicited in some patients (8). Previously normal ERG recordings may become mildly reduced with long-term follow-up (1); only occasionally will a marked reduction in ERG values be seen (8).

Weleber et al. (5) reported a family with clinically disparate phenotypes caused by a mutation in 153/154 codon of peripherin 2. A profoundly abnormal ERG was recorded in one member of the family with a retinitis pigmentosa phenotype, a moderately abnormal ERG was found in a member with a macular dystrophy phenotype, and a markedly abnormal ERG was found in another who had also a form of macular dystrophy (5).

Reduced mfERGs representing the fovea have been recorded in patients with PD, and a generalized decrease in amplitude has also been seen in a small proportion of patients (14%) (8).

DIFFERENTIAL DIAGNOSES

PD should be differentiated from Best disease, STGD-FFM, acute exudative polymorphous vitelliform maculopathy, central serous chorioretinopathy (CSR), and AMD.

In contrast to PD, in Best disease the EOG light rise is usually extinguished or severely reduced and onset occurs in childhood or early adulthood (see also Chapter 11F). Furthermore, the size of the vitelliform lesion tends to be larger.

Multifocal PD can easily be mistaken for STGD-FFM (52), particularly if there is no family history. STGD-FFM is associated with mutations in the ABCA4 gene (see also Chapter 11G), and it usually has a worse visual prognosis than PD. The presence of a dark choroid on FA and a relative peripapillary sparing in STGD-FFM will help in the differentiation. AD Stargardt-like dystrophy caused by mutations in *ELOVL4* may be part of the PD spectrum.

Acute exudative polymorphous vitelliform maculopathy (53), characterized by the presence of transient, multifocal, and numerous small yellowish lesions, may also be mistaken for PD. As in PD, affected patients may have reduced or normal amplitudes of ERG and EOG (54). Abnormalities in dark adaptometry have been found in patients with acute exudative polymorphous vitelliform maculopathy (54). Unlike lesions in PD, those in acute exudative polymorphous vitelliform maculopathy can disappear over a relatively short period of time, with gradual recovery of vision. However, this is not always the case. Also, the onset of lesions associated with acute exudative polymorphous dystrophy may be accompanied by headache, and if imaged with ICG the choriocapillaris may be abnormal, which is not seen in PD.

Old RPE changes in CSR can simulate those observed in PD (see also Chapter 13). Increased levels of AF can be seen in both conditions. However, in CSR changes are more diffuse and ill defined than in PD and, unlike PD, only very rarely will a well-delineated increased AF signal at the fovea be observed.

AVMD is often misdiagnosed as AMD, and fundus AF is very helpful in differentiating these conditions. Although weakly increased AF can be detected in patients with early AMD and drusen, the high-intensity AF signal present in PD is rarely observed in AMD. This is particularly useful in patients with large drusenoid PEDs, which clinically may look like vitelliform lesions. Because AVMD generally has a better prognosis and may be associated with an AD inheritance, it is very important to distinguish between AMD and PD.

SUMMARY

Different forms of PD have been described, with AVMD and multifocal PD simulating STGD-FFM being the most common. PD can vary in presentation even within a family with AD disease, and combinations of phenotypes can be seen in individuals in the same family. Furthermore, variable penetrance has been recognized in PD. AF imaging can be helpful in making the diagnosis of PD and in differentiating PD from other retinal diseases, such as AMD. It is likely that fundus AF will become a key tool for evaluating response to future therapies.

REFERENCES

1. Marmor MF, Byers B. Pattern dystrophy of the pigment epithelium. Am J Ophthalmol 1977:84:32–44.
2. Gass JDM. A clinicopathologic study of a peculiar foveomacular dystrophy. Trans Am Ophthal Soc 1974;72:139–155.
3. Deutman AF, van Blommestein JDA, Henkes HE, et al. Butterfly shaped pigment dystrophy of the fovea. Arch Ophthalmol 1970;83:558–569.
4. Yang Z, Li Y, Jiang L, et al. A novel RDS/peripherin gene mutation associated with diverse macular phenotypes. Ophthalmic Genet 2004;25:133–145.
5. Weleber RG, Carr RE, Murphey WH, et al. Phenotypic variability including retinitis pigmentosa, pattern dystrophy, and fundus flavimaculatus in a single family with a deletion of codon 153 or 154 of the peripherin/RDS gene. Arch Ophthalmol 1993;111:1531–1542.
6. Felbor U, Schilling H, Weber BHF. Adult vitelliform macular dystrophy is frequently associated with mutations in the peripherin/RDS gene. Hum Mutat 1997;10:301–309.

7. van Lith-Verhoeven JJC, Cremers FPM, van den Helm B, et al. Genetic heterogeneity of butterfly-shaped pigment dystrophy of the fovea. Mol Vision 2003;9:138–143.

8. Renner AB, Tillack H, Kraus H, et al. Morphology and functional characteristics in adult vitelliform macular dystrophy. Retina 2004;24:929–939.

9. Massin P, Virally Monod M, Vialettes B, et al. Prevalence of macular pattern dystrophy in maternally inherited diabetes and deafness. GEDIAM Group. Ophthalmology 1999;106:1821–1827.

10. Kimizuka Y, Kiyosawa M, Tamai M, et al. Retinal changes in myotonic dystrophy. Clinical and follow-up evaluation. Retina 1993;13:129–135.

11. Agarwal A, Patel P, Adkins T, et al. Spectrum of pattern dystrophy in pseudoxanthoma elasticum. Arch Ophthalmol 2005;123:923–928.

12. Porter N, Downes SM, Fratter C, et al. Catastrophic visual loss in a patient with Friedreich ataxia. Arch Ophthalmol 2007;125:273–274.

13. De Franceschi P, Costagliola C, Soreca E, et al. Pattern dystrophy of the retinal pigment epithelium in Crohn's disease. Opthalmologica 2000;214: 441–446.

14. Patrinely JR, Lewis RA, Font RL. Foveomacular vitelliform dystrophy, adult type: a clinicopathologic study including electron microscopic observations. Ophthalmology 1985;92:1712–1718.

15. Jaffe GJ, Schatz H. Histopathologic features of adult-onset foveomacular pigment epithelial dystrophy. Arch Ophthalmol 1988;106:958–960.

16. Dubovy SR, Hairston RJ, Schatz H, et al. Adult-onset foveomacular pigment epithelial dystrophy. Clinicopathologic correlation of three cases. Retina 2000; 20:638–649.

17. Grover S, Fishman G, Stone EM. Atypical presentation of pattern dystrophy in two families with peripherin/RDS mutations. Ophthalmology 2002;109:1110–1117.

18. Fossarello M, Bertini C, Galantuomo MS, et al. Deletion in the peripherin/RDS gene in two unrelated Sardinian families with autosomal dominant butterfly-shaped macular dystrophy. Arch Ophthalmol 1996;114:448–456.

19. Bernstein PS, Tammur J, Singh N, et al. Diverse macular dystrophy phenotype caused by a novel complex mutation in the ELOVL4 gene. Invest Ophthalmol Vis Sci 2001;42:3331–3336.

20. Seddon JM, Afshari MA, Sharma S, et al. Assessment of mutations in the Best macular dystrophy VMD2 gene in patients with adult-onset foveomacular vitelliform dystrophy, age related maculopathy and bull's eye maculopathy. Ophthalmology 2001;108:2060–2067.

21. Travis GH, Sutcliffe JG, Bok D. The retinal degeneration slow (rds) gene product is a photoreceptor disc membrane associated glycoprotein. Neuron 1991;6:61–70.

22. Lee ES, Burnside B, Flannery JG. Characterization of peripherin/rds and Rom1 transport in rod photoreceptors of transgenic and knockout animals. Invest Ophthalmol Vis Sci 2006;47:2150–2160.

23. Van Gulik PJ, Kortweg R. Susceptibility to follicular hormone and disposition to mammary cancer in female mice. Am J Cancer 1940;38:506.

24. Van Nie RD, Ivanyi D, Demant P. A new H-2 linked mutation, rds, causing retinal degeneration in the mouse. Tissue Antigens 1978;12:106–108.

25. Ali RR, Sarra G-M, Stephens C, et al. Restoration of photoreceptor ultrastructure and function in retinal degeneration slow mice by gene therapy. Nat Genet 2000;25:306–310.

26. Downes SM, Fitzke FW, Holder GE, et al. Clinical features of codon 172 RDS macular dystrophy. Arch Ophthalmol 1999;117:1373–1383.

27. Ambasudhan R, Wang X, Jablonski MM, et al. Atrophic macular degeneration mutations in ELOVL4 result in the intracellular misrouting of the protein. Genomics 2004;83:615–625.

28. Zhang K, Kniazeva M, Han M, et al. A 5-bp deletion in ELOVL4 is associated with two related forms of autosomal dominant macular dystrophy. Nat Genet 2001;2789–2793.

29. Vine AK, Schatz H. Adult-onset foveomacular pigment epithelial dystrophy. Am J Ophthalmol 1980;89:680–691.

30. Battaglia Parodi M, Da Pozzo S, Ravalico G. Photodynamic therapy for choroidal neovascularisation associated with pattern dystrophy. Retina 2003;23:171–176.

31. Zeldovich A, Beaumont P, Chang A, et al. Indocyanine green angiographic interpretation of reticular dystrophy of the retinal pigment epithelium complicated by choroidal neovascularisation. Clin Exp Ophthalmol 2002;30:383–385.

32. Marmor MF, McNamara JA. Pattern dystrophy of the retinal pigment epithelium and geographic atrophy of the macula. Am J Ophthalmol 1996;122:382–392.

33. Prensky JG, Bresnick GH. Butterfly macular dystrophy in four generations. Arch Ophthalmol 1983;101:1198–1203.

34. Sjogren H. Dystrophia reticularis laminae pigmentosae retinae: an earlier not described hereditary eye disease. Acta Ophthalmol 1950:28:279–295.

35. Deutman AF, Rumke AM. Reticular dystrophy of the retinal pigment. Dystrophia reticularis laminae pigmentosa retinae of H. Sjogren. Arch Ophthalmol 1969;82:4–9.

36. Mesker RP, Oosterhuis JA, Delleman JW. A retinal lesion resembling Sjogren's dystrophia reticularis lamiiniae pigmentosae retiniae. In: Perspectives in Ophthalmology, Vol. 2. Amsterdam: Excerpta Medical Foundation, 1970:40–45.

37. Fishman GA, Woolf MB, Goldberg MF, et al. Reticular tapeto-retinal dystrophy as a possible late stage of Sjogren's reticular dystrophy. Br J Ophthalmol 1976;60:35–40.

38. Slezak H, Hommer K. Fundus pulverentulus. Albrecht von Graefes Arch Klin Exp Ophthalmol 1969;178: 176–182.
39. O'Donnell FE, Schatz H, Reid P, et al. Autosomal dominant dystrophy of the retinal pigment epithelium. Arch Ophthalmol 1979;97:680–683.
40. Boon CJ, van Schooneveld MJ, den Hollander AI, et al. Mutations in the peripherin/RDS gene are an important cause of multifocal pattern dystrophy simulating STG1/fundus flavimaculatus. Br J Ophthalmol 2007;91:1504–1511.
41. Hittner HM, Ferrell RE, Borda RP, et al. Atypical vitelliform dystrophy in a 5 generation family. Br J Ophthalmol 1984;68:199–207.
42. Epstein GA, Rabb MF. Adult vitelliform macular degeneration: diagnosis and natural history. Br J Ophthalmol 1980;64:733–740.
43. Parodi MB, Iustuklin D, Russo D, et al. Adult-onset foveomacular vitelliform dystrophy and indocyanine green videoangiography. Graefes Arch Clin Exp Ophthalmol 1996;234:208–211.
44. Da Pozzo S, Parodi MB, Toto L, et al. Occult choroidal neovascularisation in adult-onset foveomacular vitelliform dystrophy. Ophthalmologica 2001;215:412–414.
45. Pierro L, Tremolada G, Introini U, et al. Optical coherence tomography findings in adult onset foveomacular vitelliform dystrophy. Am J Ophthalmol 2002;134:675–680.
46. Hayami M, Decock CHR, Brabant P, et al. Optical coherence tomography of adult onset vitelliform dystrophy. Bull Soc Belge Ophtalmol 2003;289; 53–61.
47. Benhamou N, Souied EH, Zolf R, et al. Adult-onset foveomacular vitelliform dystrophy: a study by optical coherence tomography. Am J Ophthalmol 2003; 135:362–367.
48. Wabbels B, Demmier A, Paunescu K, et al. Fundus autofluorescence in children and teenagers with hereditary retinal diseases. Graefes Arch Clin Exp Ophthalmol 2006;244:36–45.
49. Parodi MB, Iacono P, Pedio M, et al. Autofluorescence in adult onset foveomacular vitelliform dystrophy. Retina 2008;28:801–807.
50. Saito W, Yamamoto S, Hayashi M, et al. Morphological and functional analyses of adult onset vitelliform macular dystrophy. Br J Ophthalmol 2003;87:758–762.
51. Theischen M. Schilling H, Steinhorst UH. EOG in adult vitelliform macular degeneration, butterfly shaped pattern dystrophy and Best disease. Ophthalmologe 1997;94:230–233.
52. Aaberg TM, Han DP. Evaluation of phenotypic similarities between Stargardt flavimaculatus and retinal pigment epithelial dystrophies. Trans Am Ophthalmol Soc 1987;85:101–119.
53. Gass JD, Chuang EL, Granek H. Acute exudative polymorphous vitelliform maculopathy. Trans Am Ophthalmol Soc 1988;86:354–366.
54. Chan CK, Gass JD, Lin SG. Acute exudative polymorphous vitelliform mauculopathy syndrome. Retina 2003;23:453–462.

Fundus Autofluorescence in Best Disease

Best disease was first reported in 1905 as a disease affecting the macula (1). The initial report was on eight members of one family from Giessen with mixed bilateral and unilateral disease presenting with a clearly demarcated macular lesion below the fovea of light red to yellow-white color, which Best described as completed central "choroiditis." Various stages of the lesion were recognized as showing rectangular and crescent-shaped forms (1). These stages were later classified by Gass et al. (2). Currently, five stages are generally accepted (Fig. 11F.1):

- Previtelliform stage: No fundus abnormalities; mutation carriers are in this stage and will not be recognized if the family does not present with a history of Best disease (Fig. 11F.1A,B).
- Vitelliform stage: Prominent, yellow or light red, well-demarcated central macular lesion that, over time, increases in size to occupy the entire macular area; the lesion is circular and the color is quite uniform (Fig. 11F.1C,D). This stage was the primary stage described by Best (1).
- Pseudohypopyon stage: The yellowish material occupies predominantly the lower half of the lesion (Fig. 11F.1E,F).
- Vitelliruptive or "scrambled egg" stage: The lesion develops an elliptical shape in the vertical axis that is described in association with a loss of visual acuity and disruption of the uniform distribution of the yellowish material, which appears, at this stage, to precipitate in the subretinal space and at the margins of the lesion (Fig. 11F.1G,H).
- Fibrotic stage: Corresponds to the complete "choroiditis" described by Best (1) in which there is cicatrization of the macula and subretinal fibrosis. A minimal amount of yellow material may still be visible within the scar (Fig. 11F.1I,J).

The age of onset of the disease, the progression through the different stages, and the penetrance of the symptoms is very variable among different families. Symptoms may appear in the first decade of life or may never develop, as it occurs in carriers of the disease. The disease may initially affect one eye only, with both eyes later progressing independently. Some patients may have lesions in the vitelliform stage that remain unchanged for many years, whereas others may progress to the pseudohypopyon stage within a few months. This heterogeneity in the progression of the disease was originally recognized by Best (1) and confirmed in several later reports, including our own studies (3).

MOLECULAR BASIS AND HISTOPATHOLOGY

Human Best1 gene (*hBEST1*) codes for a protein (bestrophin) involved in transmembrane transport in membranes of the retinal pigment epithelium (RPE). The gene prod-

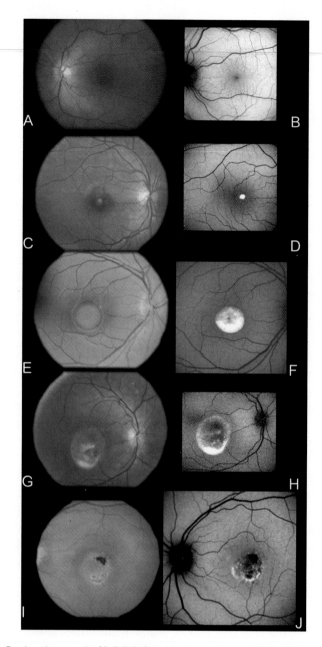

FIGURE 11F.1. Fundus photographs **(A,C,E,G,I)** and fundus AF images **(B,D,F,H,J)** of five patients with various stages of Best disease. A clinical heterogeneity with regard to the age of onset and the progression of the disease is manifested in these photographs of a 39-year-old patient in the previtelliform stage **(A,B)**, a 6-year-old patient in the vitelliform stage **(C,D)**, an 8-year-old patient in the early pseudohypopion stage **(E,F)**, a 16-year-old patient in the vitelliruptive stage **(G,H)**, and a 17-year-old patient in the fibrotic and final stage of the disease **(I,J)**.

uct is part of a Ca^{2+}-activated Cl^- channel (CACC). Bestrophin was considered to be the channel itself (4), but its functional characteristics did not support the notion that bestrophin acts as a Cl^- channel (5). Recent studies have solved the problem by showing that bestrophin interacts with β-subunits of the channel, influencing the activity of the CACC, and thus explaining the functional characteristics of bestrophin (6). Histological studies locate bestrophin on the basolateral side of the RPE, and the common notion was that the protein is part of the basolateral membrane (7). Expression is higher in the extramacular than in the macular RPE, as shown based on protein and RNA levels (8). The question of the functional impact and pathological effect remains to be resolved. As a first hypothesis. Fischmeister and Hartzell (9) proposed that bestrophin is involved in a cell volume-dependent current that decreases when the volume of the RPE cell increases. Such an increase in volume may be caused by osmotic stress in the interphotoreceptor space, or follow phagocytotic activity when the RPE clears the shaded outer segments at night. In this regard, phagocytosis may be hampered by the imbalanced osmotic equilibration caused by improper bestrophin function (9).

Best disease (VMD2) segregates in an autosomal dominant way. Reduced penetrance has been associated with certain mutations, including c.969delTCA, a very frequent in-frame deletion (3).

Patients affected by Best disease present to the ophthalmologist with decreased visual acuity and color vision deficits, or ask for an appointment for genetic counseling due to a positive family history. In carriers and in patients up to the vitelliform stage of the disease, the reduction of visual acuity may not be as prominent as the fundus changes would suggest. A rapid drop in visual acuity occurs when the patient progresses through the vitelliruptive stage, although useful visual acuity may be retained into the fibrotic stage (3). Visual acuity depends on surviving photoreceptor cells and a preserved photoreceptor cell layer on which the image can be mapped. Any change in surface, receptor density, and receptor distribution will lead to faulty image mapping. A faulty image mapping reduces visual acuity. The faulty mapping may be tolerated to a certain extent by the adaptability of the visual system and may be recognized by the patient in later stages of the disease only. Especially when photoreceptor loss becomes profound in the fibrotic stage or rearrangements of the photoreceptor layer take place in vitelliruptive stage, the visual acuity will drop (3,10).

The lesion described by Best was seen on fundus photographs to be located under the fovea and within the retinal layers (1). Histological studies dating from the 1980s reported on cases in the vitelliruptive (11) and fibrotic (12) stages. These studies localized the lesion to the level of the RPE. Weingeist et al. (12) described accumulation of vesicles in the RPE below the lesion that stained with lipophilic substances on light microscopy. These vesicles were distributed throughout the cells and identified as lipofuscin granules (11,13).

The histology of an eye from a patient in a late stage of the disease and with a known *hBEST1* mutation (T6R) supported the results of Weingeist et al. (12). The results showed that accumulation of lipofuscin granules occurred peripheral to the scar region and that, beneath the scar, the RPE was atrophic with only rare inclusions (8). Results from a 93-year-old patient with peripheral flecks carrying a Y227N mutation contradicted the findings in the T6R patient concerning lipofuscin accumulation. The Y227N mutation was associated with normal distribution of AF in the macular region. Mullins et al. (8) judged this as a variability of phenotypical expression. Lipofuscin density was studied in purified intracellular granules in a further patient carrying a homozygous missense mutation (W93C) in *hBEST1* compared with a heterozygous individual carrying the T6R mutation (8) and age-matched controls (13). The severity of the disease was no higher in the patient carrying the homozygous mutation. Both patients showed a reduction of the classical lipofuscin fraction of light dense granules. A shift to denser lipofuscin granules was noted by fluorescence measurements of fractionated RPE granules (13). The denser granules were multilobed, indicating fusion of lipofuscin granules and thus impaired trafficking of lipofuscin granules within the RPE as a result of the dysfunction of bestrophin.

Some additional features were noted, such as a reduced number of melanosomes and an increased amount of secondary lysosomes. Mitochondria showed abnormal torpedo-like shapes and small electron dense particles were shown in the extracellular space enmeshed in a fine fibrillar substance (12). Hypertrophy of the ER was reported in a further case, as well as loss of fenestration and occurrence of ghost vessels in the choriocapillaris (8).

IMAGING AND DIAGNOSTIC TECHNIQUES

Best disease is a macular disorder with prominent and characteristic features seen on fundus photography (see Introduction). The diagnosis of Best disease is usually made by slit-lamp biomicroscopy, taking into account visual acuity, color vision, and visual field findings. Functional testing, especially electro-oculography (EOG), is often obtained to confirm the diagnosis.

Fluorescein and Indocyanine Green Angiography

Angiography is only rarely used to evaluate patients with Best disease. Since fluorescein angiography (FA) displays the retinal vasculature, its application may be useful to discern elder and late-stage Best disease patients from patients with adult vitelliform macular dystrophy (AVMD) and age-related macular degeneration (AMD). The latter show leakage of retinal vessels throughout the retina by FA, whereas in patients with Best, the fluorescein leakage is restricted to the macular lesion. Few reports on the use of indocyanine green (ICG) angiography in patients with Best disease are available (14,15). Maruko et al. (14) found many hyperfluorescent spots in the peripheral and midperipheral retina on ICG angiography in patients with confirmed mutations in *hBEST1*. The hyperfluorescent spots in the periphery did not correspond to vitelliform lesions resulting from lipofuscin accumulation. This was shown by AF of the peripheral vitelliform lesions. Maruko et al. (14) concluded that the diffuse hyperfluorescent spots seen on ICG angiography were located on the RPE/Bruch's membrane level and were associated with fibrillar and drusenoid material. Quaranta et al. (15) focused their fluorescein and ICG angiography on the macular lesion, showing the diffuse hyperfluorescent spots also reported by Maruko et al. (14). Quaranta et al. (15) did not report on any mutation in *hBEST1* in the patients presented. Both groups showed that fluorescence in the macula did not occur on FA but resulted from the AF inside the lesion (15). Finally, Pollack et al. (16) reported the FA findings in a case of Best disease with positive mutation detection. In that report, hyperfluorescent spots were presented at the macula corresponding to light spots of yellowish material in the macular lesion. FA is helpful in detecting the rare occurrence of choroidal neovascularization (CNV) in patients with Best disease, especially in those in advanced stages of the disease.

Optical Coherence Tomography

Modern imaging techniques such as optic coherence tomography (OCT) imaging have shown the lesion to be a hyporeflective structure underneath the neuroretina (Fig. 11F.2) (3,10). Studies reported to date have not provided OCT imaging with a resolution sufficient to discern which retinal layer is actually involved. OCT images show the lesion splitting a layer that contains photoreceptor outer segments, RPE, and Bruch's membrane (outer retina-choroid complex [ORCC]). It is currently thought that the split occurs between RPE and choroid in Bruch's membrane (10). This contradicts the reports by Mullins et al. (8), who located the split between RPE and neuroretina. The hyporeflectivity of the lesion in OCT argues against a cellular nature of the content and points toward a uniform refractive index, which is in accordance with a substance of lipophilic nature seen in histological sections (12).

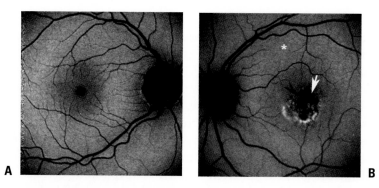

FIGURE 11F.2. **(A)** AF imaging of a control proband and **(B)** a patient in the fibrotic stage (see Fig. 11F.1J). The white arrow indicates an area of lost RPE identified by missing AF; the black arrow indicates an area of remaining RPE identified by its AF, which is comparable to the AF in the macula; and the asterisk indicates an area of background AF, which is comparable to normal AF intensity.

Functional Testing

Marked functional changes are seen on electro-oculography (EOG) in patients and carriers. EOG allows evaluation of RPE function by testing the alternating potential between the posterior pole and anterior segment of the eye during eye movements (17,18). EOG determines the maximal reduction of the standing potential of the RPE during a dark phase (dark trough) and the maximal increase of the standing potential of the RPE during a subsequent light phase (light peak). The ratio of the light peak vs. the dark trough is called the Arden ratio and is considered abnormal when it is less than 2.0 (3). Since the standing potential is measured with electrodes positioned at both canthus and a ground electrode at the forehead, the EOG measures the whole retinal potential, and thus, if abnormal, implies functional disturbances throughout the retina.

Although a few patients and carriers with normal EOG in the early stages of the disease have been reported (3,16), an Arden ratio below 2.0 is the classical feature of Best disease. Patients presenting with normal EOG were associated with *hBEST1* mutations showing reduced penetrance (3,16,19). Normal EOG recordings may be present up to the vitelliruptive stage (3,16).

Electrophysiological recordings localize the lesion to the RPE layer. Photoreceptor-generated signals and the subsequent responses from bipolar cells and other cells in the neuroretina as recorded by Ganzfeld-electroretinography (ERG) and multifocal (mf)ERG demonstrate reduced responses and prolonged latencies starting in patients within the vitelliruptive stage when the lesion begins to disintegrate, but not early on in the course of the disease (3). This suggests a secondary effect on neuroretinal function that may result from bestrophin-mediated dysfunction of the RPE. Photoreceptor degeneration as a result of RPE dysfunction is corroborated by the heterogeneous results of visual acuity tests showing reduced visual acuity starting from the vitelliform stage in some patients but sustained normal visual acuity throughout the disease up to the vitelliruptive stage in other patients (16).

Fundus Autofluorescence Imaging

The distribution of fundus autofluorescence (AF) in the different stages of Best disease is shown in Figure 11F.1. In the previtelliform stage, no abnormality in the distribution of AF is detected (Fig. 11F.1B). In the vitelliform stage, however, there is a marked and uniform increase in the AF signal at the site of the macular lesion

(Fig. 11F.1D). The high AF signal correlates well with the histopathology findings of increased lipophilic material within the lesion, which was later identified as lipofuscin (3,11,12). In the pseudohypopyon stage, the lesion reaches its maximal expansion, covering the whole macula area (Fig. 11F.1F). Background AF is unchanged outside of the lesion and it seems to be lower than normal in the pseudohypopyon stage (Fig. 11F.1F). This decrease, however, is not real but caused by the sensitivity adjustment of the recording instrument to limit the strong AF from the lesion. Since the lipofuscin granules shown in histological studies will be hardly resolved by the imaging system because their small size, a granular pattern of AF is less likely than a uniform distribution of increased AF. Of interest, no increased AF can be detected outside the macular lesion (3). The AF signal remains very high at the site of the lesion, especially inferiorly, where the remains of the yellowish material are predominantly deposited (Fig. 11F.1F). In the vitelliruptive or "scrambled egg" stage, remains of the yellowish material are found at the margins of the lesion and inferiorly (Fig. 11F.1H).

Although AF changes should be expected from the histological data throughout the retina, since *hBest1* is expressed in all RPE cells, it is interesting that fundus AF in patients with Best disease is not increased or decreased outside the macular lesion (Fig. 11F.2).

INTERPRETATION OF FUNDUS AUTOFLUORESCENCE FINDINGS

It was assumed that Best disease is caused by a generalized defect on the RPE with widespread accumulation of lipofuscin material in RPE cells, and that the *hBEST1* gene is expressed in all RPE cells. Therefore, it was unclear why areas of increased AF should be restricted to the center of the macula. A recent report by Mullins et al. (8) solved this dilemma. The authors showed less intense immunolabeling of bestrophin in the macula, indicating reduced expression of *hBEST1* compared to the regions outside of the macula. Given a function of bestrophin in phagocytosis, as indicated by Fischmeister and Hartzell (9), the accumulation of lipofuscin material in the macula area could be explained by the reduced levels of bestrophin expression and phagocytosis at that site. In this regard, the yellowish material may be considered as shed but not phagocytosed photoreceptor outer segments. AF outside of the lesion is inconspicuous, as shown by several authors (20–22), and may be understood as a result of haploinsufficiency restricted to the macula as the area presenting with the highest density of photoreceptors and lowest concentration of bestrophin. In the periphery, minimal but sufficient residual function of bestrophin results in sufficient phagocytotic activity in patients affected by mutations in *hBEST1* (8).

Further reports have supported the notion that the peripheral RPE may not be as dependent on bestrophin function as the macular RPE. Bakall et al. (13) presented a patient homozygous for a missense mutation of uncertain functionality (W93C), and Schatz et al. (23) reported on a family with two patients carrying compound heterozygous mutations in *hBEST1*, an obvious *null* mutation (T29X), and another mutation that may provide residual function (R141H). Family members carrying each of these mutations in the heterozygous state presented with Best disease that was less severe than in the compound heterozygous patients (23). Both reports provide data to evaluate a maximum loss of functionality of bestrophin. From the histological data provided by these reports, at least a normal AF can be expected (13), which argues for a great adaptability in compensating for bestrophin dysfunction in the peripheral RPE. Unfortunately, none of these reports included AF imaging (13,23).

The distribution of fundus AF abnormalities in Best disease indicates that the mutant bestrophin affects the fate of lipofuscin or its precursors within the RPE cells, as well as the fate of the RPE cells themselves. Both may well be due to impaired phagocytosis or storage of lipofuscin within the RPE cells, as indicated by Fischmeister and Hartzell (9). Degeneration will subsequently occur and the destruction of the macula will progress until the final fibrotic stage is completed. The question as to why photoreceptor cells degenerate may be at least partially answered by AF and OCT findings. The presence of spots of increased AF throughout the macular lesion and mostly along its margins from the vitelliruptive stage onward indicates residual AF material in regions of the lesion that did not reattach. This notion is in accordance with OCT findings that show disorganized RPE and neuroretina and remaining hyporeflective areas that correlate with the areas of increased AF (3,10). Thus the degeneration of the photoreceptors occurs by the missing reattachment of the split tissues, and therefore from a reduced support of oxygen and nutrients and reduced waste disposal from and to the choroid, respectively.

It remains unclear how mutations in *hBEST1* affect the RPE to produce the yellowish material in the macular lesion. The highly increased AF signal inside the macular lesion observed in the vitelliform stage decreases centrally to levels similar to those of the background in the vitelliruptive stage (Fig. 11F.1H). The fact that the AF signal inside the lesion from the vitelliruptive stage onward returns to normal or near-normal background levels indicates that the yellowish material is not inside the RPE cell layer but is extracellular (Fig. 11F.3). If the fluorescent material present in the vitelliform stage were inside RPE cells, the AF signal should not decrease in the vitelliruptive stage as long as RPE cells were present below the macular lesion. Also, the intensity of the AF signal supports the concept that the RPE does not accumulate more fluorescent material in the macula (outside the central lesion) and periphery than RPE in unaffected individuals (Fig. 11F.3). In the vitelliruptive stage, the area of the lesion that is not filled with yellowish material shows AF intensity comparable to that of the surrounding fundus (Fig. 11F.1G,H). In the same area, reduced AF intensity occurs later in the fibrotic stage (Figs. 11F.1I,J and 11F.3). This notion is supported by Mullins et al. (8), who argued that the yellowish material is located in the subretinal space, which would support the notion that Best disease is caused by

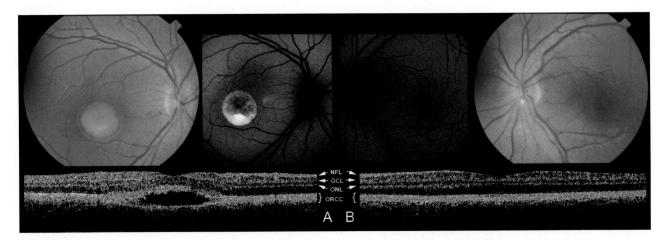

FIGURE 11F.3.   OCT imaging of a 13-year-old patient with Best disease. The right eye demonstrates a lesion **(A)**, whereas the left eye is in the previtelliform stage **(B)**. NFL, nerve fiber layer; GCL, ganglion cell layer; ONL, outer nuclear layer; ORCC, outer retina-choroid complex.

reduced phagocytotic activity of the RPE. From the histological data reported by Weingeist et al. (12) and Mullins et al. (8), RPE degeneration must be expected in late stages. Therefore, reduced AF inside the macular lesion compared to background levels outside of the lesion indicates loss of RPE cells in later stages (Fig. 11F.3).

The fate of the fluorescent material inside the lesion is still unresolved. As shown by our group (3) and others (10,24), the neuroretina overlying the lesion is not disrupted. Pianta et al. (10) showed some OCT scans that allow the interpretation of a disruption of the basolateral membrane of the RPE, which would allow leaking of the fluorescent material into the choroid (24). However, final proof of this interpretation is still lacking. Degradation of the AF material filling the lesion has not yet been shown in fundus photographs and AF images.

DIFFERENTIAL DIAGNOSIS

At the vitelliform stage, the differential diagnosis includes AVMD (see also Chapter 11E) and vitelliform detachments occurring in patients with basal laminar drusen. The former can be distinguished from Best disease by the later age of onset and the lack of progression through stages of the macular lesion; the latter is discerned by the lack of drusen in Best disease.

SUMMARY

Fundus AF imaging in Best disease can be used to provide immediate support to the clinical diagnosis made by slit-lamp biomicroscopy, given that, in most cases, the changes observed clinically, including color, size, form, and structure of the macular lesion, are characteristic of the disease. The presence of a positive family history will be helpful in confirming the diagnosis. EOG is usually used to support the diagnosis of Best disease, which is then confirmed by molecular genetic testing.

AF can assist in differentiating late stages of Best disease from other maculopathies that may cause fibrosis of the macula. AF findings correlate well with histological data and OCT findings. The presence of areas of reduced AF in advanced stages of the disease is an important factor in estimating remaining RPE cells below the lesion. However, to date, fundus AF, as well as all other ancillary studies, does not appear to provide information regarding the prognosis for progression of the disease in an individual patient.

ACKNOWLEDGMENTS

Many thanks go to Prof. Birgit Lorenz, head of the Department of Ophthalmology at the Medical Faculty of the Justus-Liebig University, Giessen, who provided the images shown in this chapter.

REFERENCES

1. Best F. Über eine hereditäre Maculaaffektion. Z Augenheik 1905;13:199–212.
2. Gass JDM. Heredodystrophic disorders affecting the pigment epithelium and retina. In: Gass JDM, ed. Stereoscopic Atlas of Macular Disease—Diagnosis and Treatment. St. Louis: Mosby, 1997:303–436.

3. Wabbels B, Preising MN, Kretschmann U, et al. Genotype-phenotype correlation and longitudinal course in ten families with Best vitelliform macular dystrophy. Graefes Arch Clin Exp Ophthalmol 2006;244:1453–1466.

4. Sun H, Tsunenari T, Yau KW, et al. The vitelliform macular dystrophy protein defines a new family of chloride channels. Proc Natl Acad Sci USA 2002;99:4008–4013.

5. Pusch M. Ca^{2+}-activated chloride channels go molecular. J Gen Physiol 2004;123:323–325.

6. Strauss O, Milenkovic VM, Striessnig J, et al. Direct interaction of Bestrophin-1 and beta-subunits of voltage-dependent calcium channels. ARVO Abstr 2008;49:5182.

7. Marmorstein AD, Marmorstein LY, Wang X, et al. Bestrophin, the protein encoded by the best macular dystrophy gene (VMD2), is a component of the plasma membrane. Invest Ophthalmol Vis Sci 2000:4:S398.

8. Mullins RF, Kuehn MH, Faidley EA, et al. Differential macular and peripheral expression of bestrophin in human eyes and its implication for best disease. Invest Ophthalmol Vis Sci 2007;48: 3372–3380.

9. Fischmeister R, Hartzell HC. Volume sensitivity of the bestrophin family of chloride channels. J Physiol 2005;562(Pt 2):477–491.

10. Pianta MJ, Aleman TS, Cideciyan AV, et al. In vivo micropathology of Best macular dystrophy with optical coherence tomography. Exp Eye Res 2003;76:203–211.

11. O'Gorman S, Flaherty WA, Fishman GA, et al. Histopathologic findings in Best's vitelliform macular dystrophy. Arch Ophthalmol 1988;106:1261–1268.

12. Weingeist TA, Kobrin JL, Watzke RC. Histopathology of Best's macular dystrophy. Arch Ophthalmol 1982;100:1108–1114.

13. Bakall B, Radu RA, Stanton JB, et al. Enhanced accumulation of A2E in individuals homozygous or heterozygous for mutations in BEST1 (VMD2). Exp Eye Res 2007;85:1;34–43.

14. Maruko I, Iida T, Spaide RF, et al. Indocyanine green angiography abnormality of the periphery in vitelliform macular dystrophy. Am J Ophthalmol 2006;141:976–978.

15. Quaranta M, Buglione M, Lo Schiavo ER, et al. Angiographie au vert d'indocyanine des drusen de la membrane basale de l'epithelium pigmentaire retinien associes a du materiel pseudo-vitelliforme. J Fr Ophtalmol 1998;21:185–190.

16. Pollack K, Kreuz FR, Pillunat LE. Morbus Best mit normalem EOG—Fallvorstellung einer familiären Makuladystrophie. Der Ophthalmologe 2005;102:891–894.

17. Marmor MF. Standardization notice: EOG standard reapproved. Electro-oculogram. Doc Ophthalmol 1998;95:91–92.

18. Marmor MF, Zrenner E. Standard for clinical electro-oculography. International Society for Clinical Electrophysiology of Vision. Arch Ophthalmol 1993;111: 601–604.

19. Krämer F, White K, Pauleikhoff D, et al. Mutations in the VMD2 gene are associated with juvenile-onset vitelliform macular dystrophy (Best disease) and adult vitelliform macular dystrophy but not age-related macular degeneration. Eur J Hum Genet 2000;8:286–292.

20. Spaide R. Autofluorescence from the outer retina and subretinal space: hypothesis and review. Retina 2008;28:5–35.

21. Spaide RF, Noble K, Morgan A, et al. Vitelliform macular dystrophy. Ophthalmology 2006;113: 1392–1400.

22. Wabbels B, Demmler A, Paunescu K, et al. Fundus autofluorescence in children and teenagers with hereditary retinal diseases. Graefes Arch Clin Exp Ophthalmol 2006;244:36–45.

23. Schatz P, Klar J, Andreasson S, et al. Variant phenotype of Best vitelliform macular dystrophy associated with compound heterozygous mutations in VMD2. Ophthalmic Genet 2006;27:51–56.

24. Aleman T, Stone EM, Hernandez R, et al. Ophthalmologic findings in a retinitis pigmentosa family with rhodopsin gene mutation Asp-190-Asn. Invest Ophthalmol Vis Sci 1996;37;S667.

Vikki McBain
Noemi Lois

Fundus Autofluorescence in Stargardt Disease

Stargardt disease (STGD) (1) (also termed fundus flavimaculatus [2]) is the most common recessively inherited macular dystrophy, affecting approximately one person in 10,000 (3). STGD can affect individuals of any gender and race (1,4–8) and there is wide variability in age of onset, visual acuity, fundus appearance, and severity of the disease (1,5–10). Visual acuity may vary between 20/20 to 20/400; rarely will it drop below 20/400 (7,11). Patients with STGD may be asymptomatic or complain of visual acuity loss, photophobia, and, less commonly, nyctalopia (5).

Fundus examination may be normal in early stages of the disease or reveal retinal pigment epithelium (RPE) mottling or a bull's-eye appearance at the macula, and active (deposition of yellow material at the level of the RPE) and/or resorbed (RPE depigmentation/atrophy) flecks and atrophy at the macula and midperipheral retina (1,5,6,9,12). Characteristically, the flecks have a pisciform ("fish-like") appearance, but they can also be round, like dots, and appear either as individual lesions or joined together (6,13). Different clinical classifications of STGD have been proposed based on the presence or absence and distribution of the fundus lesions (6,9,12); however, none of these have been widely accepted.

Electrophysiology testing in patients with STGD may demonstrate macular dysfunction alone or macular and peripheral cone or cone and rod dysfunction (10,14). These patterns of functional loss cannot be predicted by the fundus appearance (10,14). Mutations in the *ABCA4* gene, located in the short arm of chromosome 1, are responsible for all cases of STGD (15,16).

Currently, there is no treatment available for patients with STGD. However, laboratory studies suggest that progression of the disease may be slowed by protecting the eyes from light exposure (17). Additionally, new treatment strategies to reduce or prevent A2E accumulation in the RPE are also being investigated (see also Chapters 2 and 4) (Fig. 11G.1) (17–20).

MOLECULAR BASIS AND PATHOLOGY

The mechanisms by which photoreceptors degenerate in STGD are not completely understood. Recent laboratory studies investigating the function of the ABCA4 protein, as well as studies conducted in the *ABCA4* knockout mice, an animal model of the disease, have shed light on the molecular basis of STGD. The evidence suggests that the ABCA4 protein facilitates the transport of retinoids, preferentially N-retinylidene-phosphatidylethanolamine (N-retinylidene-PE) and all-*trans*-retinal (21,22), from the cytoplasmic side of the photoreceptor disc membrane to the cytosolic side, making them accessible to all-*trans*-retinol-dehydrogenase and facilitating its conver-

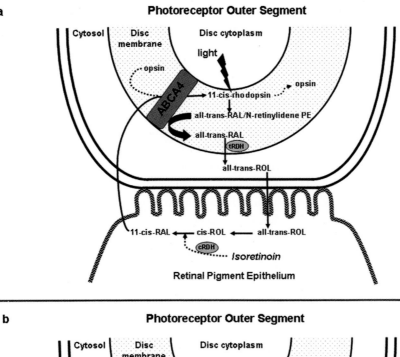

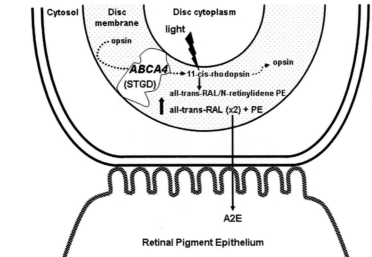

FIGURE 11G.1. **(A)** All-*trans*-retinal (all-*trans*-RAL) can react with phosphatidylethanolamine (PE) and form N-retinylidene-PE. Free all-*trans*-RAL and all-*trans*-RAL contained in N-retinylidene-PE are reduced to all-*trans*-retinol (all-*trans*-ROL) by the all-*trans*-retinol dehydrogenase (tRDH). Evidence suggests that ABCA4 transports N-retinylidene-PE and all-*trans*-RAL from the cytoplasmic side of the disc membrane to the cytosolic side, where they are reduced to all-*trans*-ROL by the all-*trans*-retinol DHase (trDH). **(B)** In patients with STGD, there is an impaired transport of all-*trans*-RAL and N-retinylidene-PE, with the subsequent accumulation of both molecules in the photoreceptor outer segment disc membrane. Condensation of all-*trans*-RAL and PE gives rise to N-retinylidene-N-retinyl-ethanolamine (A2E). A2E, the major fluorophore of lipofuscin, then accumulates in the RPE after photoreceptor outer segment disc shedding (modified from Refs. 28 and 57). CRDH, Cis-retinol DHase.

sion into all-*trans*-retinol (22,23) (Fig. 11G.1A,B). This assists in the recovery of the photoreceptor cell following light exposure, reduces photoreceptor cell noise (the result of an increase in all-*trans*-retinal and opsin, which when combined can activate the visual transduction cascade), and diminishes the accumulation of all-*trans*-retinal and N-retinylidene-PE within the disc membranes (22). The latter in turn increases the production of N-retinylidene-N-retinyl-ethanolamine (A2E), the major fluorophore of lipofuscin, in the RPE (see also Chapter 2), which has potential cytotoxic effects on RPE cells (24–27). RPE damage/loss is then followed by photoreceptor cell degeneration and loss of vision (33).

Histopathological evaluation of eyes from patients with STGD have shown RPE cells densely packed with a substance with ultrastructural, autofluorescent, and histochemical characteristics consistent with lipofuscin in both the macula and peripheral retina (29,30). Only one histopathology study failed to detect increased lipofuscin in the RPE in a case of STGD without maculopathy (31). Subretinal desquamated RPE cells, macrophages engorged with melanolipofuscin in the outer retina, RPE and choriocapillaris atrophy, and photoreceptor-cell loss at the fovea have been also observed (29,30).

DIAGNOSTIC TECHNIQUES

Fundus flecks are the hallmark of STGD. Although "active" flecks are often seen by slit-lamp biomicroscopy or indirect ophthalmoscopy (5,9,32), "resorbed" flecks are more difficult to visualize and can be missed by the examining ophthalmologist. In the latter case, the diagnosis of STGD may be difficult.

Fluorescein and Indocyanine Green Angiography

Fluorescein angiography (FA) is only rarely required for the diagnosis or evaluation of patients with STGD. In both early and late frames of FA, "active" flecks appear hypofluorescent (5). "Resorbed" flecks may appear either hypo- (5) or hyperfluorescent (9). Areas of overt macular atrophy are visualized as areas in which no choriocapillaris is present but large choroidal vessels are seen. Patients with STGD may have a "dark choroid" or "choroidal silence" sign (33), characterized by a lack of early hyperfluorescence coming from the choroid, such that the retinal blood vessels, even the small capillaries, are easily seen over a very dark background where there is no choroidal fluorescence. Not all patients with STGD will demonstrate a dark choroid. In a recent study, only 62% of patients with STGD had this FA sign (7). Similarly, the dark choroid is not a specific sign of STGD; it has also been observed in patients with cone and cone-rod dystrophy (see also Chapter 11B) (7,33,34). However, if present, this sign may be useful in the differential diagnosis of STGD (see below), especially when the diagnosis of multifocal pattern dystrophy simulating STGD is entertained (see also Chapter 11E). Of interest, the overall increase in the fundus autofluorescence (AF) signal observed in patients with STGD (see below) seems to be independent of the presence or absence of a dark choroid (35).

Indocyanine green (ICG) angiography allows the choroidal details to be seen even in patients with a dark choroid (36). It is also possible to detect choroidal vascular closure, such as that present in patients with atrophic macular lesions. Active fundus flecks appear hypofluorescent on ICG and are typically best detected in late frames of the angiogram (36).

Optical Coherence Tomography

The clinical usefulness of optical coherence tomography (OCT) in STGD remains to be elucidated. Earlier studies using OCT concentrated on evaluating the location of retinal flecks (37,38). In time-domain OCT imaging (Stratus OCT 300; Zeiss, Germany) fundus flecks are seen as hyperreflective deposits, either as dome-shaped lesions at the level of the RPE or just above the RPE, or as small, linear, highly reflective lesions at the level of the photoreceptor inner segments or outer nuclear layer (37). Fourier-domain OCT imaging (University of California–Davis, prototype), however, reveals only well-demarcated oval "bumps" within the RPE in all cases of STGD (38).

Recently, Querques et al. (39) found that the two types of highly reflective dome-shaped deposits described above did not correlate with foveal thinning or best corrected visual acuity. Ergun et al. (40) used ultra-high-resolution OCT to assess transverse photoreceptor cell loss and compared the results with visual acuity and changes detected on AF and FA imaging. They found that a lower visual acuity corresponded to a greater transverse photoreceptor cell loss, which also correlated with the extent of reduced AF (transverse diameter) and atrophy seen on FA. OCT thus may provide valuable structural information in patients with STGD.

Electrophysiology

Electrophysiology alone cannot be used to establish the diagnosis of STGD. However, it is essential for gathering information on the location and extent of retinal dysfunction in patients with this disease.

The degree of functional loss can be assessed by using the pattern electroretinogram (PERG) and the full-field electroretinogram (ERG) (5,6,9,12,13,41–43). Patients may demonstrate macular dysfunction alone (abnormal PERG with normal full-field ERG), macular and peripheral cone dysfunction (abnormal PERG and photopic ERG responses), or macular and peripheral cone and rod dysfunction (abnormal PERG and scotopic and photopic ERG responses) (10). It is important to note that these patterns of functional loss cannot be predicted by the fundus appearance (10). There seems to be a high degree of intrafamilial homogeneity with respect to the pattern of functional loss present as determined by electrophysiology (9,42).

Electrophysiology is a valuable prognostic tool that can help the clinician to identify, early on in the course of the disease, those patients with peripheral cone and rod involvement who will likely have a higher chance of developing not only central but also peripheral visual loss and a more severe form of the disease.

Fundus Autofluorescence

To date, fundus autofluorescence (AF) seems to be the most effective clinical adjunct for the diagnosis and evaluation of patients with STGD (10,42,44). On fundus AF imaging, both "active" and "resorbed" flecks and areas of outer retinal atrophy can be easily identified (Fig. 11G.2) (44). Active flecks appear as foci of high AF signal (Fig. 11G.2B), indicating an increased lipofuscin content at the site of the fleck. In contrast, resorbed flecks are seen as foci of low AF signal on AF imaging (Fig. 11G.2B) (42,44). Given that resorbed flecks seem to occur most commonly at sites previously occupied by active flecks, the low AF signal observed on AF imaging could represent damaged/lost RPE, probably as a direct or indirect result of the previously increased lipofuscin content in the RPE at the site of the fleck (44). Both resorbed and active

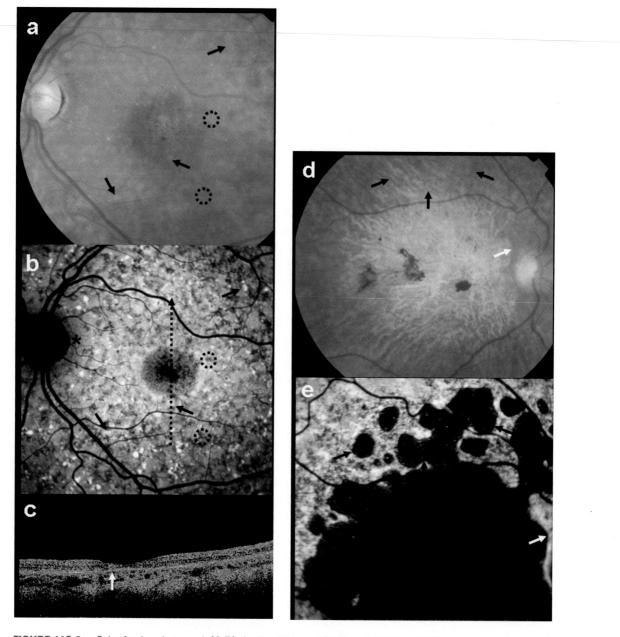

FIGURE 11G.2. Color fundus photograph **(A,D)**, fundus AF image **(B,E)**, and OCT image **(C)** from two patients with STGD showing active **(A–C**, *black arrows)* and resorbed **(A,B**, *circles)* flecks. Active flecks appear on slit-lamp examination as white-yellowish lesions formed by accumulation of material in the outer retina **(A**, *black arrows)*. On AF images **(B**, *black arrows)* the active flecks are seen as foci of increased AF signal. Resorbed flecks **(B**, *circles)*, which appear as small areas of depigmentation in the RPE, are difficult to detect on slit-lamp biomicroscopy but are easily visualized on AF images as foci of low AF signal **(B**, *circles)*. Fundus AF is helpful in demonstrating peripapillary sparing **(B**, *asterisks*; Fig. 11G.3C). Active flecks are seen on OCT imaging as dome-shaped bumps at the level of RPE **(C**, *black arrow*, 90 degree section). Well-defined areas of low AF signal **(E**, *white arrow)* corresponding to areas of clinically detectable **(D**, *white arrow)* or undetectable **(A**, *black arrows)* retinal atrophy can be seen at the macula and midperipheral retina.

flecks can be seen either confined to the macula or distributed throughout and beyond the posterior pole (10,28,35,42,44,45) with a particular predominance nasally (45). A normal retinal sensitivity, as determined by fundus microperimetry, has been detected over areas of increased AF corresponding to active flecks. In contrast, reduced retinal sensitivity has been found over areas of reduced AF signal that corresponded to patches of atrophy observed clinically (46).

When resorbed flecks are present in patients with advanced disease and atrophic macular lesions but no active flecks, the diagnosis of STGD may represent a challenge to the clinician. In these circumstances, AF imaging can be extremely useful by demonstrating multiple, small foci of decreased AF signal at the macula or midperipheral retina corresponding to resolved flecks. It has also been noted that in STGD there is a typically relative peripapillary sparing (lack of flecks and atrophy around the optic nerve head), even in cases with diffuse RPE abnormalities and atrophy (Figs. 11G.2B and 11G.E,F) (36,44,47,48). This preservation of the retinal tissue around the optic nerve is easily appreciated on fundus AF imaging and is a very useful sign when establishing the diagnosis in patients with advanced disease in whom fundus flecks are no longer visible (44).

Well-defined areas of low AF signal corresponding to areas of clinically detectable or undetectable retinal atrophy are typically seen at the macula but may also be present in some patients in the midperipheral retina (Fig. 11G.2D,E) (42,44). The presence of multiple well-defined areas of low AF signal in the midperipheral retina has been observed only in patients with reduced macular and peripheral cone and rod function (10), and thus seems to indicate a poorer prognosis. Furthermore, a diffuse very high AF signal can be detected in some patients throughout the macula, where no fundus changes are evident on slit-lamp biomicroscopy. This finding seems to indicate a faster speed of progression of atrophy and a poorer prognosis (see below).

Quantitative evaluations of fundus AF have demonstrated high levels of AF in the majority of patients with this disease (35,44,49,50), independently of whether a dark choroid was present on FA (35). More recently, fundus AF levels across the macula in patients with STGD were found to be high, normal, or even low compared to those in age-matched normal volunteers (44). Furthermore, there seems to be a relation between levels of AF across the macula and the peripheral retinal function, as demonstrated by full-field ERG. Low levels of AF across the macula, including the fovea, were detected in all patients with peripheral cone and rod dysfunction (44). Although quantitative evaluation of AF levels appears to be important, since in many cases clinicians cannot predict high or low levels of AF simply by looking at the AF images (49); it appears that an accurate quantitative evaluation of AF levels cannot be achieved with current commercially available instruments (see also Chapters 5 and 8).

Fundus AF imaging is very useful for monitoring the progression of the disease. Serial imaging can demonstrate the development of new foci of increased AF signal (active flecks) over time, even in patients with long-standing disease (Fig. 11G.3A–D). The appearance of new active flecks tends to follow a centrifugal pattern. In contrast, resorbed flecks tend to appear more centrally and with a smaller dispersion radius than active flecks (51). Enlargement of preexisting areas of atrophy can be also documented (Fig. 11G.3A–H). Areas of atrophy seem to expand uniformly, with no quadrantic preference (51), and more often toward areas with previously increased AF signal, suggesting that, as in AMD (53–55) (see also Chapter 10C), increased AF and thus lipofuscin may presage directly or indirectly photoreceptor-RPE cell demise. Long-term follow-up AF data from our group (unpublished results) suggest that the development of new areas of low AF signal

FIGURE 11G.3. Serial fundus AF images obtained from four patients with STGD at baseline **(A,C,E,G)** and at follow-up **(B,D,F,H**; **A,B, C,D, E,F**: 3-year follow-up; **G,H**: 2-year follow-up). AF imaging demonstrates development of new foci of increased AF signal (active flecks, *white arrows*) and the disappearance of foci of increased AF (*black arrows*) over time **(A–D)**. The development of new areas of atrophy and the enlargement of existing ones can also be documented **(A–H)**. The speed of enlargement of pre-existing areas of low AF signal may be determined by the pattern of fundus AF observed. When homogeneous background AF was detected surrounding areas of low AF signal (atrophy), a slow rate of enlargement was documented (**A,B,** 55-year-old male, age at onset = 19 years, duration of disease = 34 years, 3-year follow-up, rate of progression LE = 1.13 mm²/year; **C,D,** 43-year-old female, age at onset = 11 years, duration of disease = 32 years, 3-year follow-up, rate of progression LE = 0.51 mm²/year). In contrast, when a widespread pattern of increased background AF signal interspersed with foci of low and high AF signals was identified, multiple new areas of low AF signal (atrophy) and/or a rapid enlargement of preexisting areas of low AF signal were detected (**E,F,** 41-year-old female, age at onset = 37 years, duration of disease = 4 years, 3-year follow-up, rate of progression 5.79 mm²/year; **G,H,** 40-year-old male, age at onset 31 years, duration of disease = 10 years, AF 2-year follow-up, rate of progression LE = 4.37 mm²/year).

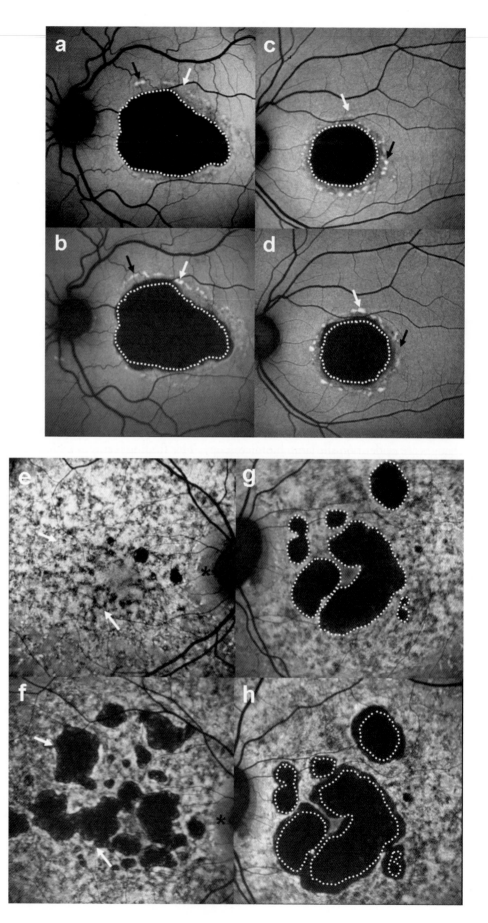

(atrophy) and the speed of enlargement of preexisting areas of low AF signal may be determined by the pattern of fundus AF observed. Thus, when homogeneous background AF was detected surrounding areas of low AF signal (atrophy) a slow rate of enlargement was documented (Fig. 11G.3A–D). In contrast, when a widespread pattern of increased background AF signal intersperse with foci of low and high AF signals was identified, multiple new areas of low AF signal (atrophy) developed and/or a rapid enlargement of preexisting areas of low AF signal was detected (Fig. 11G.3E–H).

Although to date there is no available treatment for patients with STGD, pharmacological strategies aimed at reducing the synthesis and accumulation of A2E and other retinoids are under investigation (17–20). Isotretinoin (13-*cis*-retinoic acid or Accutane, a drug commonly used to treat patients with acne) was found to biochemically suppress the accumulation of A2E in the RPE, and also inhibited the accumulation of lipofuscin granules in the RPE as detected by electron microscopy in the rodent model of STGD (abcr$^{-/-}$ mice) (Fig. 11G.1A) (see also Chapter 4) (19). Future clinical trials with these or other agents would need to identify objective outcome measures to evaluate the response to these treatments. Electrophysiology testing is unlikely to be useful for this purpose, since most patients with STGD have normal full-field ERG responses and a flat, unrecordable PERG (10). Furthermore, it is expected that long follow-up and a high number of patients will be required to detect statistically significant variations in electrophysiology recordings. Under these circumstances, fundus AF images would provide objective and measurable data on the development of new areas of increased or decreased AF at the macula and midperipheral retina and/or on the speed of enlargement of preexisting ones (see Fig. 11G.3).

It is possible that the new imaging technique of near-infrared autofluorescence (NIA) will also be very helpful in the evaluation of patients with STGD (see Chapter 6).

DIFFERENTIAL DIAGNOSIS OF STGD

The differential diagnosis of STGD includes autosomal dominant Stargardt-like macular dystrophy, Best disease, cone and cone-rod dystrophy, central areolar choroidal dystrophy, age-related maculopathy (ARM)/age-related macular degeneration (AMD), pattern dystrophy, and retinitis pigmentosa (RP). A detailed family history should be obtained and can be helpful in establishing this differentiation. The dominant pattern of inheritance in Stargardt-like disease can help distinguish it from the recessive mode of inheritance in patients with STGD. As in STGD, in advanced Best disease (see also Chapter 11F), cone dystrophy (see also Chapter 11B), central areolar choroidal dystrophy, and AMD (see also Chapter 10), a central area of atrophy at the macula is often seen. However, in contrast to STGD, active and resolved flecks are not present in these retinal diseases. Drusen in patients with ARM may simulate the round flecks observed in some patients with STGD; fundus AF can help differentiate between the two by demonstrating a very high AF signal at the site of the round flecks and no abnormality or a mildly increased or decreased AF signal in the case of drusen. Like patients with STGD, patients with multifocal pattern dystrophy simulating fundus flavimaculatus (56) present with multiple pisciform lesions at the macula and midperipheral retina (see also Chapter 11E). In both retinal diseases, these lesions will demonstrate a high AF signal on AF imaging. However, the mode of inheritance (dominant in pattern dystrophy) and the absence of peripapillary sparing will assist the differential diagnosis. Furthermore, most patients with STGD will demonstrate a flat PERG, which only very rarely will be obtained in patients with pattern dystrophy. Severe forms of STGD can simulate cone-rod dystrophy (see also Chapter 11B) and RP (see also Chapter 11A). Multiple foci of decreased AF signal at the macula and midperipheral retina, indicating the presence of resorbed flecks, will be observed in patients with STGD but not in those with cone-rod dystrophy or RP.

SUMMARY

Fundus AF imaging provides a rapid and noninvasive way to evaluate patients with STGD. AF imaging allows a clear visualization of both active and resorbed flecks, areas of macular and midperipheral atrophy, and the presence of the relative peripapillary sparing, helping to establish the diagnosis of the disease. AF imaging is exceptionally helpful in the diagnosis of patients with advanced disease, in whom active fundus flecks are no longer visible and only resolved flecks are present. Fundus AF imaging may have also a prognostic value by demonstrating areas of low AF signal in the midperipheral retina in patients with the most severe form of the disease, and widespread increased AF signal at the macula interspersed with foci of low and high AF signals in patients with a faster rate of atrophy progression. It is likely that fundus AF imaging will become the imaging technique of choice to evaluate the response to future treatments for patients with STGD.

REFERENCES

1. Franceschetti A. Ueber tapeto-retinale Degenerationen im Kindesalter (Kongenitale Form (Leber), amaurotische Idiotie, rezessive-geschlechtsgebundene tapeto-retinale Degenerationen, Fundus albipunctatus cum Hemeralopia, Fundus flavimaculatus). Dritter Fortbildungskurs der Deutschen Ophthalmologischen Gesellschaft, Hamburg 1962, herausgegeben von Prof. Dr. H. Sautter. In: Enke F, ed. Entwicklung und Fortschritt in der Augenheilkunde. Stuttgart: Verlag, 1963:107–120.
2. Franceschetti A, Francois J. Fundus flavimaculatus. Arch Ophthalmol 1965;25:505–530.
3. Blacharski PA. Fundus flavimaculatus. In: Newsome DA, ed. Retinal Dystrophies and Degenerations. New York: Raven Press, 1988:135–159.
4. Armstrong JD, et al. Long-term follow-up of Stargardt's disease and fundus flavimaculatus. Ophthalmology 1998;105:448–458.
5. Hadden OB, Gass JDM. Fundus flavimaculatus and Stargardt's disease. Am J Ophthalmol 1976;82:527–539.
6. Klien BA, Krill AE. Fundus flavimaculatus. Clinical, functional, and histopathologic observations. Am J Ophthalmol 1967;64:3–23.
7. Rotenstreich Y, Fishman GA, Anderson RJ. Visual acuity loss and clinical observations in a large series of patients with Stargardt disease. Ophthalmology 2003; 110:1151–1158.
8. Stargardt K. Uber familiare progressive degeneration in der makulagegend des auges. Albrecht von Graefes Arch Klin Ophthalmol 1909;71:534–550.
9. Aaberg TM. Stargardt's disease and fundus flavimaculatus: evaluation of morphologic progression and intrafamilial co-existence. Trans Am Ophthalmol Soc 1986;84:453–487.
10. Lois N, et al. Phenotypic subtypes of Stargardt macular dystrophy-fundus flavimaculatus. Arch Ophthalmol 2001;119:359–369.
11. Fishman GA, et al. Visual acuity loss in patients with Stargardt's macular dystrophy. Ophthalmology 1987;94:809–814.
12. Fishman GA. Fundus flavimaculatus. Arch Ophthalmol 1976;94:2061–2067.
13. Franceschetti A. A special form of tapetoretinal degeneration: fundus flavimaculatus. Trans Am Acad Ophthalmol Otolaryngol 1965;69:1048–1053.
14. Oh KT, et al. Clinical phenotype as a prognostic factor in Stargardt disease. Retina 2004;24:254–262.
15. Allikmets R, et al. A photoreceptor cell-specific ATP-binding transporter gene (ABCR) is mutated in recessive Stargardt macular dystrophy. Nat Genet 1997; 15:236–246.
16. Kaplan J, et al. A gene for Stargardt's disease (fundus flavimaculatus) maps to the short arm of chromosome 1. Nat Genet 1993;5:308–311.
17. Radu RA, et al. Light exposure stimulates formation of A2E oxiranes in a mouse model of Stargardt's macular degeneration. Proc Natl Acad Sci USA 2004;101:5928–5933.

18. Maiti P, et al. Small molecule RPE65 antagonists limit the visual cycle and prevent lipofuscin formation. Biochemistry 2006;45:852–860.
19. Radu RA, et al. Treatment with isotretinoin inhibits lipofuscin accumulation in a mouse model of recessive Stargardt's macular degeneration. Proc Natl Acad Sci USA 2003;100:4742–4747.
20. Radu RA, et al. Reductions in serum vitamin A arrest accumulation of toxic retinal fluorophores: a potential therapy for treatment of lipofuscin-based retinal diseases. Invest Ophthalmol Vis Sci 2005; 46:4393–4401.
21. Beharry S, Zhong M, Molday RS. N-retinylidene-phosphatidylethanolamine is the preferred retinoid substrate for the photoreceptor-specific ABC transporter ABCA4 (ABCR). J Biol Chem 2004;52:53972–53979.
22. Sun H, Molday RS, Nathans J. Retinal stimulates ATP hydrolysis by purified and reconstituted ABCR, the photoreceptor-specific ATP-binding cassette transporter responsible for Stargardt disease. J Biol Chem 1999;274:8269–8281.
23. Weng J, et al. Insights into the function of Rim protein in photoreceptors and etiology of Stargardt's disease from the phenotype in abcr knockout mice. Cell 1999;98:13–23.
24. Eldred GE, Lasky MR. Retinal age pigments generated by self-assembling lysosomotropic detergents. Nature 1998;361:724–726.
25. Holz FG, et al. Inhibition of lysosomal degradative functions in RPE cells by a retinoid component of lipofuscin. Invest Ophthalmol Vis Sci 1999;40:737–743.
26. Sparrow JR, Nakanishi K, Parish CA. The lipofuscin fluorophore A2E mediates blue light-induced damage to retinal pigmented epithelial cells. Invest Ophthalmol Vis Sci 2000;41:1981–1989.
27. Suter M, et al. Age-related macular degeneration. The lipofuscin component N-retinyl-N-retinylidene ethanolamine detaches proapoptotic proteins from mitochondria and induces apoptosis in mammalian retinal pigment epithelial cells. J Biol Chem 2000;275:39625–39630.
28. Lois N. New perspectives in Stargardt's disease. In: Holz FG, Spaide RF, eds. Essentials in Ophthalmology: Medical Retina. Berlin: Springer-Verlag, 2007:166–177.
29. Birnbach CD, et al. Histopathology and immunocytochemistry of the neurosensory retina in fundus flavimaculatus. Ophthalmology 1994;101:1211–1219.
30. Eagle RCJ, et al. Retinal pigment epithelial abnormalities in fundus flavimaculatus: a light and electron microscopic study. Ophthalmology 1980;87:1189–1200.
31. McDonnell PJ, et al. Fundus flavimaculatus without maculopathy. A clinicopathologic study. Ophthalmology 1986;93:116–119.
32. Irvine AR, Wergeland FLJ. Stargardt's hereditary progressive macular degeneration. Br J Ophthalmol 1972;56:817–826.
33. Bonnin P. Le signe du silence choroidien dans les degenerescences tapeto-retiniennes centrales examinees sous fluoresceine. Bull Soc Ophthalmol Fr 1971;71:1423–1427.
34. Uliss AE, Moore AT, Bird AC. The dark choroid in posterior retinal dystrophies. Ophthalmology 1987;94:1423–1427.
35. Von Rückmann A, Fitzke FW, Bird AC. In vivo fundus autofluorescence in macular dystrophies. Arch Ophthalmol 1997;115:609–615.
36. Wroblewski JJ, et al. Indocyanine green angiography in Stargardt's flavimaculatus. Am J Ophthalmol 1995;120:208–218.
37. Querques G, et al. Analysis of retinal flecks in fundus flavimaculatus using optical coherence tomography. Br J Ophthalmol 2006;90:1157–1162.
38. Gerth, C. Visualization of lipofuscin accumulation in Stargardt macular dystrophy by high-resolution Fourier-domain optical coherence tomography. Arch Ophthalmol 2007;125:575.
39. Querques G, et al. Correlation of visual function impairment and OCT findings in patients with Stargardt disease and fundus flavimaculatus. Eur J Ophthalmol 2008;18:239–247.
40. Ergun E, et al. Assessment of central visual function in Stargardt's disease/fundus flavimaculatus with ultrahigh-resolution optical coherence tomography. Invest Ophthalmol Vis Sci 2005;46:310–316.
41. Carr RE. Fundus flavimaculatus. Arch Ophthalmol 1965;74:163–168.
42. Lois N, et al. Intrafamilial variation of phenotype in Stargardt macular dystrophy-fundus flavimaculatus. Invest Ophthalmol Vis Sci 1999;40:2668–2675.
43. Stavrou P, et al. Electrophysiological findings in Stargardt's-fundus flavimaculatus. Eye 1998;12:953–958.
44. Lois N, et al. Fundus autofluorescence in Stargardt macular dystrophy-fundus flavimaculatus. Am J Ophthalmol 2004;138:55–63.
45. Boon CJ, Jeroen Klevering B, Keunen JE, et al. Fundus autofluorescence imaging in retinal dystrophies. Vision Res 2008;48:2569–2577.
46. Gomes NL, et al. Visual function, fundus autofluorescence and structure in Stargardt disease. ARVO 2008;2041.
47. De Laey JJ, Verougstraete C. Hyperlipofuscinosis and subretinal fibrosis in Stargardt's disease. Retina 1995;15:399–406.
48. Klein R, et al. Subretinal neovascularization associated with fundus flavimaculatus. Arch Ophthalmol 1978;96:2054–2057.
49. Delori FC, et al. In vivo measurement of lipofuscin in Stargardt's disease-fundus flavimaculatus. Invest Ophthalmol Vis Sci 1995;36:2327–2331.

50. Von Ruckmann A, Fitzke FW, Bird AC. Distribution of fundus autofluorescence with a scanning laser ophthalmoscope. Br J Ophthalmol 1995;79:407–412.

51. Smith, T, et al. Autofluorescence metrics in Stargardt disease. ARVO 2008;2203.

52. Lois, N, et al. Quantitative evaluation of fundus autofluorescence "in vivo" in eyes with retinal disease. Br J Ophthalmol 2000;84:741–745.

53. Holz FG, et al. Progression of geographic atrophy and impact of fundus autofluorescence patterns in age-related macular degeneration. Am J Ophthalmol 2007;143:463–472.

54. Hwang JC, et al. Predictive value of fundus autofluorescence for development of geographic atrophy in age-related macular degeneration. Invest Ophthalmol Vis Sci 2006;47:2655–2661.

55. Schmitz-Valckenberg S, et al. Correlation between the area of increased autofluorescence surrounding geographic atrophy and disease progression in patients with AMD. Invest Ophthalmol Vis Sci 2006;47:2648–2654.

56. Gass JDM. Heredodystrophic disorders affecting the pigment epithelium and retina. In: Gass JDM, ed. Stereoscopic Atlas of Macular Disease, Diagnosis and Treatment. St. Louis: Mosby, 1997:314–325.

57. Molday RS. ATP-binding cassette transporter ABCA4: molecular properties and role in vision and macular degeneration. J Bioeng Biomembr 2007;39:507–517.

Caren Bellmann
Pamela Rath

Fundus Autofluorescence in Maternal Inherited Diabetes and Deafness

Mitochondria are ubiquitous in eukaryotes and are essential for survival. Their primary function is to support aerobic respiration and provide energy to the cell. Mitochondria also play an important role in cell signaling for apoptotic cell death. Genes located in the mitochondrial DNA (mtDNA) encode subunits of the mitochondrial respiratory chain where ATP is generated. Because pathogenic mutations of mtDNA usually do not affect all mtDNA within a cell, the clinical phenotype of the mitochondrial disease depends on the relative proportion of mutant and wild-type mtDNA in different tissues. Furthermore, depending on the energy demand of a particular cell, the level of mutated genomes required to produce a phenotypic expression will vary. Disease is expressed when, at a particular threshold, ATP production falls below the energy demand. Until relatively recently, there was a general lack of awareness of mitochondrial disease. Maternal inherited diabetes and deafness (MIDD) was first reported only in 1992 (1,2).

The prevalence of MIDD described in the general population is 0.06%; the disease is found in about 1.5% of diabetic populations in different countries and people of different ethnic backgrounds (1–4). MIDD is considered to be a subtype of diabetes mellitus that cosegregates with the most common mitochondrial DNA point mutation, an adenine-to-guanine transition at position 3243 of the mitochondrial DNA (A3243G) (1).

Clinically, mitochondrial diabetes is typically combined with neurosensory hearing loss and retinal dystrophy. Therefore, this disease is easily distinguishable from the idiopathic forms of diabetes (4). Additional findings, such as a progressive defect in insulin secretion and neuromuscular signs, may be helpful in identifying the disease. The final diagnosis is made by detecting the mitochondrial DNA point mutation A3243G in peripheral blood leukocytes by molecular-genetic procedures using DNA from oral mucosa cells, hair follicles, or muscle biopsy.

Diabetic retinopathy changes are seldom found in patients with MIDD, whereas retinal dystrophy changes are very common. The latter have been described with a prevalence of up to 85.7% (5,6), and they may lead to a diagnosis of the condition. These retinal changes are concentrated on the posterior pole and range from mildly abnormal pigmentation at the posterior pole to extensive atrophy of the retinal pigment epithelium (RPE) with a symmetric distribution between both eyes (Fig. 11H.1) (5–19). Different patterns of pigmentary retinopathy have been observed within the same family, which suggests that the particular pattern present in a patient may change over time (11). Furthermore, in a recent study of seven patients with MIDD, 10 out of 34 maternal relatives presented the typical retinal changes of MIDD with abnormal pigmentation at the posterior pole. All of them tested positive for the A3243G mutation, suggesting that retinal abnormalities may be a reliable clinical indicator for a positive mutation (20). Despite the retinal changes, visual prognosis is generally good in patients with MIDD. In a multicenter study, 80% of patients presented with visual acuity of 6/7.5 or better in

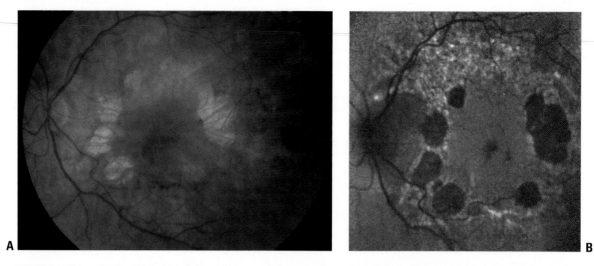

FIGURE 11H.1.   Fundus photograph **(A)** and AF image **(B)** obtained from the left eye of a patient with MIDD. Patches of RPE atrophy preserving the fovea were observed on fundus examination **(A)**. AF images disclosed well-defined areas of reduced AF signal **(B)**. AF images defined more clearly areas of RPE loss. In fact, at a location where clinically there seemed to be RPE atrophy (superior to the fovea), AF images disclosed a background AF signal, indicating preserved AF and thus RPE in this area. Very small foci of increased and decreased AF signal are also visible outside the fovea and in between areas of atrophy.

both eyes (5). No correlation has been found among the severity of retinal changes, the patient's age, and the percentage of mutant mtDNA (11). Moreover, there is no known correlation between the proportion of mutant mtDNA and the clinical features of family members (14). However, the percentage of mutant mtDNA may vary from one tissue to another and may not correspond to the percentage of mutant mtDNA in retinal tissue in a patient with this disease.

MOLECULAR BASIS AND PATHOLOGY

The pathogenesis of the retinal dystrophy in MIDD is not clear. Retinal pigmentary abnormalities commonly occur in other mitochondrial disorders, such as Kearns-Sayre syndrome, a neuromuscular disorder that is characterized by, in addition to retinal changes, chronic progressive external ophthalmoplegia, and heart disease. In MELAS syndrome, the combination of mitochondrial myopathy, encephalomyopathy, lactate acidosis, and stroke-like episodes leads to a high prevalence of retinal changes (21). Both syndromes are caused by the same mitochondrial A3243G mutation as described for MIDD. Morphological studies in patients with Kearns-Sayre and MELAS syndromes revealed ultrastructural changes in the RPE with enlarged mitochondria (22). Pathologic abnormalities were most marked posteriorly and included both hypo- and hyperpigmentation (23–26). These studies showed further degeneration of photoreceptor outer segments as well as complete atrophy of photoreceptor cells. It was suggested that these changes were most likely secondary to RPE degeneration. Chang and coworkers (24) reported ocular histopathologic and ultrastructural changes in two patients who suffered from Kearns-Sayre and MELAS syndromes. In one of the patients studied, fluorescein angiography (FA) had been obtained 3 years before the patient's death. The blocked fluorescence described on FA was thought to be due to the accumulation of lipofuscin in RPE cells. Pathologic evaluation of the same eye revealed a degenerated RPE with overlying photoreceptor cell atrophy in the central retina. In adjacent areas, there was intact RPE containing melanin granules, lipofuscin globules, and large melanolipofuscin conglomerates with overlying disorganized photoreceptor outer segments. However, McKechnie and coworkers (23) could not confirm an increased amount of lipofuscin in RPE cells in a case with Kearns-Sayre syndrome.

The mechanisms by which the RPE is affected in MIDD are not completely understood. An age-dependent somatic selection favors the persistence of mitochondria carrying the mutation in mitochondrial disease, which explains why patients with MIDD typically are not identified before the fourth decade of life (5). Defective mitochondria may be not properly autophagocytosed. Their components may undergo further oxidative modification within the lysosomes, resulting in the formation of additional undegradable material, such as the lipofuscin in RPE cells, and progressively less mitochondrial recycling. Consequently, compensatory mechanisms may fail with time, followed by dysfunction and cell death, particularly in relation to postmitotic tissues with high energy demands, such as photoreceptors and RPE cells (27). In this regard, fundus autofluorescence (AF) findings have shed some light on the pathogenesis of the retinal changes that occur in MIDD (see below).

IMAGING TECHNIQUES

Fluorescein Angiography

Fluorescein angiography (FA) is rarely, if ever, required in the evaluation of patients with MIDD and has been replaced by AF imaging (see below). FA may disclose mottled hyper- and hypofluorescence at the macula from RPE window defects and increased RPE pigmentation, respectively (5). In this regard, FA may be a useful tool to establish the diagnosis of MIDD. However, the very distinct phenotypic appearance of patients with MIDD on AF imaging, and the fact that AF is noninvasive have made AF the preferred imaging technique for evaluating patients with a possible diagnosis of MIDD.

Fundus Autofluorescence

AF is a useful tool for evaluating retinal changes in MIDD. AF imaging in MIDD can clearly demonstrate RPE involvement (Figs. 11H.1–11H.4) (19). A decreased

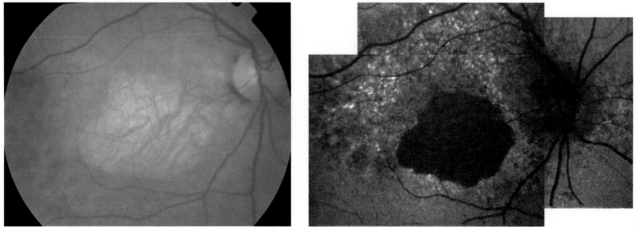

A   B

FIGURE 11H.2.   Fundus photograph **(A)** and fundus AF **(B)** image obtained from the right eye of a patient with MIDD with advanced macular atrophy involving the fovea. A characteristic speckled pattern of AF is observed outside the area of atrophy.

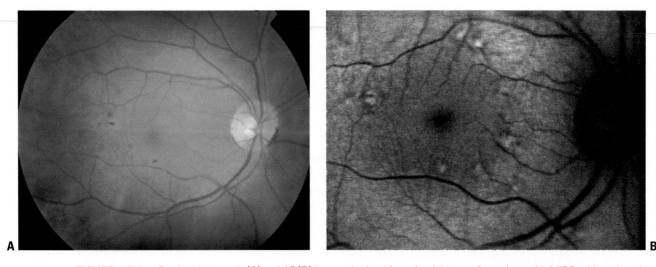

FIGURE 11H.3. Fundus photograph **(A)** and AF **(B)** image obtained from the right eye of a patient with MIDD with early retinal changes in the parafoveal region. Small areas of increased pigmentation clinically **(A)** corresponded to areas on increased AF signal **(B)**.

AF signal is observed corresponding to areas of RPE atrophy detected clinically, by slit-lamp biomicroscopy and fundus photography. However, a reduced AF signal indicating RPE loss may also be observed in areas that are not clearly identified clinically. An increased AF signal is found adjacent to areas of RPE atrophy, where no changes are detected clinically. Increased AF is thought to be the result of a high metabolic turnover of photoreceptor outer segments leading to lipofuscin accumula-

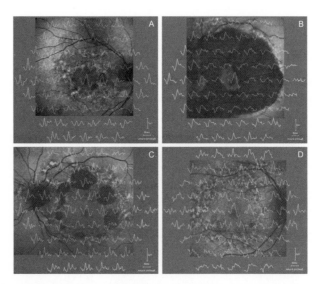

FIGURE 11H.4. Multifocal ERG stimuli superimposed on fundus AF images obtained from four different patients **(A–D)** with MIDD. Extensive RPE atrophy with decreased fundus AF is visible at the posterior pole in patients **B** and **C**. In adjacent areas the AF signal is irregularly increased. Patients **A** and **D** present a more speckled AF appearance. In all subjects, mfERG trace array amplitude changes are present. These changes are not limited to the zones of RPE atrophy but are present in areas of increased AF, using the 61-hexagon stimulus. No distinction can be made between areas of RPE atrophy and areas with increased AF. (Reprinted from Ref. 19 with permission from the Association for Research in Vision and Ophthalmology as the copyright holder.)

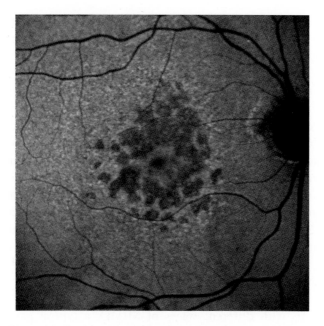

FIGURE 11H.5. AF image obtained from the right eye of a patient with geographic atrophy due to AMD. In areas of atrophy the AF signal is decreased, and in adjacent areas at the posterior pole the AF signal is increased.

tion in RPE cells, with subsequent retinal impairment (19,28). Similarities between the pattern of AF observed in MIDD and that described in patients with macular dystrophies and geographic atrophy due to age-related macular degeneration (AMD) (Figs. 11H.5 and 11H.6) (29,30) suggest a common pathogenic pathway in the development of RPE atrophy in retinal degenerations, which may be explained by the fact that mitochondrial abnormalities are present not only in cells of patients with

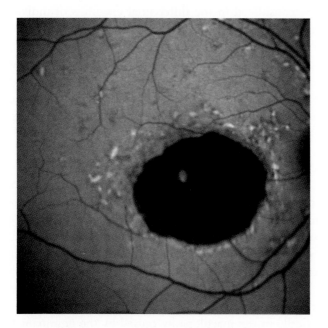

FIGURE 11H.6. AF image obtained from the right eye of a patient with Stargardt disease. A central area of atrophy with reduced AF signal is observed, surrounded by small foci of increased AF corresponding to fundus flecks.

maternally inherited diseases, but also in any aging postmitotic cells (31). Retinal changes associated with mitochondrial disease thus may reflect the acceleration of an age-related process. The recent finding that a variant of a mitochondrial protein is associated with the development of AMD supports this hypothesis (32).

The location of AF abnormalities in MIDD, with preferential paracentral retinal involvement, is striking (19). The observation of a restricted area of damage in MIDD correlates with the electrophysiological results obtained from a small cohort of patients, which demonstrated restricted rather than generalized photoreceptor cell dysfunction. Ganzfeld full-field electroretinogram (ERG) abnormalities were not observed in the majority of patients tested, whereas amplitude changes in multifocal electroretinograms (mfERGs) corresponded well with the area of abnormality detected on AF imaging (Fig. 11H.4) (19). These findings demonstrate nonuniform retinal damage (19) and suggest damage to the cone photoreceptor outer segments in MIDD. Functional findings also support the hypothesis that both photoreceptor outer segments and RPE cells are involved in the pathogenesis of MIDD, consistent with the histological data described in Kearns-Sayre and MELAS syndromes (see above).

In 12 patients with different stages of MIDD, a typical pattern of AF was found with very small foci of highly increased AF signal combined with small foci and larger patches of reduced AF signal (Figs. 11H.1 and 11H.2). The small foci of highly increased AF signal corresponded, in some cases, to small pale deposits visible on fundus examination. However, in many cases the diffuse speckled appearance of the macula on AF imaging did not correspond to any obvious changes on slit-lamp biomicroscopy (33). In fact, the area of abnormal AF at the posterior pole in MIDD is significantly larger than that expected from the fundus appearance (33). These findings underline the usefulness of AF imaging in MIDD.

DIFFERENTIAL DIAGNOSIS

MIDD should be considered in the differential diagnosis of individuals presenting with macular pigmentary abnormalities, especially when combined with paracentral areas of atrophy (33). MIDD should be differentiated from atrophic AMD (see also Chapter 11C), central areolar choroidal sclerosis, Stargardt disease (see also Chapter 11G), and pattern dystrophy (see also Chapter 11E). In atrophic AMD, areas of decreased AF signal corresponding to areas of atrophy may be surrounded by adjacent areas of increased AF (Fig. 11H.5), but may be similar to AF changes described in MIDD (Figs. 11H.1 and 11H.2). However, the speckled AF signal observed throughout the macula, which is characteristic of patients with the A3243G mtDNA mutation, is not usually present in patients with atrophic AMD. Unlike MIDD, central areolar choroidal sclerosis affects the fovea and, in the latter, no abnormalities in the distribution of background AF, outside areas of reduced AF, are found. Similarly to MIDD, Stargardt disease may present with multiple foci of increased and reduced AF signal at the macula (Fig. 11H.6). However, in most cases of Stargardt disease, the very small foci of increased and decreased AF do not coalesce, as occurs in MIDD. In the very few cases in which this may occur, it usually happens in patients with advanced disease in whom, unlike MIDD, no foveal preservation will be present. Findings similar to those observed in MIDD can be detected in patients with pattern dystrophy, specifically in the maculopathy caused by the dominant R172W peripherin mutation (33). The AF results from such patients appear to depend on the stage of the disease (34). In the early symptomatic stages, patients with the R172W peripherin mutation present a diffuse macular abnormality on AF imaging, described as speckled areas of increased and decreased AF within the macula. Later in the course of the disease, areas of atrophy develop within the areas of abnormal AF, although this does not occur perifoveally, as is observed in patients with MIDD. Unlike A3243G maculopathy, the changes seen in R172W patients appear to be confined to the macula and peripapillary regions until very late in the disease, when atrophic changes can extend beyond the arcades (33,34).

SUMMARY

The prevalence of macular changes in MIDD is higher than was assumed until recently. Pigmentary or atrophic retinal changes may be an early sign of the disease. The combination of retinal changes typical of MIDD with diabetes and/or deafness should lead to screening for a mitochondrial DNA mutation to establish the diagnosis of MIDD. Careful fundus examination combined with AF imaging is needed to guide genetic testing. In addition to helping in the diagnosis of MIDD, AF imaging can provide valuable information regarding the degree of retinal involvement and thus the expected functional loss in these patients.

ACKNOWLEDGMENTS

The fundus photographs and fundus AF images presented in this chapter were obtained during the Medical Retina Fellowship of the authors at Moorfields Eye Hospital, London, UK.

REFERENCES

1. van den Ouweland JMW, Lemkes HHPJ, Ruitenbeek W, et al. Mutation in mitochondrial tRNA Leu (UUR) gene in a large pedigree with maternally transmitted type II diabetes mellitus and deafness. Nat Genet 1992;1:368–377.
2. Ballinger SW, Shoffner JM, Hedaya EV, et al. Maternal transmitted diabetes and deafness associated with a 10.4kb mitochondrial DNA deletion. Nat Genet 1992;1:11–15.
3. Guillausseau PJ, Massin P, Dubois-La Forgue D, et al. Maternal inherited diabetes and deafness: a multicenter study. Ann Intern Med 2001;134:721–728.
4. Gerbitz KD, van den Ouweland JM, Maassen JA, et al. Mitochondrial diabetes mellitus: a review. Biochim Biophys Acta 1995;1271:253–260.
5. Massin P, Virally-Monod M, Vialettes B, et al. Prevalence of macular pattern dystrophy in maternally inherited diabetes and deafness. GEDIAM Group. Ophthalmology 1999;106:1821–1827.
6. Fukui M, Nakano K, Obayashi H, et al. High prevalence of mitochondrial diabetes mellitus in Japanese patients with major risk factors. Metabolism 1997;46:793–795.
7. Massin P, Guillausseau PJ, Vialettes B, et al. Macular pattern dystrophy associated with a mutation of mitochondrial DNA. Am J Ophthalmol 1995;120:247–248.
8. Bonte CA, Matthijs GL, Cassiman JJ, et al. Macular pattern dystrophy in patients with deafness and diabetes. Retina 1997;17:216–221.
9. Latkany P, Ciulla TA, Cacchillo PF, et al. Mitochondrial maculopathy: geographic atrophy of the macula in the MELAS associated A to G 3243 mitochondrial DNA point mutation. Am J Ophthalmol 1999;128:112–114.
10. Smith PR, Bain SC, Good PA, et al. Pigmentary retinal dystrophy and the syndrome of maternally inherited diabetes and deafness caused by the mitochondrial DNA 3243 tRNA(Leu) A to G mutation. Ophthalmology 1999;106:1101–1108.
11. Harrison TJ, Boles RG, Johnson DR, et al. Macular pattern retinal dystrophy, adult-onset diabetes, and deafness: a family study of A3243G mitochondrial heteroplasmy. Am J Ophthalmol 1997;124:217–221.
12. Souied EH, Sales MJ, Soubrane G, et al. Macular dystrophy, diabetes, and deafness associated with a large mitochondrial DNA deletion. Am J Ophthalmol 1998;125:100–103.

13. Andrews RM, McNeela BJ, Reading P, et al. Mitochondrial DNA disease masquerading as age-related macular degeneration. Eye 1999;13:595–596.
14. Chen YN, Liou CW, Huang CC, et al. Maternally inherited diabetes and deafness (MIDD) syndrome: a clinical and molecular genetic study of a Taiwanese family. Chang Gung Med J 2004;27:66–73.
15. Bonte CA, Matthijs GL, Cassiman JJ, et al. Macular pattern dystrophy in patients with deafness and diabetes. Retina 1997;17:216–221.
16. Latkany P, Ciulla TA, Cacchillo PF, et al. Mitochondrial maculopathy: geographic atrophy of the macula in the MELAS associated A to G 3243 mitochondrial DNA point mutation. Am J Ophthalmol 1999;128:112–114.
17. Smith PR, Bain SC, Good PA, et al. Pigmentary retinal dystrophy and the syndrome of maternally inherited diabetes and deafness caused by the mitochondrial DNA 3243 tRNA(Leu) A to G mutation. Ophthalmology 1999;106:1101–1108.
18. Latvala T, Mustonen E, Uusitalo R, et al. Pigmentary retinopathy in patients with the MELAS mutation 3243A—>G in mitochondrial DNA. Graefes Arch Clin Exp Ophthalmol 2002;240:795–801.
19. Bellmann C, Neveu MM, Scholl HPN, et al. Localized retinal electrophysiological and fundus autofluorescence imaging abnormalities in maternal inherited diabetes and deafness. Invest Ophthalmol Vis Sci 2004;45:2355–2360.
20. Michaelides M, Jenkins SA, Bamiou DE, et al. Macular dystrophy associated with the A3243G mitochondrial DNA mutation. Distinct retinal and associated features, disease variability, and characterization of asymptomatic family members. Arch Ophthalmol 2008;126:320–328.
21. Sue CM, Mitchell P, Crimmins DS, et al. Pigmentary retinopathy associated with the mitochondrial DNA 3243 point mutation. Neurology 1997;49:1013–1017.
22. Newell FW, Polascik MA. Mitochondrial disease and retinal pigmentary degeneration. In: Proceedings of the 3rd International Congress of Ophthalmology, Kyoto, Japan. New York: Elsevier Science Publishing, 1979:1613–1617.
23. McKechnie NM, King M, Lee WR. Retinal pathology in the Kearns-Sayre syndrome. Br J Ophthalmol 1985;69:63–75.
24. Chang TS, Johns DR, Walker D, et al. Ocular clinicopathologic study of the mitochondrial encephalomyopathy overlap syndrome. Arch Ophthalmol 1993;111:1254–1262.
25. Rummelt V, Folberg R, Ionescu V, et al. Ocular pathology of MELAS syndrome with mitochondrial DNA nucleotide 3243 point mutation. Ophthalmology 1993;100:1757–1766.
26. Eagle RC, Hedges TR, Yanoff M. The atypical pigmentary retinopathy of Kearns-Sayre syndrome: a light and electron microscopic study. Ophthalmology 1982;89:1433–1440.
27. Wallace DC. Diseases of the mitochondrial DNA. Annu Rev Biochem 1992;61:1175–1212.
28. Rückmann Av, Fitzke FW, Bird AC. Distribution of fundus autofluorescence with a scanning laser ophthalmoscope. Br J Ophthalmol 1995;79:407–412.
29. Holz FG, Bellmann C, Margaritidis M, et al. Patterns of increased in vivo fundus autofluorescence in the junctional zone of geographic atrophy of the retinal pigment epithelium associated with age-related macular degeneration. Graefes Arch Clin Exp Ophthalmol 1999;237:145–152.
30. Bindewald A, Schmitz-Valckenberg S, Jorzik JJ, et al. Classification of abnormal fundus autofluorescence patterns in the junctional zone of geographic atrophy in patients with age related macular degeneration. Br J Ophthalmol 2005;89:874–878.
31. Wallace DC. Mitochondrial diseases in man and mouse. Science 1999;283:1482–1488.
32. Kanda A, Chen W, Othman M, et al. A variant of mitochondrial protein LOC387715/ARMS2, not HTRA1, is strongly associated with age-related macular degeneration. Proc Natl Acad Sci USA 2007;104:16227–16232.
33. Rath PP, Jenkins S, Michaelides M, et al. Characterisation of the macular dystrophy in patients with the A3243G mitochondrial DNA point mutation with fundus autofluorescence. Br J Ophthalmol 2008;92:623–629.
34. Downes SM, Fitzke FW, Holder GE, et al. Clinical features of codon 172 RDS macular dystrophy. Similar phenotype in 12 families. Arch Ophthalmol 1999;117:1373–1383.

Fundus Autofluorescence in Choroideremia

C horoideremia (CHM) is a progressive retinal dystrophy with an X-linked mode of inheritance (1–3) caused by mutations in the *CHM* gene (4). The name "choroideremia" means an absence (eremia) of the choroid and points out the typical findings in advanced stages of the disease: a complete atrophy of the choroid and visible bare sclera. CHM is characterized by a progressive degeneration of the photoreceptors and retinal pigment epithelium (RPE), followed by a degeneration of the choroid (5). Full-field electroretinogram (ERG) is reduced early on in the disease, showing a rod-cone dysfunction, and with disease progression the ERG becomes nonrecordable (6). Fundus changes are visible during the first decade of life, with mottled RPE alterations in the periphery being the first manifestations of the disease. Subsequently, areas of RPE and choroid atrophy develop in the far periphery and midperiphery. The atrophic lesions increase in size and become confluent, spreading toward the center over the years; however, the macula remains spared for decades of life. Finally, bare sclera is seen throughout the fundus. Nyctalopia is one of the first symptoms in CHM patients. Visual field defects develop in the midperiphery, followed by progression to concentric visual field loss, color vision defects, photophobia, and loss of visual acuity.

Because of the X-linked inheritance, only males are affected. Female carriers who manifest CHM are very rare (2,5,7–10). Normally, all female carriers show patchy fundus changes, including various grades of mottled RPE alterations, RPE stippling, or spotty pigment atrophy in the periphery. Lyonization, i.e., a random X-inactivation, explains the various phenotypes observed in carriers of the disease (7). The full-field ERG is mostly normal in carriers of CHM.

In addition to a complete eye examination, important diagnostic tools include detailed case and family histories, tests of color vision and visual field, recording of full-field ERG, and fundus autofluorescence (AF). Family members should be examined and, in suspected CHM, a genetic analysis of the *CHM* gene should be provided. To date, no treatment for CHM is available.

MOLECULAR BASIS/PATHOLOGY

The gene underlying CHM was first described in 1990 (4) and encodes Rab escort protein 1 (REP-1). More than 70 *CHM* gene mutations have been revealed so far (for details, see http://www.retina-international.org/sci-news/repmut.htm). All *CHM* mutations lead to complete loss of the gene product REP-1. Of interest, the gene is ubiquitously expressed; however, mutations affect only the eye (11). This phenomenon is currently explained by a specific gene substrate in the retina and choroid: Rab_{27a} (12). REP-1 is necessary for transferring geranylgeranyl groups to Rab proteins, which are small GTP-binding proteins (4,13,14). Rab proteins are involved in functions such as protein trafficking, endocytosis, intracellular vesicle transportation, and signal transduction (15). For a detailed overview of REP-1 functions, see Preising et al. (16).

CHM gene expression has been shown in rods and RPE cells (5), indicating the origin of the disease in rods and/or RPE cells. Therefore, the degeneration of the cones and choroid seems to be secondary to the demise of rods and RPE. Only a few histopathologic studies of CHM have been published, and those dealt mainly with the eyes of female carriers (5,17–19); the data regarding affected males are scarce (20). These studies showed patchy degeneration of the retina in female carriers, with mixed areas of normal photoreceptors, photoreceptors that had lost their outer segments, and areas of loss of the entire photoreceptor cells. In addition, RPE changes were found, including abnormal RPE cells with irregularities in thickness, various amounts of melanin and lipofuscin granules with some clumping of melanin granules, and areas with focal RPE hypertrophy or thinning (5). The choriocapillaris was normal except in areas with severe retinal degeneration (5).

IMAGING TECHNIQUES

Fluorescein Angiography

Fluorescein angiography (FA) facilitates the visualization of areas of RPE and choroidal atrophy. In these areas, the remaining large choroidal vessels can be easily identified (21–23). Patchy fundus changes and RPE mottling in female carriers can be demonstrated with FA (7) (Fig. 11I.1). In the case of suspected subretinal neovascularization, a very rare complication of CHM, FA is essential (9,24,25). Similarly, FA is needed to detect the very rare occurrence of intraretinal neovascularization in CHM (26).

Indocyanine Green Angiography

Indocyanine green (ICG) angiography is not routinely used in clinical practice for diagnosing CHM. Only limited data exist regarding the use of ICG in patients with CHM. Forsius et al. (27) reported that ICG shows the choroidal vessels in areas where RPE and choriocapillaris are still present, whereas RPE atrophy and remaining

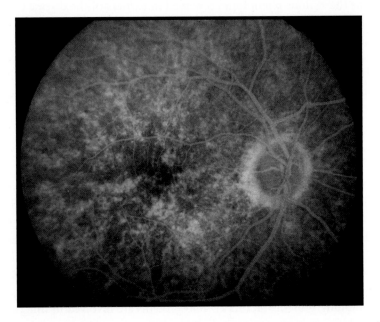

FIGURE 11I.1.   FA of the right eye of a female CHM carrier, 26 years of age. There are patchy changes of the RPE throughout the fundus.

choriocapillaris are less well visualized by ICG. The choroidal blood circulation was slow in advanced stages of CHM.

Optical Coherence Tomography

Several retinal changes can be detected by optical coherence tomography (OCT) imaging in patients with CHM. Retinal thickening, which may be due to Müller cell activation and hypertrophy, has been claimed to be a marker of the earliest stage of the disease (28). As the disease progresses, loss of photoreceptor nuclei and shortening of the outer and inner segments of the photoreceptors, followed by disorganization and subsequent slow thinning of the retina over decades, and abnormal laminar architecture have been reported (28–30).

Fundus Autofluorescence

Over the past few years, AF has become a very useful tool for the diagnosis and follow-up of patients with inherited retinal dystrophies. Data on AF in CHM and female carriers demonstrate the usefulness of AF as a diagnostic tool in this disease (10,31,32). In young CHM patients, the peripheral retina shows only RPE mottling, which is often difficult to detect clinically. AF imaging demonstrates these RPE irregularities well, in the form of densely packed small areas with reduced AF signal sparing the fovea; at the fovea, AF remains homogeneous. Under these circumstances, the diagnosis of CHM may be missed, but AF findings will point toward the diagnosis of CHM (Fig. 11I.2). The extent of RPE alterations can be evaluated more precisely with AF than with any other imaging technique. Furthermore, AF is noninvasive and is faster and easier to perform than FA. These advantages of AF imaging are especially important when evaluating children suspected to have CHM. In areas of RPE atrophy, a low AF signal is ob-

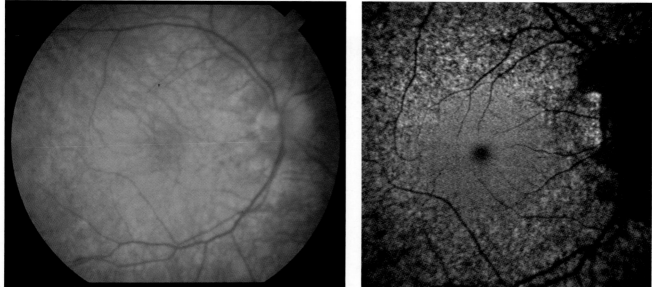

FIGURE 11I.2.   Fundus photography **(A)** and fundus AF **(B)** of the right eye of a male, 16 years of age, with CHM. Visual acuity was 1.0. Slit-lamp biomicroscopy disclosed what could be considered a normal, although very mildly pigmented, fundus **(A)**. Only a very fine and subtle mottling in the RPE was present. AF imaging demonstrated marked abnormalities in the distribution of AF, with a characteristic diffuse pattern of multiple, coalescent areas of reduced and increased AF sparing the fovea, where AF was still homogeneous.

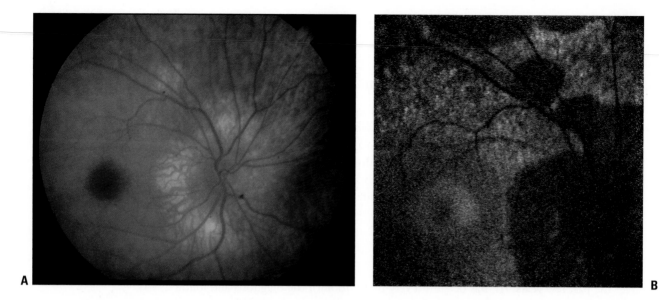

FIGURE 11I.3. Fundus photography **(A)** and fundus AF **(B)** of the right eye of a male, 17 years of age, with CHM. Visual acuity was 1.0. The optic nerve and retinal blood vessels appeared normal. The RPE showed multiple large areas of RPE depigmentation around the optic disc and in the midperiphery. The fovea appeared darker. AF imaging demonstrated a coalescent pattern of small foci of increased and decreased AF sparing the fovea, and an absent AF signal in large areas of RPE atrophy around the optic disc and in the midperiphery.

served (Figs. 11I.2 and 11I.3). In advanced stages of the disease, when RPE and choroid atrophy reaches the macula, AF can be used successfully to visualize remaining islands of preserved RPE (Fig. 11I.4).

Female carriers show, funduscopically, mottled areas of RPE or spotty pigment atrophy in the periphery. In these cases, AF imaging shows a specific speckled pattern with small areas of reduced AF corresponding to the mottled RPE irregularities (Fig. 11I.5). In female carriers of the disease, as in affected males, AF imaging is very use-

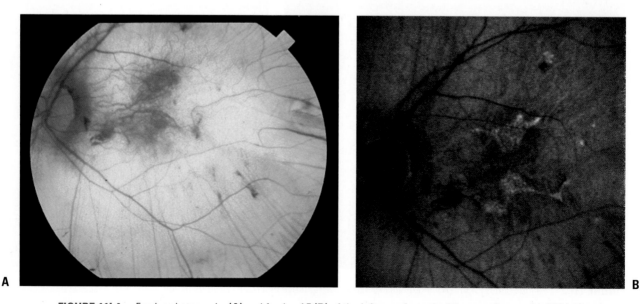

FIGURE 11I.4. Fundus photography **(A)** and fundus AF **(B)** of the left eye of a male, 38 years of age, with CHM. Visual acuity was 0.4. Complete atrophy of the RPE and choroid was observed, with the exception of some residual tissue at the macula. Bare sclera could be seen throughout the fundus. AF was still detectable in the remaining RPE at the macula.

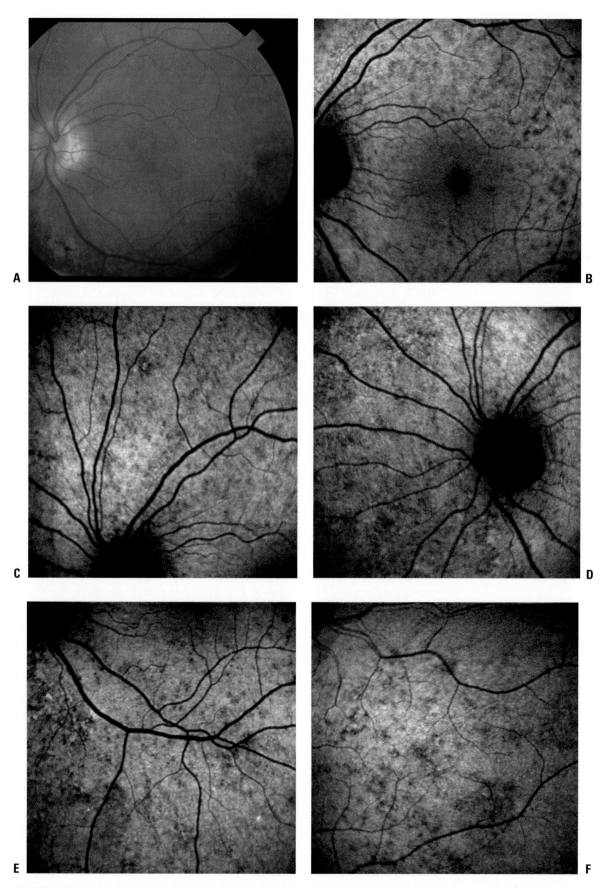

FIGURE 11I.5. Fundus photography **(A)** and fundus AF **(B–F)** of the left eye of a female carrier (37 years old) of CHM. Visual acuity was 1.0. Mottling in the RPE in the peripheral retina was observed by slit-lamp biomicroscopy **(A)**. AF imaging showed a specific speckled pattern with small areas of reduced AF corresponding to the mottled RPE irregularities **(B–F)**.

ful for detecting RPE irregularities, and it reveals more widespread changes in the RPE than can be observed funduscopically. The characteristic AF pattern in female carriers of CHM is very useful for detecting the disease.

DIFFERENTIAL DIAGNOSIS

The diagnosis of CHM can be difficult to establish in early stages of the disease. The most important differential diagnosis in these cases is X-linked retinitis pigmentosa (RP). In cases of suspected CHM, female carriers in the affected family have to be examined. This is important to exclude the diagnosis of X-linked RP, in which females carriers have no fundus changes but a reduced full-field ERG, in contrast to CHM, where female carriers show fundus changes but mostly a normal full-field ERG. A further important differential diagnosis is gyrate atrophy, which can be treated with a special diet. Like CHM, gyrate atrophy shows atrophic alterations of RPE and choroid beginning in the periphery and spreading toward the center. However, the inheritance is autosomal recessive, and a thorough family history can help differentiate between the two diseases. In addition, gyrate atrophy is accompanied by an increased blood level of ornithine acid, which should be measured to confirm or exclude the diagnosis of gyrate atrophy. To date, there are no published data on AF in gyrate atrophy, likely because of the extreme rareness of the condition. It is possible that AF may help in differentiating between CHM and gyrate atrophy. The atrophic areas in gyrate atrophy are very sharply demarcated, and there are no mottled RPE changes between the lesions or patchy RPE changes on FA. Therefore, the speckled pattern in AF should be seen only in CHM and not in gyrate atrophy.

SUMMARY

AF imaging is an excellent method for obtaining information about the RPE and its alterations in vivo. In contrast to FA, AF is fast and noninvasive. Because RPE alterations are common in CHM and, in general, most of the hereditary retinal dystrophies, AF imaging should be accepted as a standard diagnostic tool and can be used instead of FA in the majority of cases. The AF pattern in female CHM carriers seems to be specific to female carriers of CHM and may provide an additional phenotypic criterion for diagnosis in carriers of this disease (10). In affected males, AF imaging is very helpful in demonstrating the extent of RPE defects at first examination and, over time, the increasing RPE loss, which is useful for evaluating the progression of the disease.

REFERENCES

1. Krill AE, Archer D. Classification of the choroidal atrophies. Am J Ophthalmol 1971;72:562–585.
2. Kärnä J. Choroideremia. A clinical and genetic study of 84 Finnish patients and 126 female carriers. Acta Ophthalmol 1986;(Suppl)176:1–68.
3. Roberts MF, Fishman GA, Roberts DK, et al. Retrospective, longitudinal, and cross sectional study of visual acuity impairment in choroideraemia. Br J Ophthalmol 2002;86:658–662.
4. Cremers FPM, van de Pol DJR, van Kerkhoff LPM, et al. Cloning of a gene that is rearranged in patients with choroideraemia. Nature 1990;347:674–677.
5. Syed N, Smith JE, John SK, et al. Evaluation of retinal photoreceptors and pigment epithelium in a female carrier of choroideremia. Ophthalmology 2001;108:711–720.

6. Sieving PA, Niffenegger JH, Berson EL. Electroretinographic findings in selected pedigrees with choroideremia. Am J Ophthalmol 1986;101:361–367.
7. Rudolph G, Preising M, Kalpadakis P, et al. Phenotypic variability in three carriers from a family with choroideremia and a frameshift mutation 1388delCCinsG in the REP-1 gene. Ophthalmic Genet 2003;24:203–214.
8. Cheung MC, Nune GC, Wang M, et al. Detection of localized retinal dysfunction in a choroideremia carrier. Am J Ophthalmol 2004;137:189–191.
9. Potter MJ, Wong E, Szabo SM, et al. Clinical findings in a carrier of a new mutation in the choroideremia gene. Ophthalmology 2004;111:1905–1909.
10. Renner AB, Kellner U, Cropp E, et al. Choroideremia: variability of clinical and electrophysiological characteristics and first report of a negative electroretinogram. Ophthalmology 2006;113:2066–2073.
11. Shi W, van den Hurk JAJM, Alamo-Bethencourt V, et al. Choroideremia gene product affects trophoblast development and vascularization in mouse extra-embryonic tissues. Dev Biol 2004;272:53–65.
12. Seabra MC, Ho YK, Anant JS. Deficient geranylgeranylation of Ram/Rab27 in choroideremia. J Biol Chem 1995;270:24420–24427.
13. Seabra MC, Brown MS, Slaughter CA, et al. Purification of component A of Rab geranylgeranyl transferase: possible identity with the choroideremia gene product. Cell 1992;70:1049–1057.
14. Seabra MC, Brown MS, Goldstein JL. Retinal degeneration in choroideremia: deficiency of rab geranylgeranyl transferase. Science 1993;259:377–381.
15. Seabra MC. New insights into the pathogenesis of choroideremia: a tale of two REPs. Ophthalmic Genet 1996;17:43–46.
16. Preising M, Ayuso C. Rab escort protein 1 (REP1) in intracellular traffic: a functional and pathophysiological overview. Ophthalmic Genet 2004;25:101–110.
17. Ghosh M, McCulloch C, Parker JA. Pathological study in a female carrier of choroideremia. Can J Ophthalmol 1988;23:181–186.
18. Flannery JG, Bird AC, Farber DB, et al. A histopathologic study of a choroideremia carrier. Invest Ophthalmol Vis Sci 1990;31:229–236.
19. MacDonald IM, Chen MH, Addison DJ, et al. Histopathology of the retinal pigment epithelium of a female carrier of choroideremia. Can J Ophthalmol 1997;32:329–333.
20. Rodrigues MM, Ballintine EJ, Wiggert BN, et al. Choroideremia: a clinical, electron microscopic, and biochemical report. Ophthalmology 1984;91:873–883.
21. Hayakawa M, Fujiki K, Hotta Y, et al. Visual impairment and REP-1 gene mutations in Japanese choroideremia patients. Ophthalmic Genet 1999;20:107–115.
22. Itabashi T, Wada Y, Kawamura M, et al. Clinical features of Japanese families with a 402delT or a 555-556delAG mutation in choroideremia gene. Retina 2004;24:940–945.
23. Kellner U. Choroideremie. In: Heimann H, Kellner U, Foerster MH, eds. Atlas of fundus angiography. Stuttgart: Thieme, 2006.
24. Robinson D, Tiedeman J. Choroideremia associated with a subretinal neovascular membrane. Case report. Retina 1987;7:70–74.
25. Endo K, Yuzawa M, Ohba N. Choroideremia associated with subretinal neovascular membrane. Acta Ophthalmol Scand 2000;78:483–486.
26. Sawa M, Tamaki Y, Klancnik JR JM, et al. Intraretinal foveal neovascularization in choroideremia. Retina 2006;26:585–588.
27. Forsius H, Hyvarinen L, Nieminen H, et al. Fluorescein and indocyanine green fluorescence angiography in study of affected males and in female carriers with choroideremia. A preliminary report. Acta Ophthalmol (Copenh) 1977;55: 459–470.
28. Jacobson SG, Cideciyan AV, Sumaroka A, et al. Remodeling of the human retina in choroideremia: rab escort protein 1 (REP-1) mutations. Invest Ophthalmol Vis Sci 2006;47:4113–4120.
29. Katz BJ, Yang Z, Payne M, et al. Fundus appearance of choroideremia using optical coherence tomography. Adv Exp Med Biol 2006;572:57–61.
30. Mura M, Sereda C, Jablonski MM, et al. Clinical and functional findings in choroideremia due to complete deletion of the CHM gene. Arch Ophthalmol 2007;125:1107–1113.
31. Wegscheider E, Poloschek CM, Preising M, et al. Fundus autofluorescence in carriers for choroideremia. Invest Ophthalmol Vis Sci 2005;46:e-abstract 4088.
32. Poloschek CM, Kloeckener-Gruissem B, Hansen LL, et al. Syndromic choroideremia: sublocalization of phenotypes associated with Martin-Probst deafness mental retardation syndrome. Invest Ophthalmol Vis Sci 2008;49:4096–4104.

Lucia Kuffová
Vikki McBain
John V. Forrester
Noemi Lois

CHAPTER 12

Fundus Autofluorescence in Posterior Uveitis

Posterior segment intraocular inflammation (PSII, uveitis affecting the posterior segment of the eye) comes in many forms (1). These range from mild, chronic, low-grade intermediate uveitis affecting the peripheral retinal vessels with occasional inflammatory cells in the vitreous to acute, severe, sight-threatening ocular inflammation (STOI) with occlusive retinal vasculitis and/or optic disc swelling. In addition, STOI may occur because of the consequences of inflammation, particularly edema (macular or retinal edema with or without neurosensory retinal detachment) and neovascularization (retinal and choroidal with hemorrhage at either site).

Fundus imaging is of great value in the diagnosis and evaluation of patients with PSII. In particular, it may help in the assessment of STOI. However, since clear media are required for fundus imaging, there are limitations to the use of fundus imaging in PSII. In particular, patients with panuveitis and posterior synechiae with seclusio pupillae, or with dense vitreitis and vitreous hemorrhage are excluded from these investigations.

Despite these caveats, there are many cases of PSII and STOI that are amenable to and can benefit from good fundus imaging. Cystoid macular edema (CMO) and choroidal neovascularization (CNV) are two of the possible mechanisms by which STOI leads to registrable blindness. Moreover, many cases of chronic STOI escape detection because the clinical signs are not very obvious and the cause of the poor level of vision is not fully appreciated. As a result, patients lose sight unnecessarily.

There are many methods of fundus imaging: slit-lamp biomicroscopy, color and red-free fundus photography, fluorescein angiography (FA), indocyanine green angiography (ICGA), optical coherence tomography (OCT), and, most recently, fundus autofluorescence (AF) and near-infrared autofluorescence (NIA). Each of these imaging modalities has advantages and deficiencies for evaluating STOI; these will be reviewed in this chapter.

HISTOPATHOLOGY

In ocular inflammatory disease, one of the first events is the breakdown of the blood–retinal barrier (BRB). Experimentally, this is manifested by a reduction in shear flow in the large retinal vessels, occlusion of small capillaries, adhesion of leukocytes to the lining cells of the BRB, and extravasation of fluid and cells into the extravascular space. The extravascular space in the retina includes the retinal parenchyma and the subretinal space. In addition, the lining cells of the BRB include not only the retinal endothelium but also the RPE cells. Consequently, cells and fluid can accumulate on either side of the RPE and produce effects that have consequences for retinal imaging (Fig. 12.1).

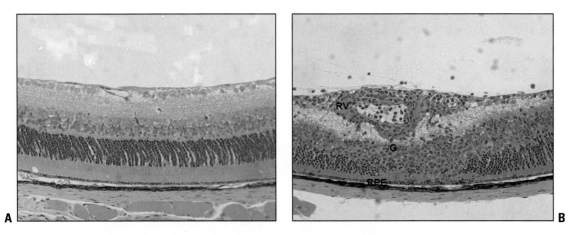

FIGURE 12.1.   Experimental autoimmune uveoretinitis (EAU) in the mouse. **(A)** Normal retina. **(B)** EAU. Note the intense retinal vasculitis (RV), granuloma (G), and RPE swelling. Fluid and inflammatory cells accumulate on either side of the RPE, indicating breakdown of the BRB.

CLINICAL FINDINGS AND IMAGING TECHNIQUES

Retinal edema (specifically macular edema, including CMO), inflammatory cell infiltration in choroid and retina, neovascularization, and subretinal fibrosis occur in patients with PSII. The following imaging systems can be used to evaluate these changes:

Fluorescein Angiography and Indocyanine Green Angiography

In fluorescein angiography (FA) and indocyanine green angiography (ICGA), the most obvious effect of inflammation is leakage of dye from the vessels into the extracellular space. In the retina, any leakage of dye is a sign of abnormality because the retinal vessels are normally impermeable through tight junctions to protein-bound fluorescein. Choroidal vessels are normally leaky through physiological fenestrations; however, in inflammation, dye leakage can be increased, leading to intense fluorescence, whereas cellular extravasation into the normally paucicellular choroidal stroma can lead to blockage of the dye signal. Thus, on FA and ICGA, accumulation of inflammatory cells can interfere with the signal and produce hypofluorescence in early frames of the angiogram and hyperfluorescence in late frames, as dye accumulates around inflammatory lesions. Similarly, as the RPE layer becomes "leaky," fluorescent dye will accumulate at this level in a "pericellular" distribution on FA (Fig. 12.2). Images of the macula and mid-peripheral retina can be obtained with FA and ICGA using conventional fundus cameras or wide-angle systems. This is important because inflammatory lesions can occur at any site in the posterior segment.

Macular edema, particularly CMO, is the most immediate direct cause of STOI in PSII. Detection and, more importantly, evaluation of macular edema in PSII clinically is highly subjective. Stereoscopic fundus photography is used to assess clinically significant macular edema in diabetic retinopathy, and similar methods are useful in PSII, but studies have shown a lack of correlation between observers, particularly regarding the degree of CMO (2,3). More objective and reproducible measures of macular edema can be obtained with FA (4–6). Macular edema can be demonstrated readily on

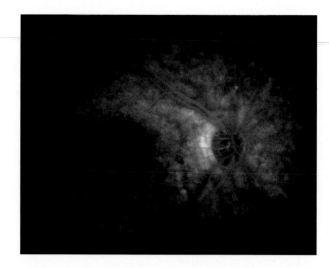

FIGURE 12.2. Late frame of an FA obtained from a patient with sympathetic ophthalmia (SO). Note the diffuse leakage from the RPE/choroid.

FA by increased fluorescence at the macula in the late phases of the angiogram. When CMO is present, a cystoid or petalloid appearance is seen. Although FA cannot directly provide quantitative information regarding the amount of edema present, computer software programs are available for that purpose (7,8).

FA is required and remains the gold standard for the evaluation of inflammatory CNV, a feature of several forms of PSII, including multifocal choroiditis, presumed ocular histoplasmosis syndrome (POHS), punctuate inner choroidopathy (PIC), birdshot choroidopathy, and infectious disease (e.g., at the edge of toxoplasma lesions). It is important to obtain accurate FA images because CNV is a major cause of visual loss in patients with these disorders. FA is necessary not only to confirm the presence of the CNV, but also to estimate its size, its location with respect to fixation, and the degree of activity of the lesion. This information is required when selecting an appropriate treatment. Similarly, FA can demonstrate areas of subretinal fibrosis with staining of dye at the site of fibrosis in late phases of the FA.

ICGA does not seem to be as useful as FA for evaluating CMO, CNV, or subretinal fibrosis.

Optical Coherence Tomography

OCT has undoubted value in the detection of retinal edema. This imaging technique allows the clinician to determine not only the presence or absence of increased retinal thickness due to macular edema, but also to evaluate quantitatively the amount of fluid present. Time-domain OCT imaging has been used for several years now in most clinics and provides a two-dimensional "cut" of the region of interest; however, it is difficult to assess the surface area of the edema without sampling several fields. The more recently developed Fourier-domain OCT method allows three-dimensional imaging of the macula and therefore computer-based quantification of the area of edema.

OCT is also an excellent imaging modality to reveal CMO; even small cystic structures can be detected in what is in effect an in vivo "section" of the retina. Antcliff and colleagues (9) reported a 96% sensitivity and 100% specificity for OCT in detecting CME in patients with uveitis when compared with FA. However, false positives can occur when this imaging technique is used (e.g., in cases of foveal retinoschisis, Goldmann-Favre, and enhanced S-cone syndrome), and should be taken into account during interpretation of the images. Tran et al. (3) recently demonstrated the value of OCT as well, and indicated a poor visual prognosis for diffuse macular edema compared to a better prognosis in cases of serous retinal detachment as seen on OCT.

Active chorioretinal lesions occurring as a result of infiltration of inflammatory cells, particularly the small round lesions observed in many forms of PSII (e.g., Dalen-Fuchs nodules in sympathetic ophthalmia, and granulomas in sarcoidosis), are well demonstrated on FA and ICGA (see above) but are difficult to see by OCT; therefore, OCT is not usually applied to specifically evaluate these lesions.

OCT has been proposed in recent years as a useful method to evaluate patients with CNV and to monitor the need for treatment in patients with exudative age-related macular degeneration (AMD; see Chapter 10B). The value of OCT as a diagnostic tool for inflammatory CNV has not been elucidated to date, and it remains unclear in which proportion of patients OCT may fail to demonstrate activity of the CNV when present. This may be particularly relevant for cases of inflammatory CNV, where a minimal amount of subretinal or intraretinal fluid is often detected in the presence of active neovascularization. Furthermore, data from studies in noninflammatory CNV have shown a weak correlation between OCT parameters and visual function (10).

Increased reflectivity at the site of subretinal fibrosis can be easily demonstrated in OCT images, although its extent may not be adequately shown by this method. Furthermore, findings may not be specific (e.g., accumulation of material in the subretinal space may elicit a similar signal).

Although OCT provides an excellent evaluation of the macular area, it does not allow an adequate visualization of mid-peripheral retinal changes, which are often observed in patients with PSII.

Fundus Autofluorescence

It is believed that the majority of the AF signal derives from lipofuscin and other fluorophores in the RPE; this signal increases with age (see Chapter 3). Experimental studies have demonstrated, however, that part of the AF signal may also arise from lipofuscin-rich microglia and macrophages (11). These also increase with age (12) but may present as a sudden entrant into a site of inflammation, producing a "recent onset" increased AF signal (see Chapter 4) . Therefore, changes in the distribution of AF in a patient with macular edema may also reflect the accumulation of cellular and fluid components of inflammation.

Changes in the normal RPE AF signal might also be expected in PSII. It is well recognized, both clinically and experimentally, that the RPE is the site of marked inflammation in PSII (Fig. 12.1). In this process, melanin is lost and lipofuscin and/or autofluorescent material may appear in both the RPE cells and associated macrophages (13–17). However, the RPE is also a major target for attack because it contains many autoantigens (18–21) and engulfs organisms, such as viruses, through specific receptors (22–26), and it may be directly damaged and destroyed. The end-stage of many clinical uveitic conditions is severe RPE atrophy, which may be diffuse and mottled (as in birdshot choroidopathy) (Fig. 12.3) or extend to large patches of RPE and choroidal atrophy (as in toxoplasmosis or serpiginous chorioretinopathy) (Fig. 12.4). Alternatively, there may be considerable subretinal fibrosis (Fig. 12.5). Thus, the consequences for the AF signal may vary significantly depending on the stage and level of activity of the disease.

CMO is easily revealed by AF imaging (Fig. 12.3) (27). AF is helpful in demonstrating CMO when there is thinning, depigmentation, or incipient atrophy of the foveal

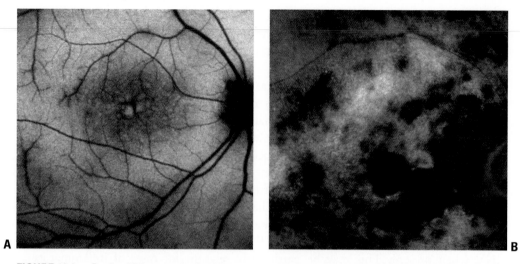

FIGURE 12.3. Fundus AF images obtained from a patient with birdshot choroidopathy in **(A)** early and **(B)** advanced stages of the disease. **(A)** Marked CMO is detected by AF imaging. **(B)** Widespread areas of reduced AF signal due to diffuse RPE atrophy are also easily visualized. An ERG obtained from the patient shown in Figure 12.3A disclosed reduced amplitude in rod and cone responses with increased implicit time in photopic and 30-Hz flicker; the a-wave of the mixed rod-cone response was also delayed.

RPE. Under these circumstances, CMO may be missed clinically and angiographically. Fundus AF allows evaluation of the entire area of edema, which can be captured noninvasively in one image in a few seconds (Fig. 12.3). Moreover, fundus AF allows an evaluation of the RPE and, indirectly, photoreceptors, thus providing essential information to balance the aggressiveness of treatment against the possibility for functional recovery (Fig. 12.3). AF imaging can also be used to noninvasively monitor the effect of immunosuppressive therapies and to guide treatment in patients with PSII (Fig. 12.6).

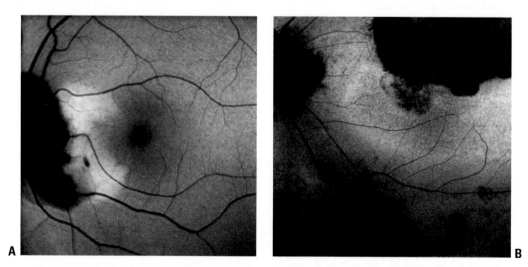

FIGURE 12.4. Fundus AF images obtained from patients with serpiginous chorioretinopathy **(A)** and toxoplasma chorioretinitis **(B)**. **(A)** A large area of increased AF signal is observed extending from a patch of reduced AF, suggesting active disease. **(B)** A patch of reduced AF signal is observed superior to the fovea, with abnormal, predominantly low AF signal at the fovea. Note the presence of an area of increased AF signal occupying most of the inferior aspect of the macula and extending toward the temporal mid periphery, indicating active disease.

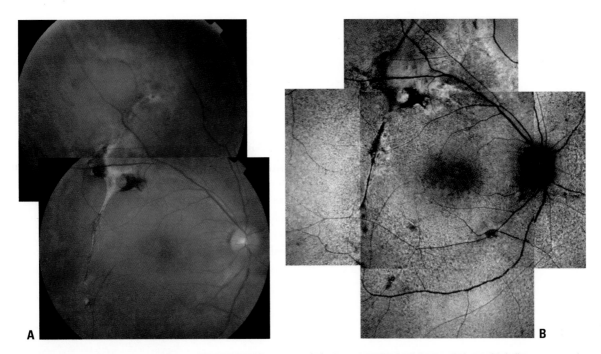

FIGURE 12.5. Composite of **(A)** color fundus photographs and **(B)** AF images obtained from a patient with inflammatory subretinal fibrosis syndrome. Note the extensive changes in the distribution of AF present; in contrast, fundus photographs demonstrate abnormalities only at the site where subretinal fibrosis is observed.

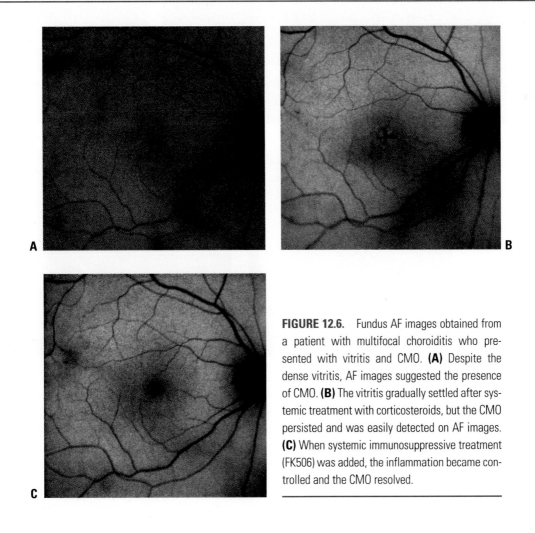

FIGURE 12.6. Fundus AF images obtained from a patient with multifocal choroiditis who presented with vitritis and CMO. **(A)** Despite the dense vitritis, AF images suggested the presence of CMO. **(B)** The vitritis gradually settled after systemic treatment with corticosteroids, but the CMO persisted and was easily detected on AF images. **(C)** When systemic immunosuppressive treatment (FK506) was added, the inflammation became controlled and the CMO resolved.

When one compares findings on FA, OCT, and AF in patients with macular edema and posterior uveitis, interesting differences in areas of RPE "leakage" and patches of choroidal nonperfusion can be seen (see legend of Fig. 12.7 to compare corresponding areas). The RPE signal detected in OCT images is usually quite distinct (Fig. 12.7) and thus it might be presumed that defects in the RPE as a result of inflammation are readily detectable. However, this is predicated in part by the amount of retinal thickness and edema in the pre-RPE layers. Therefore, OCT changes in the RPE might not correlate directly with changes in the distribution of fundus AF. Thus, complementary information obtained by combining these imaging techniques is valuable when managing patients with posterior uveitis.

Preliminary data using fundus AF images to evaluate chorioretinal infiltration in PSII suggest that this imaging technique may be of value for evaluating patients with this group of disorders. A recent report on AF in birdshot choroidopathy suggested that this technique might reveal the true extent of RPE cell atrophy, which is not evidenced by slit-lamp biomicroscopy (Fig. 12.3) (28). In addition, similar findings

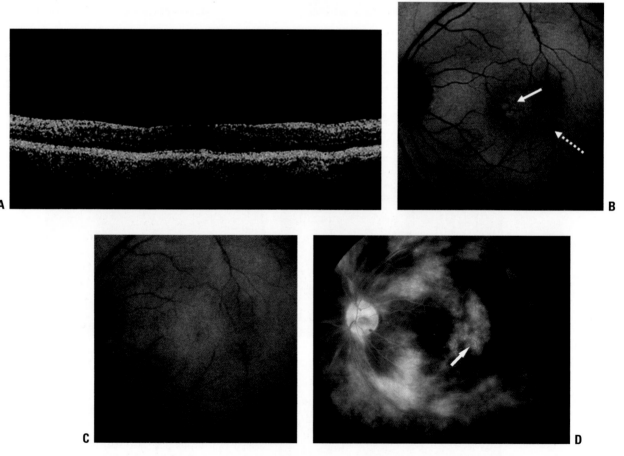

FIGURE 12.7. **(A)** OCT (90 degree cut), **(B)** AF, **(C)** NIA, and **(D)** late frame of FA obtained from a patient with multifocal choroiditis affecting predominantly the macular area. **(A)** OCT demonstrated retinal thickening/edema and prominent RPE signal. **(B)** On AF imaging an increased AF signal was observed at the fovea (*white full arrow*) and a reduced AF signal was seen in the temporal parafoveal area (*dotted white arrow*), with normal AF surrounding this area (*black arrow*). **(C)** On NIA, a reduced AF signal was also observed in the temporal parafoveal area. **(D)** The area of reduced AF and NIA signal appears to correspond to an area demonstrating late leakage (*white full arrow*) on FA; choroidal nonperfusion was also observed temporally (*black arrow*).

were obtained in a series of cases of multifocal choroiditis and panuveitis (29). Of interest, AF revealed small incipient lesions that were not always visible on fundus photographs. Hence, it is possible that fundus AF can be used for early detection and screening of active disease in patients with these disorders, without the need to resort to invasive FA or ICGA methods. We have observed similar findings, for instance, in serpiginous chorioretinopathy. Fundus AF often reveals larger patches of RPE atrophy than can be observed on slit-lamp biomicroscopy. Additionally, an increased AF signal can be detected at the edge of atrophic lesions, likely indicating the presence of active disease (Fig. 12.4). Therefore, it is possible that fundus AF can be used to evaluate the risk of lesion extension and encroachment onto the fovea, with resultant visual loss.

Although FA remains the gold standard in the evaluation of patients with inflammatory CNV, useful information can also be obtained in these cases by AF imaging. On AF images, a CNV most often appears as an area of reduced AF signal, which can be surrounded by a complete or incomplete halo of increased AF (Fig. 12.8). Areas of recent onset or long-standing subretinal fluid appear as areas of reduced (Fig. 12.8) or increased AF signal, respectively. However, it is not always possible to determine whether the CNV is active based on AF imaging. In CNV associated with AMD, a relatively normal distribution of AF at the fovea appears to have prognostic significance with regard to the potential for visual acuity improvement following treatment (see Chapter 10B). This may also be the case in inflammatory CNV, although to date there are no data available to support this.

In areas of subretinal fibrosis, where presumably the RPE is atrophic, has lost its melanin, or is packed with lipofuscin-like material or other fluorophores, changes to

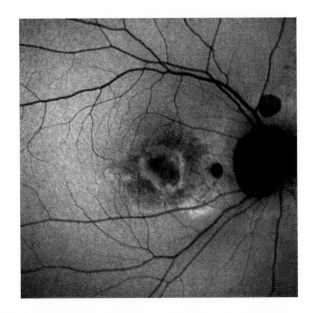

FIGURE 12.8.   AF image obtained from a patient with inflammatory CNV. A decreased AF signal is observed at the site of the CNV, surrounded by a halo of increased AF; the latter is likely the result of proliferation of RPE cells and/or macrophages around the neovascular process. Ill-defined reduced AF signal is also observed around the CNV, likely related to the presence of subretinal fluid. Note the increased AF signal around the optic nerve; interestingly, in this area two patches of reduced AF signal compatible with RPE atrophy are also observed.

the normal AF signal occur. The extent of the subretinal fibrosis can be clearly delineated and shown to be more widespread than suspected on color fundus imaging (Fig. 12.5). In addition, differences in the level of AF signal in different regions of the fundus in these cases may also relate to differences in "activity" of the disease throughout the fundus (Fig. 12.5). Assuming that the AF signal represents lipofuscin accumulation inside RPE cells or macrophages, areas with increased AF signal may indicate activated RPE cells or macrophages in those regions. Clearly, longitudinal studies of these lesions would be required to confirm their changing nature.

ELECTROPHYSIOLOGY

The functional abnormalities ascertained by electrophysiological testing in patients with PSII may correlate with the fundal changes observed on clinical examination. Patients with chorioretinitis typically have normal or only mildly reduced amplitude in full-field electroretinogram (ERG, both a- and b-wave), but normal implicit times (30). Similarly, patients with localized inflammatory disease, such as toxoplasmosis, can also have a normal or only very mild reduction in full-field ERG with normal implicit times (30,31). However, in diffuse and generally chronic inflammatory conditions of the retina and choroid, full-field ERG findings more commonly show both an amplitude reduction and an implicit time delay of the full-field ERG responses (31). Inflammatory conditions that lead to pigmentary degenerative changes can mimic the fundus appearance of retinitis pigmentosa (RP) (see below); however, full-field ERG abnormalities tend to be less marked (30). Furthermore, full-field ERG abnormalities in patients with PSII may be unilateral or bilateral, in which case they are often substantially asymmetric, in contrast to the typically symmetrical ERG reduction and implicit time delay seen in RP.

The majority of patients with birdshot choroidopathy have abnormal scotopic and photopic ERGs and, in addition, the amplitude of the b-wave is frequently reduced to a greater extent than that of the a-wave (electronegative ERG), suggesting dysfunction of the inner retina (30,32). The presence of delay in the 30-Hz flicker ERG response in all patients with birdshot choroidopathy suggests that it is the most sensitive indicator of retinal dysfunction (32). Electrophysiological assessment of patients with birdshot choroidopathy is extremely useful for monitoring the response to treatment (e.g., normalization of the b:a ratio and flicker implicit time). Subjective and clinical signs are, in contrast, poorer indicators of a therapeutic response (32,33). However, pattern ERG recovery after treatment does not always mirror the improvement in the full-field ERG, due to the possible presence of persistent macular edema (32).

DIFFERENTIAL DIAGNOSIS

Although visualization of inflammatory cells in the anterior chamber and vitreous cavity on slit-lamp examination suggests the diagnosis of PSII, this finding is not always present. Similarly, a typical "pattern" of inflammatory infiltration such as that observed in POHS, PIC, birdshot choroidopathy, or other forms of PSII may not always be seen. Under these circumstances, the diagnosis of PSII may represent a challenge. This is particularly true when PERG and scotopic and photopic ERGs are reduced (Fig. 12.3A). In the latter cases, there might be a misdiagnosis of inherited retinal dystrophy, and no treatment would then be considered for the patient. The opposite might also occur and patients could be treated unnecessarily. Fundus AF

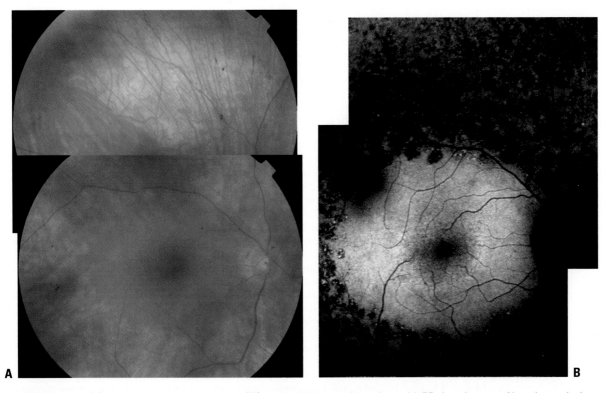

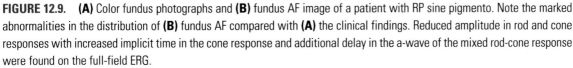

FIGURE 12.9. **(A)** Color fundus photographs and **(B)** fundus AF image of a patient with RP sine pigmento. Note the marked abnormalities in the distribution of **(B)** fundus AF compared with **(A)** the clinical findings. Reduced amplitude in rod and cone responses with increased implicit time in the cone response and additional delay in the a-wave of the mixed rod-cone response were found on the full-field ERG.

may be helpful in establishing the correct diagnosis by demonstrating preservation of the mid-peripheral AF signal (Fig. 12.3A) or well-defined patches of reduced AF (Fig. 12.3B) in cases of PSII and multiple smaller areas of reduced AF throughout the mid periphery in patients with inherited retinal dystrophies (Fig. 12.9).

SUMMARY

Fundus AF is a relatively new modality for fundus imaging based on a well-recognized phenomenon from the early days of FA. Interpretation of the AF signal should be based on a clear understanding of the pathology of the condition under investigation. In the case of uveitis, recent information about lipofuscin in microglial cells and macrophages has added a new dimension to what was already understood about RPE cell damage and loss in this condition. Fundus AF may be useful in monitoring disease progression and establishing, noninvasively, the activity of disease in PSII. Furthermore, AF may also be helpful for evaluating patients who are allergic to FA or ICGA.

REFERENCES

1. Forrester JVF, Okada A, BenEzra D, et al. Posterior Segment Intraocular Inflammation: Guidelines. The Hague: Kugler, 1998.
2. Arend O, Remky A, Elsner AE, et al. Quantification of cystoid changes in diabetic maculopathy. Invest Ophthalmol Vis Sci 1995;36:608–613.

3. Tran TH, de Smet MD, Bodaghi B, et al. Uveitic macular oedema: correlation between optical coherence tomography patterns with visual acuity and fluorescein angiography. Br J Ophthalmol 2008;92:922–927.

4. Kiss CG, Barisani-Asenbauer T, Maca S, et al. Reading performance of patients with uveitis-associated cystoid macular edema. Am J Ophthalmol 2006;142:620–624.

5. Markomichelakis NN, Halkiadakis I, Pantelia E, et al. Patterns of macular edema in patients with uveitis: qualitative and quantitative assessment using optical coherence tomography. Ophthalmology 2004;111: 946–953.

6. Kang SW, Park CY, Ham DI. The correlation between fluorescein angiographic and optical coherence tomographic features in clinically significant diabetic macular edema. Am J Ophthalmol 2004;137:313–322.

7. Phillips RP, Ross PG, Tyska M, et al. Detection and quantification of hyperfluorescent leakage by computer analysis of fundus fluorescein angiograms. Graefes Arch Clin Exp Ophthalmol 1991;229:329–335.

8. Phillips RP, Ross PG, Sharp PF, et al. Use of temporal information to quantify vascular leakage in fluorescein angiography of the retina. Clin Phys Physiol Meas 1990;11(Suppl A):81–85.

9. Antcliff RJ, Stanford MR, Chauhan DS, et al. Comparison between optical coherence tomography and fundus fluorescein angiography for the detection of cystoid macular oedema in patients with uveitis. Ophthalmology 2000;107:593–599.

10. Moutray T, Alarbi M, Mahon G, et al. Relationships between clinical measures of visual function, fluorescein angiographic and optical coherence tomography features in patients with subfoveal choroidal neovascularisation. Br J Ophthalmol 2008;92:361–364.

11. Xu H, Chen M, Mayer EJ, et al. Turnover of resident retinal microglia in the normal adult mouse. Glia 2007;55:1189–1198.

12. Xu H, Chen M, Manivannan A, et al. Age-dependent accumulation of lipofuscin in perivascular and subretinal microglia in experimental mice. Aging Cell 2008;7:58–68.

13. Forrester JVF. Intermediate and posterior uveitis. Chem Immunol Allergy 2007;92:228–243.

14. Jiang HR, Hwenda L, Makinen K, et al. Sialoadhesin promotes the inflammatory response in experimental autoimmune uveoretinitis. J Immunol 2006;177:2258–2264.

15. Jiang HR, Lumsden L, Forrester JVF. Macrophages and dendritic cells in IRBP-induced experimental autoimmune uveoretinitis in B10RIII mice. Invest Ophthalmol Vis Sci 1999;40:3177–3185.

16. Lim WK, Chee SP, Sng I, et al. Immunopathology of progressive subretinal fibrosis: a variant of sympathetic ophthalmia. Am J Ophthalmol 2004;138:475–477.

17. Jakobiec FA, Marboe CC, Knowles II DM, et al. Human sympathetic ophthalmia. An analysis of the inflammatory infiltrate by hybridoma-monoclonal antibodies, immunochemistry, and correlative electron microscopy. Ophthalmology 1983;90:76–95.

18. Deeg CA, Raith AJ, Amann B, et al. CRALBP is a highly prevalent autoantigen for human autoimmune uveitis. Clin Dev Immunol 2007;39245.

19. Wang M, Bai F, Pries M, et al. Identification of MHC class I H-2 Kb/Db-restricted immunogenic peptides derived from retinal proteins. Invest Ophthalmol Vis Sci 2006;47:3939–3945.

20. Umeda S, Suzuki MT, Okamoto H, et al. Molecular composition of drusen and possible involvement of anti-retinal autoimmunity in two different forms of macular degeneration in cynomolgus monkey (*Macaca fascicularis*). FASEB J 2005;19:1683–1685.

21. Janssen JJ, Janssen BP, van Vugt AH. Characterization of monoclonal antibodies recognizing retinal pigment epithelial antigens. Invest Ophthalmol Vis Sci 1994;35:189–198.

22. Wang D, Yu QC, Schroer J, et al. Human cytomegalovirus uses two distinct pathways to enter retinal pigmented epithelial cells. Proc Natl Acad Sci USA 2007;104:20037–20042.

23. Cai S, Brandt CR. Induction of interleukin-6 in human retinal epithelial cells by an attenuated *Herpes simplex* virus vector requires viral replication and NFkappaB activation. Exp Eye Res 2008;86:178–188.

24. Liu B, Li Z, Mahesh SP, et al. HTLV-1 infection of human retinal pigment epithelial cells and inhibition of viral infection by an antibody to ICAM-1. Invest Ophthalmol Vis Sci 2006;47:1510–1515.

25. Haamann P, Kessel L, Larsen M. Monofocal outer retinitis associated with hand, foot, and mouth disease caused by coxsackievirus. Am J Ophthalmol 2000;129:552–553.

26. Kadrmas EF, Buzney SM. Coxsackievirus B4 as a cause of adult chorioretinitis. Am J Ophthalmol 1999;127:347–349.

27. McBain VA, Forrester JV, Lois N. Fundus autofluoresence in the diagnosis of cystoid macular oedema. Br J Ophthalmol 2008;92:946–949.

28. Koizumi H, Pozzoni MC, Spaide RF. Fundus autofluorescence in birdshot chorioretinopathy. Ophthalmology 2008;115:e15–20.

29. Haen SP, Spaide RF. Fundus autofluorescence in multifocal choroiditis and panuveitis. Am J Ophthalmol 2008;145:847–853.

30. Fishman GA, Birch DG, Holder GA, et al. Electrophysiologic Testing in Disorders of the Retina, Optic Nerve and Visual Pathway. 2nd ed. San Francisco: American Academy of Ophthalmology, 2001.

31. Scholl HPN, Zrenner E. Electrophysiology in the investigation of acquired retinal disorders. Surv Ophthalmol 2000;45:29–47.

32. Holder GE, Robson AG, Pavesio C, et al. Electrophysiological characterisation and monitoring in the management of birdshot chorioretinopathy. Br J Ophthalmol 2005;89:709–718.

33. Sobrin L, Lam BL, Liu M, et al. Electroretinographic monitoring in birdshot chorioretinography. Am J Ophthalmol 2005;140:52–64.

Fundus Autofluorescence in Central Serous Chorioretinopathy

Central serous chorioretinopathy (CSC) is a common retinal disease characterized by an idiopathic flat retinal detachment within the macula (1,2). It typically affects young and middle-aged adults between 20 to 50 years of age and often reveals a shallow, round, and serous detachment of the neurosensory retina; however, small detachments of the retinal pigment epithelium (RPE) may also occur (2). Primarily male patients (male:female ratio about 10:1) are affected and typically a type-A behavior in these patients can be observed. Moreover, emotional stress frequently accompanies the visual disturbances. CSC has also been associated with vasoconstrictive agents, endogenous hypercortisolism, and systemic corticosteroid use (3).

When the serous detachment involves the foveal region, patients become symptomatic and usually complain about blurred vision, scotoma, micropsia, or metamorphopsia. This can easily be detected by Amsler Grid testing. Decreased visual acuity can be improved by the addition of small hyperopic correction, focusing the light bundles to the detached central region. Of interest, visual acuity remains largely preserved despite the prolonged separation of the neurosensory layer from the RPE. The long-term visual prognosis for most patients is excellent and improvement can usually be achieved without specific treatment. However, about 20% to 30% of patients will have one or more recurrences, and a small percentage (about 5%) will develop choroidal neovascularization or chronic detachment with cystoid macular edema from this condition (4,5). Chronic forms of CSC are characterized by multiple sites of prolonged and recurrent serous retinal detachments in one or both eyes, and are particularly seen in Latin and Oriental people (5). Such patients may be asymptomatic for a prolonged time if the localized areas of retinal detachment are outside the foveal area. On biomicroscopy, multiple areas of RPE atrophic tracts, particularly in the inferior site of the macula and in the peripapillary regions, are observed (6,7). Angiography then reveals multiple sites of staining that correspond to the areas of RPE atrophy; however, no significant leakage is observable in these areas. Even though in these patients the macula is usually attached, the photoreceptors are chronically damaged due to previous long-term dysfunction. Thus, these patients usually suffer from significant loss of vision and paracentral visual field defects. In the case of chronic detachment, lipid exudates and cystoid macular edema may occur, complicating the disease (5). Whereas focal laser photocoagulation is recommended in acute CSC if no resolution of exudates appears after 4–6 weeks, in the atrophic stages of the disease no treatment can be offered. However, in chronic recurrences with prolonged or repetitive serous retinal detachments, laser photocoagulation can improve the visual course. A faster resolution of the edema and a faster rehabilitation of visual acuity are then observable; however, there is often no substantial benefit with regard to visual acuity following laser photocoagulation. Usually laser treatment is directed to the site of leakage. Laser therapy induces damage of the RPE layer with migration and proliferation of neighboring RPE cells to cover the defect, resulting in a restoration of the outer blood–retina barrier (8–10). As a result of this biologic tissue reaction from the laser photocoagulation, the neurosensory retinal detachment disappears and the visual acuity recovers.

PATHOLOGY OF CSC

In contrast to the well-defined clinical appearance of CSC, a clear understanding of the exact pathogenesis of accumulation of subretinal fluid is lacking. It is widely accepted that the origin of the subretinal fluid is the choroid. Because of a defect in the RPE layer, choroidal fluid enters the subretinal space and leads to the detachment of the neurosensory layer (1). CSC was induced in monkeys by repeated injections of epinephrine (11). Histologic examination of the monkeys' eyes revealed focal RPE degeneration and endothelial cell destruction in the underlying choriocapillary layer (12). This supports the generally adopted opinion that the RPE plays a crucial role in the development of CSC. Measurements of the metabolic activity of RPE cells also revealed significant changes in CSC (13). The cause of the focal leak is unclear. It was initially proposed that a simple breakdown of the RPE layer is responsible for the leak (14). Later, the theory of pathologically hypersecreting RPE was proposed (15); however, this did not explain the observation of widespread hyperpermeability in the areas of neurosensory detachment seen with indocyanine green (ICG) angiography (16,17). In fact, ICG suggested impaired choroidal circulation as a cause of CSC by showing delayed choroidal capillary filling in areas of hyperpermeability (18). It was proposed that localized capillary and venous congestion in distinct areas leads to ischemia, increased choroidal exudation, and a focally hyperpermeable choroid. Because of this excessive choroidal fluid extravasation, the RPE detaches and after further accumulation of fluid, breaks within the RPE appear, allowing the fluid to create a neurosensory retinal detachment (19). However, earlier but limited histopathologic examinations in humans showed no abnormalities in the choriocapillaris underlying the RPE detachment (20). On the other hand, it was noted that the gray-white exudates contained fibrin, which was taken as evidence that serum proteins escaped from the choriocapillaris. This supports the hypothesis that a focal increase in the permeability of the choriocapillaris is the primary cause of damage to the overlying RPE leading to distinct breaks and subsequent neurosensory detachment (2,5).

IMAGING TECHNIQUES IN THE DIAGNOSIS OF CENTRAL SEROUS CHORIORETINOPATHY

Biomicroscopy

The diagnosis of CSC is primarily clinical and usually confirmed by angiography. Biomicroscopically, and best seen with a narrow light beam from the slit-lamp, a well-defined round or oval area of shallow elevation of the retina, which usually presents a slightly darker color than the surrounding normal retina (5), can be observed. The detached retina is usually transparent and of normal thickness, and the subretinal fluid is also usually clear; however, sometimes gray-white serofibrinous exudates can be seen. Because of the retinal detachment, the visibility of the xanthophyll pigment within the center of the fovea may be enhanced, presenting as a central yellow spot. Also, through gravity, the subretinal fluid often pools inferiorly within the area of retinal detachment (5). Sometimes small dot-like deposits on the inner side of the retina or on the RPE surface within the detached area can be seen, most likely representing protein precipitates (2).

Fluorescein Angiography

Fluorescein angiography (FA) plays an important role in the evaluation of CSC. It is used to detect the distinct site of one or more RPE breaks and to determine the amount of leakage, which can be very heterogeneous. Thus, some patients reveal only small detachments and less angiographic leakage, whereas others present with large detachments and heavy leakage. In FA, usually the dye from the choroid leaks through the focal RPE defect and pools in the subretinal space. In more than 95% of patients with CSC, at least one leaking point can be seen. Typically, the dye spreads symmetrically in the subretinal space but does not extend outside the borders of the detachment. Sometimes the classic "smokestack phenomenon" can be observed showing the dye percolating upward in the subretinal space with subsequently pooling into the whole space. This pattern, first described in 1971 (21), is thought to result from an osmotic pressure gradient generated by differences between the protein concentration of the subretinal fluid under the detachment and the fluorescein dye entering the detachment (13).

Indocyanine Green Angiography

Together with FA, ICG angiography is an important imaging technique for the diagnosis and follow-up of patients with CSC. For cases in which FA findings are not typical of CSC, ICG angiography may be helpful in establishing the diagnosis, often revealing multifocal choroidal hyperfluorescence in affected and unaffected regions of active and fellow eyes (17,22). These hyperfluorescence areas have been hypothesized to be causative factors in the pathogenesis of CSC and may not be observed by FA alone. The ICG is a larger molecule highly bound to proteins and therefore does not leak extensively through the fenestrations of the choriocapillaris (13). Thus, choroidal vasculature can be observed in detail, in contrast to fluorescein, which leaks rapidly and easily through the fenestrations, immediately obscuring the choroidal vasculature. One study (13) reported that all patients with CSC examined had multiple bright areas of choroidal hyperfluorescence up to three disc areas around the leakage points and elsewhere, and the boundaries were independent of the neuroretinal detachment. Of interest, these areas of hyperfluorescence were also noted in eyes with inactive disease (22) and after resolution of the disease (13). Frequently observed detachments of the RPE (PED) accompanying CSC showed distinct characteristics in ICG angiography as a pooling of the dye in the late phase in the particular area of PED forming a hyperfluorescent ring (13).

Optical Coherence Tomography

Optical coherence tomography (OCT) has been found to be a useful tool in the diagnosis of CSC (23). Sometimes a slight elevation of the neurosensory retina is not detectable on slit-lamp biomicroscopy; however, such elevations can easily be detected by OCT and usually overlie an optically clear fluid-filled cavity. The mostly attached underlying RPE can be observed as a highly reflective band at the base of the cavity. Furthermore, additional PEDs can be easily seen on OCT as localized elevations of the highly reflective band over a clear cavity. The detached RPE then causes attenuation of the reflected light, resulting in extensive shadowing of the underlying choroidal signal (24). OCT may also be helpful in defining anatomic changes of the detached neurosensory retina as thickening of the retina or intraretinal cystic changes in CSC (23). Moreover, OCT is able to distinguish between serous retinal detachment and other pathologies, such as choroidal neovascular membrane, seen as a distinct thickening of the outer retinal layers in the latter condition (24). However, a clear differential diagnosis for this condition should be obtained by angiography. OCT is best used to monitor the disease during the follow-up period because it can reveal the resolution of the subretinal fluid by a reattachment of the neurosensory layer. For study purposes, the retinal thickness can even be measured to obtain quantitative follow-up values after interventions. When changes from acute to chronic CSC appear, enhanced OCT signals at the outer surface of the neurosensory retina can be observed, indicating fibrinous precipitates accumulating in this area (25).

Fundus Autofluorescence

In patients with acute CSC, a focal area of decreased autofluorescence (AF) is typically seen at the site of the focal leakage on FA, and a reduced AF signal is also observed within the entire area of serous retinal detachment (Fig. 13.1) (25–27).

In chronic-recurrent CSC, the focal leakage point and/or the area of angiographic hyperfluorescence most commonly demonstrates a decreased AF signal (27). In some patients, these areas of reduced AF signal are surrounded by zones with mottled, irregular AF, with foci of increased or decreased AF. In a small group of patients, no abnormal AF, in comparison with that of the background, can be detected at the leakage point. However, an increased AF signal is most often seen in

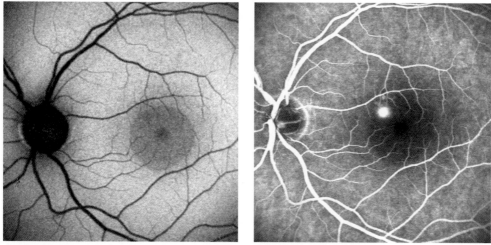

A   B

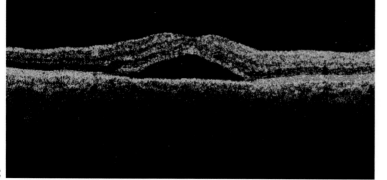

C

FIGURE 13.1. A 36-year-old male presented with acute visual loss in his left eye for 3 weeks. Visual acuity was 0.8. Fundus AF revealed a sharply demarcated area of decreased AF **(A)** corresponding to the angiographically visible blockage of fluorescence **(B)**. **(C)** A neurosensory retinal detachment is confirmed by OCT (vertical scan). An area of further decreased AF is also observed corresponding to the RPE leaking point on FA.

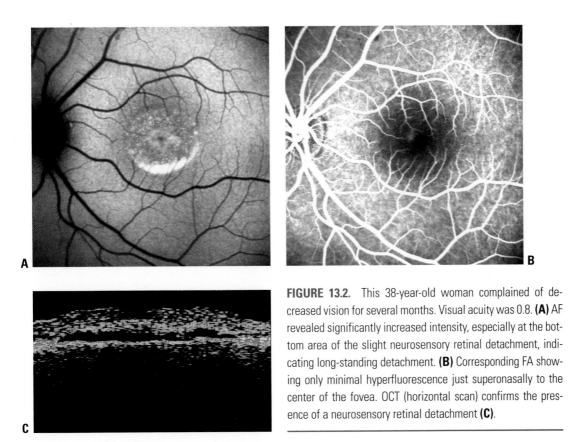

FIGURE 13.2. This 38-year-old woman complained of decreased vision for several months. Visual acuity was 0.8. **(A)** AF revealed significantly increased intensity, especially at the bottom area of the slight neurosensory retinal detachment, indicating long-standing detachment. **(B)** Corresponding FA showing only minimal hyperfluorescence just superonasally to the center of the fovea. OCT (horizontal scan) confirms the presence of a neurosensory retinal detachment **(C)**.

the area of presumed former or residual neurosensory retinal detachment (Fig. 13.2) (25,27). Fundus AF is extremely helpful in the noninvasive diagnosis of chronic CSC, demonstrating multiple areas of mottled, increased, or decreased AF suggestive of previous episodes of active disease (25,27,28). In these cases, only minimal ophthalmoscopic changes may be present, and OCT imaging usually shows only slight abnormalities as little subretinal fluid (Fig. 13.3).

INTERPRETATION OF AF FINDINGS IN CSC

In the acute phase of CSC, the reduced AF signal observed at the leaking point could be the result of the presence of damaged RPE, which may, at least partially, explain the occurrence of leakage from the choroid into the subretinal space. Alternatively, it could be related to a blockage of the AF signal by the presence of subretinal fluid. The reduced AF signal at the site of the subretinal fluid is most likely related to the blockage of the AF signal caused by the subretinal fluid.

In chronic-recurrent CSC, RPE atrophy may contribute to the decreased AF observed at the former leaking point. The increased AF observed in areas of presumed former neurosensory retinal detachment may be the result of a higher metabolic activity of the RPE leading to a higher phagocytosis rate of debris from the subretinal space (27,28) and shed photoreceptor outer segments (25). However, an accumulation of fluorophores within the serous fluid may also contribute to this enhanced AF. The low AF signal observed in cases of chronic-recurrent CSC in some areas (Fig. 13.3) may be the result of reduced metabolic activity, presumably due to photoreceptor cell loss in areas of chronic neurosensory retinal detachment (25,28).

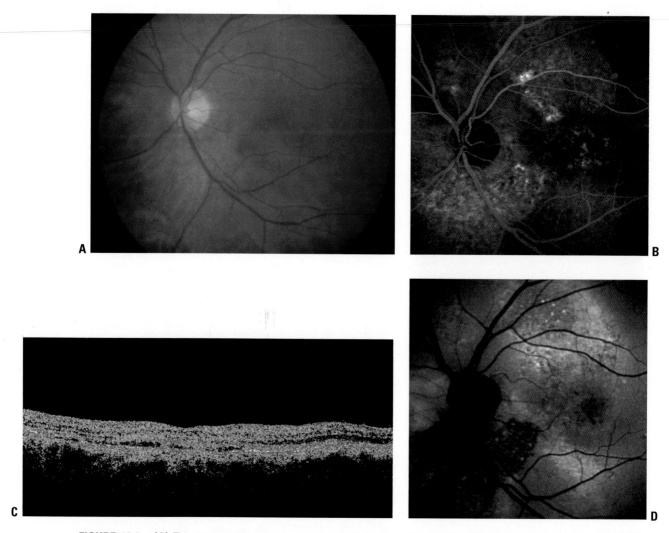

FIGURE 13.3. **(A)** This 51-year-old male presented with decreased visual acuity of 0.3 in both eyes with only minimal changes in ophthalmoscopy. The patient had experienced recurrent visual disturbances throughout the past years. **(B)** FA revealed hyperfluorescence in the peripapillary region and centrally, but no active leakage. **(C)** In OCT sections, no significant edema was noted. **(D)** Fundus AF disclosed reduced AF signal in the peripapillary area, compatible with RPE atrophy, at the site of angiographic hyperfluorescence. Perifoveolar increased AF was also observed, suggesting former areas of neurosensory retinal detachments that led to RPE changes. The diagnosis of chronic-recurrent CSR was made.

RELATIVE IMPORTANCE OF ANGIOGRAPHY, OCT, AND AF FOR THE DIAGNOSIS OF CSC

From a clinical point of view, in most cases, the correct diagnosis of acute CSC can be established by history and slit-lamp biomicroscopy, showing the typical significant round or oval shaped neurosensory retinal detachment within the macular area. In the absence of other techniques, fundus photography may provide some objective basis for follow-up of the natural history of CSC. However, FA is an appropriate and necessary investigation to confirm the diagnosis of CSC and to determine the location of the RPE leak(s) during the first episode of the disease, especially when treatment is considered, and also to obtain information on the presence of active disease as judged by the leakage of dye at the area(s) of RPE damage. ICG angiography is less informative concerning the activity and prognosis of the disease. OCT allows evaluation of the amount and extent of subretinal fluid, and is a useful tool for follow-up in patients with CSC, allowing monitoring of the resolution of the neurosensory retinal detachment and PED(s) if present. In patients with worsening symptoms, a repeat FA may be useful to detect possible new areas of RPE leakage.

In cases of acute CSC, AF may be able to detect the distinct leakage point(s) by demonstrating focal areas of reduced AF levels. In chronic-recurrent CSC, AF imaging is of significant value, especially considering that these cases often represent a diagnostic challenge. As shown in Figure 13.2, well-defined areas of increased AF can be detected in chronic cases. Similarly, multiple areas of mottled, increased, or decreased AF can also be observed, unilaterally or bilaterally, strongly suggesting the diagnosis of chronic-recurrent CSC (Fig. 13.3). These findings are important, particularly when no subretinal fluid is present, since in these cases OCT might fail to establish the diagnosis of CSC. In the latter cases, AF is invaluable as noninvasive diagnostic tool to establish the diagnosis of CSC. In the presence of subretinal fluid in chronic cases, which can be observed on OCT images, precipitates that demonstrate increased AF signal can often be seen at the level of the outer retinal layer (25). Further evidence of long-term chronic CSC can be provided by the presence of areas of reduced AF signal in the peripapillary zone and extending inferiorly, indicating damage and atrophy of the RPE from the previous presence of subretinal fluid in these areas.

DIFFERENTIAL DIAGNOSIS

In principle, serous elevations of the neurosensory retina in the macular area can be produced by diseases of the choroid, the RPE, and the retina itself. The following diseases can produce localized serous detachments similar to those observed in CSC: congenital pit of the optic nerve, malignant hypertension, toxemia of pregnancy, Harada disease, idiopathic uveal effusion, vitreomacular tractional syndrome, and age-related macular degeneration (AMD) (5). One of the most important diseases to rule out, particularly in older patients, is neovascular AMD, especially now when more effective treatments for this condition are available. The presence of a drusen supports the diagnosis of AMD rather than CSC. FA will allow the differentiation between CSC and exudative AMD.

SUMMARY

Distinct AF patterns can be observed in patients with acute and chronic-recurrent CSC. Whereas acute CSC is usually suspected by slit-lamp biomicroscopy and diagnosed using FA, the diagnosis of chronic-recurrent CSC is often challenging. Combined AF and OCT may have the potential to replace invasive angiography in the diagnosis of acute CSC. AF may allow recognition, in some patients, of the point of RPE leakage, which cannot be distinguished in OCT. If that is not possible, FA will still be needed. AF seems to be particularly helpful in the diagnosis of chronic-recurrent stages of the disease, which sometimes may be difficult to differentiate from other pathologic conditions because of the poorly defined and mottled, partly multifocal angiographic leakage. The AF patterns of increased AF levels and findings of RPE atrophy (mottled and decreased AF), as described above, provide strong evidence to support the diagnosis of chronic-recurrent CSC. Follow-up changes after treatment can also be easily detected by AF and usually correlate well with OCT findings (Fig. 13.4). Thus, fundus AF also serves as an appropriate tool to monitor the resolution of CSC during follow-up.

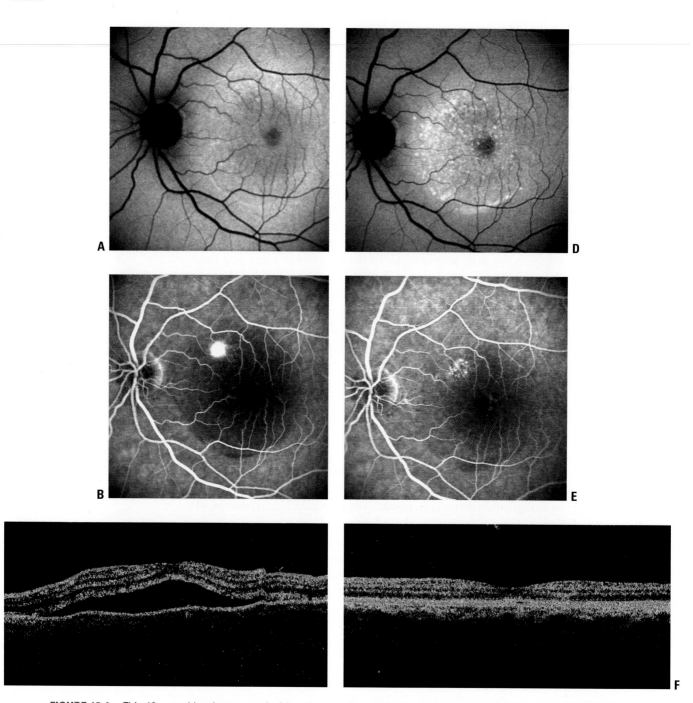

FIGURE 13.4. This 49-year-old male presented with a visual acuity of 0.4 in the left eye for about 3 months. Fundus AF **(A)** revealed slightly decreased AF in the area of angiographic visible edema **(B)**, but also showed a slight ring of increased AF at the border of the well-demarcated neurosensory detachment **(A,B)**, which was confirmed by OCT (vertical scan) **(C)**. Three months after laser treatment, AF in the area of former neurosensory retinal detachment showed small foci of increased AF **(D)**, whereas angiography showed only hyperfluorescence at the site of the laser scars in the area of former leakage **(E)**. OCT (horizontal scan) confirmed attached retina **(F)**. Visual acuity increased to 0.6.

ACKNOWLEDGMENTS

Images 13.1, 13.2, and 13.4 were taken from Reference 27 with friendly permission of the publisher.

REFERENCES

 1. Bennet G. Central serous retinopathy. Br J Ophthalmol 1955;39:605–618.
 2. Gass JDM. Pathogenesis of disciform detachment of the neuroepithelium, II: idiopathic central serous choroidopathy. Am J Ophthalmol 1967;63:587–615.
 3. Polak BCP, Baarsma GS, Snyers B. Diffuse retinal pigment epitheliopathy complicating systemic corticosteroid treatment. Br J Ophthalmol 1995;79:922–925.
 4. Gomolin JES. Choroidal neovascularization and central serous chorioretinopathy. Can J Ophthalmol 1989;24:20–23.
 5. Gass JDM. Stereoscopic Atlas of Macular Diseases—Diagnosis and Treatment. 4th ed. St. Louis: Mosby, 1997.
 6. Castro-Correia J, Coutinho MF, Rosas V, et al. Long-term follow-up of central serous retinopathy in 150 patients. Doc Ophthalmol 1992;81:379–386.
 7. Yannuzzi LA, Shahin JL, Fisher YL, et al. Peripheral retinal detachments and retinal pigment epithelial tracts secondary to central serous pigment epitheliopathy. Ophthalmology 1984;91:1554–1572.
 8. Wallow IH. Repair of the pigment epithelial barrier following photocoagulation. Arch Ophthalmol 1984;102:126–135.
 9. Marshall J, Clover G, Rothery S. Some new findings on retinal irradiation by krypton and argon lasers. Doc Ophthalmol 1984;36:21–37.
10. Del Priore LV, Glaser BM, Quigley HA, et al. Response of pig retinal pigment epithelium to laser photocoagulation in organ culture. Arch Ophthalmol 1989;107:119–122.
11. Yoshioka H, Katsume Y, Akune H. Experimental central serous chorioretinopathy in monkey eyes: fluorescein angiographic findings. Ophthalmologica 1982;185:168–178.
12. Yoshioka H, Katsume Y. Experimental central serous retinopathy. III. Ultrastructural findings. Jpn J Ophthalmol 1982;26:397–409.
13. Hall LS, Guyer DR, Yannuzzi LA. Central serous retinopathy. In: Guyer DR, Yanuzzi LA, Chang S, Shields JA, Green WR, eds. Retina-Vitreous-Macula. Vol. 1. 1999:206–216.
14. Leuenberger A, Gasche A. Lichtkoagulation der Retinopathia serosa centralis. Ophthalmologica 1972;165:366–372.
15. Spitznas M. Pathogenesis of central serous retinopathy: a new working hypothesis. Graefes Arch Clin Exp Ophthalmol 1986;224:321–324.
16. Piccolino FC, Borgia L. Central serous chorioretinopathy and indocyanine green angiography. Retina 1994;14:231–242.
17. Guyer DR, Yannuzzi LA, Slakter JS, et al. Digital indocyanine green videoangiography of central serous chorioretinopathy. Arch Ophthalmol 1994;112:1057–1062.
18. Prunte C, Flammer J. Choroidal capillary and venous congestion in central serous choroidopathy. Am J Ophthalmol 1996;121:26–34.
19. Marmor MF. New hypothesis on the pathogenesis and treatment of serous retinal detachment. Graefes Arch Clin Exp Ophthalmol 1988;226:548–552.
20. Gass JDM. Stereoscopic Atlas of Macular Diseases—Diagnosis and Treatment. 2nd ed. St. Louis: Mosby, 1987:40.
21. Shimizu K, Tobari I. Central serous retinopathy dynamics of subretinal fluid. Mod Probl Ophthalmol 1971;9:152–157.
22. Spaide RF, Hall L, Haas A, et al. Indocyanine green videoangiography of older patients with central serous chorioretinopathy. Retina 1996;16:203–213.
23. Hee MR, Puliafito CA, Wong C. Optical coherence tomography of central serous chorioretinopathy. Am J Ophthalmol 1995;120:65–74.
24. Mavrofrides EC, Puliafito CA, Fujimoto JG. Central serous chorioretinopathy. In: Schuman JS, Puliafito CA, Fujimoto JG, eds. Optical Coherence Tomography in Ocular Diseases. 2nd ed. Thorofare, NJ: Slack Inc., 2004.
25. Spaide RF, Klancnik Jr JM. Fundus autofluorescence and central serous chorioretinopathy. Ophthalmology 2005;112:825–833.
26. Eandi CM, Ober M, Iranmanesh R, et al. Acute central serous chorioretinopathy and fundus autofluorescence. Retina 2005;25:989–993.
27. Framme C, Walter A, Gabler B, et al. Autofluorescence in acute and chronic-recurrent central serous chorioretinopathy. Acta Ophthalmol Scand 2005;83:161–167.
28. von Rückmann A, Fitzke FW, Fan J, et al. Abnormalities of fundus autofluorescence in central serous retinopathy. Am J Ophthalmol 2002;133:780–786.

Fundus Autofluorescence in Full-Thickness Macular Holes

A n idiopathic full-thickness macular hole (FTMH) is a defect in the neurosensory retina at the fovea, from the internal limiting membrane to the outer segment of the photoreceptors. The first reported case of a macular hole, described by Knapp (1) in 1869, occurred in a patient who had sustained prior blunt trauma to the eye. Subsequent case reports and series pointed to an antecedent episode of ocular trauma prior to FTMH formation, such that the two were linked to each other. It later became clear that most cases occur spontaneously (idiopathic FTMH) and few are associated with trauma to the eye.

Patients with FTMH usually complain of blurred vision and/or metamorphopsia. As the FTMH becomes larger, patients become aware of a central scotoma. Some, however, may be asymptomatic, and the FTMH will be diagnosed during a routine eye examination.

The visual acuity of a patient with FTMH varies according to the size, location, and stage of the macular hole. Patients with small, eccentric holes may retain excellent visual acuity in the range of 20/25 to 20/40. However, in most cases the visual acuity varies from 20/80 to 20/400, with an average vision of 20/200.

A FTMH visualized with direct ophthalmoscopy appears as a well-defined round or oval lesion in the center of the macula, often with yellow-white deposits at the base. On slit-lamp biomicroscopy, a round or oval excavation with well-defined borders interrupting the beam of the slit-lamp can be observed, surrounded in most cases by a cuff of subretinal fluid (neurosensory retinal detachment). An overlying semitranslucent tissue representing a true operculum or a pseudo-operculum can be seen over the hole. Cystic changes of the retina may be evident at the margins of the hole. The retinal pigment epithelium (RPE) is usually intact at the site of the hole, although in long-standing FTMH it may appear atrophic or hyperplastic. Fine wrinkling of the inner retinal surface caused by the presence of an epiretinal membrane may also be detected.

The Watzke-Allen test (2) has been widely used as a diagnostic test to distinguish FTMH from other lesions, such as lamellar macular holes (LMHs) and macular pseudoholes (MPHs). In this test, a thin beam of light is projected over the area of the hole while the patient is asked whether he sees the beam being broken or intact. It was assumed that most patients with FTMH would see a broken beam of light, because of the corresponding lack of tissue at the site of the macular hole. However, a recent study suggested that, in fact, most patients with FTMH did not report a broken beam of light but instead just thinning of the beam of light (3).

In 1988, Johnson and Gass (4) described a classification for idiopathic FTMH. Gass (5) recently updated this biomicroscopic classification as follows: In the first stage (stage 1a) a yellow spot 100–200 μm in diameter, resulting from a foveolar detachment secondary to spontaneous tangential traction by the prefoveolar vitreous cortex, is observed on slit-lamp biomicroscopy. The yellow spot is presumed to be caused by the presence of intraretinal xanthophyll pigment, which becomes more visible as a result of the foveolar detachment. In stage 1b (occult hole), the yellow spot is transformed into a doughnut-shaped yellow ring of approximately 200–300 μm in size centered on the foveola. The visual acuity in stage 1 lesions ranges typically from 20/25 to 20/70 and there is often some degree of metamorphopsia. The first evidence of the presence of a full-thickness retinal defect occurs in stage 2 holes, which are defined as holes ≤400 μm. Most stage 2 holes progress to stage 3 holes (>400 μm). In both stages 2 and 3 there is an absence of complete posterior vitreous detachment. When complete separation of the vitreous from the entire macula and optic disc occurs, the hole is classified as a stage 4 FTMH, independently of its size.

HISTOPATHOLOGY AND PATHOGENESIS

Histopathology studies frequently have demonstrated cystic spaces in the outer plexiform and inner nuclear layers in patients with FTMH (6). There is also frequent glial proliferation from the edges of the macular hole over the inner retinal surface around the hole (5). Nodular proliferations of the RPE, at the RPE level, can be also found at the site of the hole (5). In the majority of cases, associated epiretinal membranes are seen (6). A variable degree of photoreceptor cell degeneration at the margins of the hole has also been observed (6).

One immunocytochemistry study (7) demonstrated that, in addition to glial cells, photoreceptor cells (cones) were usually present in the operculum lying in front of the macular hole (true operculum). In some cases, however, only glial tissue was present (pseudo-operculum). It was also shown that eyes with opercula containing more than five photoreceptors were associated with higher anatomical failure (the macular hole remained open after surgery) compared to those in which less than five photoreceptor cells were found (7).

Anteroposterior and tangential vitreomacular traction has been suggested as a possible mechanism in idiopathic FTMH formation (8–11). Furthermore, the role of the internal limiting membrane facilitating the proliferation of cellular components, which could cause tangential traction around the fovea and FTMH formation, has also been postulated (for review see Abdelkader and Lois [12]).

IMAGING TECHNIQUES

Fluorescein Angiography

The diagnosis of FTMH is usually made by history and slit-lamp biomicroscopy with a noncontact or contact lens. However, occasionally it may be difficult to differentiate between a FTMH and an MPH or LMH (see also Chapter 14B). In such cases fluorescein angiography (FA) can be used to help in this differentiation. FA in FTMH stages 2 and 3 typically discloses hyperfluorescence in early frames, with no leak in late frames (window defect). However, FA is invasive and carries potential risks for adverse reactions (13). Optical coherence tomography (OCT) and fundus autofluorescence (AF) images have now replaced FA in the evaluation of patients with FTMH (see below).

Optical Coherence Tomography

OCT allows the physician to noninvasively detect the presence of an FTMH and changes in the surrounding retina (Fig. 14A.1) (14). Cystic spaces in the retina and

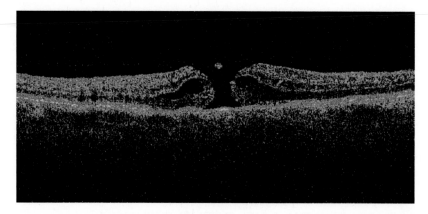

FIGURE 14A.1.   OCT (90 degree cut) obtained from an eye with an FTMH. Cystic spaces in the retina and an operculum/pseudo-operculum overlying the area of the defect are seen.

a neurosensory retinal detachment surrounding the hole are usually visualized (Fig. 14A.2). In addition, the status of the vitreomacular interface can be evaluated (Fig. 14A.2) (10,14).

OCT can be used to determine early macular hole closure following surgery (24 hours postoperatively) (15). However, in many cases it may be difficult to obtain appropriate images because of the presence of gas in the eye, especially in pseudophakic eyes.

Three different OCT patterns were described after what was considered to be a successful surgical repair of an FTMH (macular hole no longer visible or macular hole still visible but with disappearance of the neurosensory retinal detachment around it), which correlated with postoperative vision (16). These were described as a U pattern (normal foveal contour), a V pattern (steep foveal contour), and a W pattern (persistence of a neurosensory retinal defect at the site of the hole but with lack of associated neurosensory retinal detachment). Postoperatively, the highest levels of vision were recorded in the former, and the lowest were recorded in the latter (16). Similarly, it was recently shown that the presence of a normal inner segment and outer segment junction in OCT images at the site of the hole postoperatively was associated with good visual recovery following surgery (17).

OCT can also provide information in addition to that gathered by slit-lamp biomicroscopy, especially in early stages of macular hole formation. In early stages of

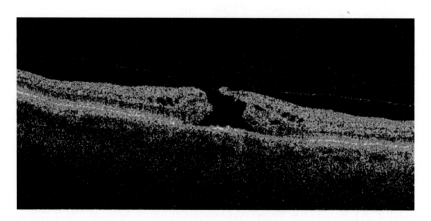

FIGURE 14A.2.   OCT (330 degree cut) obtained from an eye with an eccentric FTMH. The vitreous remains adherent to the retina at the edge of the hole. Small cystic changes around the hole are present.

development (stage 1), OCT demonstrates in most cases a macular cyst, rather than a foveolar detachment, as proposed by Gass (18). Furthermore, the presence of a normal foveal contour and normal retinal thickness but a preretinal, minimally reflective, thin band inserting obliquely on at least one side of the fovea (which has been termed a stage 0 macular hole) was found to be a significant risk factor in fellow eyes for the development of an FTMH (19).

Although OCT demonstrates very well the full-thickness neurosensory retinal defect in patients with FTMH, in some cases it may not be able to detect whether loss of inner retina has occurred, and thus whether an LMH is present (see Chapter 14B).

Fundus Autofluorescence

In the first study ever published on the distribution of fundus AF in patients with macular holes (20), were evaluated AF images and the corresponding color fundus photographs and FAs of the affected eye and AF images of the unaffected, contralateral eye. The AF intensity at the site of the macular hole was compared with that at the corresponding area in the unaffected eye. It was found that in some patients with stage 1 FTMH the distribution of AF and the corresponding FA was normal; in some, however, the foveal AF signal appeared slightly increased compared to the contralateral eye. Similarly, the FA in these latter cases showed mild central hyperfluorescence in the mid phase of the angiogram. All stage 2 FTMH demonstrated an increased AF signal at the site of the hole (Fig. 14A.3); a window defect that corresponded exactly in location, size, and shape with that seen on AF imaging was detected on FA. This was also the case in stage 3 and 4 FTMHs. These findings can be explained as follows: It has been demonstrated that the AF signal derives predominantly from the lipofuscin in the RPE (see Chapters 3 and 9) (21–23). This signal is attenuated at the center of the macula by the presence of the luteal pigment (see also Chapter 14B) (23). In FTMH, there is no neurosensory retina at the site of the hole, and thus there is no luteal pigment overlying the defect. An intense AF signal is subsequently observed at the hole.

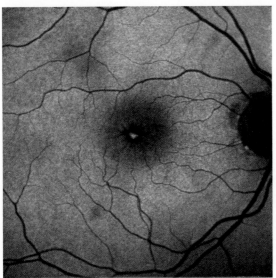
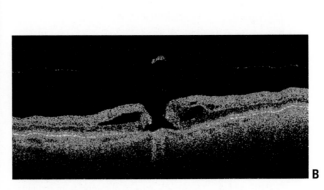

FIGURE 14A.3. Fundus AF image of a patient with FTMH **(A)**. Note the increased AF signal at the site of the hole and a mildly increased AF signal around the hole in a "petalloid" pattern. The latter is due to the presence of cystoid spaces in the retina, as demonstrated by OCT (180 degree cut) **(B)**.

The cuff of neurosensory retinal detachment surrounding the macular hole demonstrated a reduced AF signal (Fig. 14A.4A). In contrast, on FA the cuff of subretinal fluid appeared hyperfluorescent in the majority of cases; in about a third it disclosed hypofluorescence. Color photographs and FA were examined to determine whether any retinal elevation could be detected beyond the cuff of the subretinal fluid surrounding the macular hole. Shallow retinal elevation extending beyond the cuff was seen in about half of the cases; at this site, reduced AF signal was observed, although to a lesser extent than at the site of the cuff of subretinal fluid. The cuff of subretinal fluid and the retinal elevation extending beyond this cuff demonstrated reduced AF, likely due to the effect caused by the presence of subretinal fluid and/or thickening of the neurosensory retina, which would attenuate the AF signal coming from the RPE.

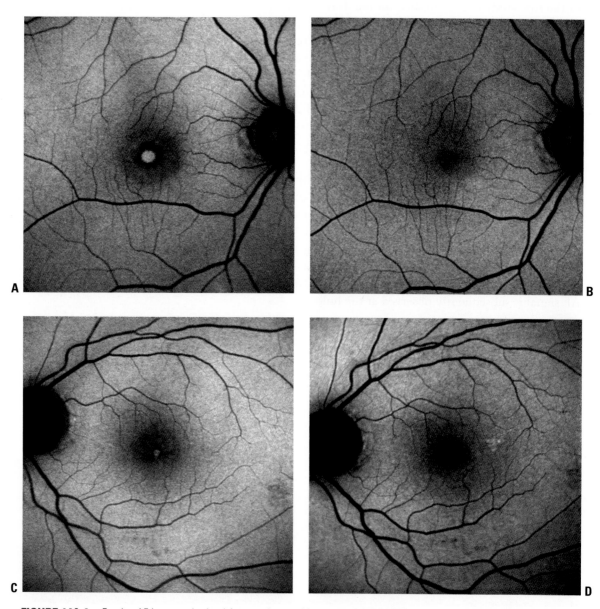

FIGURE 14A.4.   Fundus AF images obtained from patients with a stage 3 FTMH **(A)** and a stage 2 FTMH **(B)**. Note the increased AF signal at the site of the hole **(A,C)** and a ring of reduced AF signal around the hole that corresponds to a cuff of subretinal fluid **(A)**. **(C)** A mildly increased AF signal around the hole with a "petalloid" appearance is also seen that corresponds to cystic spaces in the retina. **(B,D)** After successful macular hole surgery, the normal AF signal is restored.

The presence of a preretinal operculum or pseudo-operculum was demonstrated by the presence of a mobile disc-like area of reduced AF signal overlying the area of increased AF signal corresponding to the macular hole or its surroundings. This was interpreted as the shadow casted by the operculum on the RPE. The presence of the operculum or pseudo-operculum could not be documented by FA.

After successful surgery, the high-intensity AF signal and the hyperfluorescence on FA at the hole disappeared (Fig. 14A.4). This suggested that the RPE was covered by retina and/or glial tissue, as previously demonstrated histologically (24), again blocking the AF signal from this layer. Similarly, the cuff of subretinal fluid was no longer visible on AF imaging or FA after successful surgery.

Our findings on the distribution of fundus AF in FTMH, as described above, were confirmed more recently by other researchers (25,26).

There is one limitation of fundus AF in the diagnosis of FTMH: the differentiation between a LMH and a FTMH. As explained in detail in Chapter 14B, in both LMH and FTMH, an increased AF signal would be detected because of the complete or partial loss of neurosensory retina and, subsequently, of luteal pigment at the site of the FTMH and LMH, respectively. However, the presence of a cuff of subretinal fluid around the defect visualized on fundus AF as a well-defined area of reduced AF signal would point toward the diagnosis of FTMH.

COMPARISON OF AVAILABLE IMAGING TECHNIQUES

Patients with FTMH can be imaged before and after surgery. The most widely used imaging techniques for FTMH include color fundus photography, FA, OCT, and fundus AF. The resolution of color fundus photographs may be insufficient to allow for a consistent and reliable recognition of small macular holes or to demonstrate the presence of a preretinal operculum/pseudo-operculum. On FA, FTMH is usually imaged appropriately; however, the disadvantage of this imaging technique is that it is an invasive procedure that carries a small but significant risk of morbidity. In addition, it is time-consuming and requires the presence of an experience photographer and a nurse or doctor. The images may not be instantly available unless a digitized imaging system is used. The combination of fundus AF and OCT appears to be the best available method to evaluate patients for whom a diagnosis of FTMH, MPH, or LMH is entertained (see also Chapter 14B).

SUMMARY

In most patients with FTMH, the diagnosis can be reliably established with the use of slit-lamp biomicroscopy and a noncontact or contact lens; however, occasionally difficulties may be encountered, even by experienced ophthalmologists, in diagnosing this condition (see also Chapter 14B) (27). In such cases OCT and AF imaging will be helpful in establishing the diagnosis of FTMH. Although FA is also an important tool for evaluating eyes with FTMH (28,29), with the advent of OCT and AF it is now only rarely needed.

ACKNOWLEDGMENTS

I thank Dr. Vikki McBain and Dr. Noemi Lois for providing the photographs that illustrate this chapter. I also thank Prof. Alan C Bird, Prof. Fredrick W. Fitzke, and Dr. Zdenek J. Gregor for their cooperation in the initial study on AF of macular holes.

REFERENCES

1. Knapp H. Über isolierte Zerreissungen der Aderhaut in Folge von Traumen auf den Augenapfel. Arch Augeheilkd 1869;1:6–29.
2. Watzke RC, Allen L. Subjective slit-beam sign for macular disease. Am J Ophthalmol 1969;68:449–453.
3. Tanner V, Williamson TH. Watzke-Allen slit beam test in macular holes confirmed by optical coherence tomography. Arch Ophthalmol 2000;118:1059–1063.
4. Johnson RN, Gass JDM. Idiopathic senile macular holes: observations, stages of formation, and implications for surgical intervention. Ophthalmology 1988;95:917–924.
5. Gass JDM. Macular dysfunction caused by vitreous and vitreoretinal interface abnormalities. In: Gass JDM, ed. Stereoscopic Atlas of Macular Diseases: Diagnosis and Treatment. 4th ed. St Louis: Mosby, 1997.
6. Guyer DR, Green WR, de Bustros S, et al. Histopathologic features of idiopathic macular holes and cysts. Ophthalmology 1990;97:1045–1051.
7. Ezra E, Fariss RN, Possin DE, et al. Immunocytochemical characterization of macular hole opercula. Arch Ophthalmol 2001;119:223–231.
8. Gass JD. Idiopathic senile macular hole. Its early stages and pathogenesis. Arch Ophthalmol 1988;106:629–639.
9. Gass JD. Reappraisal of biomicroscopic classification of stages of development of a macular hole. Am J Ophthalmol 1995;119:752–759.
10. Gaudric A, Haouchine B, Massin P et al. Macular hole formation: new data provided by optical coherence tomography. Arch Ophthalmol 1999;117:744–751.
11. Johnson MW, van Newkirk MR, Meyer KA. Perifoveal vitreous detachment is the primary pathogenic event in idiopathic macular hole formation. Arch Ophthalmol 2001;119:215–222.
12. Abdelkader E, Lois N. Internal limiting membrane peeling in vitreo-retinal surgery. Surv Ophthalmol 2008;53:368–396.
13. Yannuzzi LA, Rohrer KT, Tindel LJ, et al. Fluorescence angiography complication survey. Ophthalmology 1986;93:611–617.
14. Hee MR, Puliafito CA, Wong C, et al. Optical coherence tomography of macular holes. Ophthalmology,1995;102:748–756.
15. Kasuga Y, Arai J, Akimoto M, et al. Optical coherence tomography to confirm early closure of macular hole. Am J Ophthalmol 2000;130:675–676.
16. Imai M, Iijima H, Gotoh T, et al. Optical coherence tomography of successfully repaired idiopathic macular holes. Am J Ophthalmol 1999;128:621–627.
17. Baba T, Yamamoto S, Arai M, et al. Correlation of visual recovery and presence of photoreceptor inner/outer segment junction in optical coherence images after successful macular hole repair. Retina 2008;28:453–458.
18. Azzolini C, Patelli F, Brancato R. Correlation between optical coherence tomography data and biomicroscopic interpretation of idiopathic macular hole. Am J Ophthalmol 2001;132:348–355.
19. Chan A, Duker JS, Schuman JS, et al. Stage 0 macular holes: observations by optical coherence tomography. Ophthalmology 2004;111:2027–2032.
20. von Rückmann A, Fitzke FW, Gregor ZJ. Fundus autofluorescence in patients with macular holes imaged with a laser scanning ophthalmoscope. Br J Ophthalmol 1998;82:346–351.
21. von Rückmann A, Fizke FW, Bird AC. Distribution of fundus autofluorescence with a scanning laser ophthalmoscope. Br J Ophthalmol 1995;119:543–562.
22. von Rückmann A, Fizke FW, Bird AC. Fundus autofluorescence in age related macular disease imaged with a laser scanning ophthalmoscope. Invest Ophthalmol Vis Sci 1997;38:478–486.
23. Delori FC, Dorey K, Staurenghi G, et al. In vivo fluorescence of the ocular fundus exhibits retinal pigment epithelial lipofuscin characteristics. Invest Ophthalmol Vis Sci 1995;36:718–729.
24. Funata M, Wedel RT, De La Cruz Z, et al. Clinicopathologic study of bilateral macular holes treated with pars plana vitrectomy and gas tamponade. Retina 1992;12:289–298.
25. Framme C, Roider J. Fundus autofluorescence in macular hole surgery. Ophthalmic Surg Lasers 2001;32:383–390.
26. Wakabayashi T, Ikuno Y, Sayanagi K, et al. Fundus autofluorescence related to retinal morphological and functional changes in idiopathic macular holes. Acta Ophthalmol 2008;86:897–901.
27. Martinez J, Smiddy WE, Kim J, et al. Differentiating macular holes from macular pseudoholes. Am J Ophthalmol 1994;117:762–767.
28. Thompson JR, Hiner CJ, Glaser BM, et al. Fluorescein angiographic characteristics of macular holes before and after vitrectomy with transforming growth factor beta-2. Am J Ophthalmol 1994;117:291–301.
29. Fish RH, Anand R, Izbrand DJ. Macular pseudoholes. Clinical features and accuracy of diagnosis. Ophthalmology 1992;99:1665–1670.

Fundus Autofluorescence in Lamellar Macular Holes and Pseudoholes

DEFINITION OF PSEUDOHOLE AND LAMELLAR MACULAR HOLE

The definitions of macular pseudohole (MPH) and lamellar macular hole (LMH) have been a matter of great debate in the past. Today there is a general consensus to define an MPH as a macular lesion that has the appearance of a full-thickness macular hole (FTMH) but does not have a loss of foveal tissue. By contrast, a loss of foveal tissue is mandatory for a diagnosis of LMH (1,2). However, and in contrast to FTMH, in LMH only part of the foveal tissue is lost (there is no full-thickness defect).

Before optical coherence tomography (OCT) was available, the definitions of MPH and LMH were based on certain characteristic history and examination findings, which were shown to be not sensitive enough for a clear differential diagnosis. Clinically, both MPH and LMH have a similar appearance, with a round and well-circumscribed reddish lesion at the center of the fovea (1,3–10). Functional tests, such as the Watzke-Allen test (11) and microperimetry (12), in which no scotoma is detected in either MPH and LMH are not useful for differentiating between these conditions, and both clinical entities can lead to similarly impaired vision (median 20/40) (1–3).

OCT evaluation has proved valuable in the diagnosis of macular holes, as it is able to visualize retinal anatomy with near microscopic resolution ($\approx$10 μm for STRATUS OCT™ [Carl Zeiss Meditec]; $\approx$5–7 μm for spectral domain OCT). However, although OCT studies have added valuable information regarding the definition, pathogenesis, and progression of macular holes (6–10), it is not always possible to differentiate between MPH and LMH. In particular, when there is residual tissue at the bottom of the foveal defect, as occurs with macular holes in stage 2 (according to the OCT classification of Azzolini et al. [9]), OCT imaging may not be able to indicate with certainty whether there is loss of retinal tissue. In such cases, the diagnosis of MPH or LMH is often a matter of speculation.

PATHOGENESIS

The pathogenesis of MPH and LMH is not fully understood, but they have always been considered to be quite different processes. It has been hypothesized that MPH is attributable to the centripetal contraction of an epiretinal membrane (3). In contrast, LMH is thought to be the result of an abortive process in the formation of an FTMH. Posterior vitreous detachment is the main initiating process of the latter, but epiretinal membrane contraction has been suggested as a likely secondary factor (2). This mechanism is supported by two findings: (i) 62% to 89% of LMHs may present with an epiretinal membrane (1,2); and (ii) pseudo-opercula, suggestive of an aborted macular hole, have been reported in only 24% of patients with LMH (1), Therefore, it seems that the pathogenesis of LMH cannot simply be attributed to an abortive process in FTMH formation.

FUNDUS AUTOFLUORESCENCE

It is believed that fundus autofluorescence (AF) derives mainly from the lipofuscin-laden retinal pigment epithelium (RPE; see Chapter 3) (13). It is generally accepted that lipofuscin represents the product of degradation of photoreceptor outer segments. In a normal fundus, the distribution of AF is diffuse, with decreased intensity at the optic nerve head, the retinal blood vessels, and the macula (13,14). Macular AF is attenuated by the presence of luteal pigment, which has a higher concentration along the outer plexiform layer at the fovea (Fig. 14B.1) (15). Any foveal defect, including an LMH that spares the photoreceptors (2), may alter the degree of foveal AF by decreasing the amount of masking luteal pigment and thus increasing the foveal AF.

IMAGING TECHNIQUES

Slit-Lamp Biomicroscopy

Slit-lamp biomicroscopy in patients with MPH and LMH may simply show the common feature of a round, reddish lesion at the center of the macula, but it is not sensitive enough to detect a small loss of foveal tissue, which is present in LMH with preserved visual acuity. Additionally, the presence of an epiretinal membrane is not definitive in the differential diagnosis of LMH and MPH; as mentioned above, 62% to 89% of patients with LMH may have an associated epiretinal membrane (1,2), which will always be present in MPH (3).

In a study by Haouchine et al. (1), only 28% of LMH cases diagnosed with OCT were diagnosed as LMH on fundus examination. Likewise, Witkin et al. (2) reported that only 37% of LMH cases diagnosed using ultrahigh-resolution OCT were detected clinically on fundus examination. These data show the limitation of slit-lamp biomicroscopy in the diagnosis of LMH.

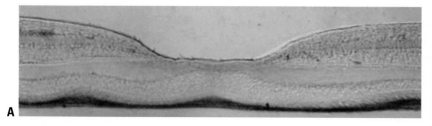

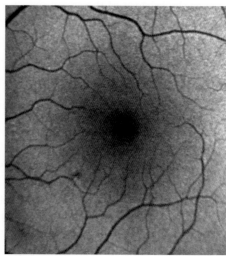

FIGURE 14B.1. **(A)** Macular pigment distribution (*yellow*) in a macaque. (From Snodderly DM, Auran JD, Delori FC. The macular pigment. II. Spatial distribution in primate retinas. Invest Ophthalmol Vis Sci 1984;25:674–685.) **(B)** Normal distribution of fundus AF.

Optical Coherence Tomography

Recently, Haouchine et al. (1) defined new criteria for the OCT diagnosis of MPH and LMH, and Witkin et al. (2) further expanded this topic using ultrahigh-resolution OCT, a not yet commercially available technology capable of ≈ 3 μm axial image resolution in the human eye. Haouchine et al.'s (1) OCT criteria were established by quantitative image analysis of six radial macular images obtained using a standardized STRATUS OCT™ imaging protocol. Briefly, retinal thickness was measured manually with software calipers at the foveal center and 750 μm temporally and nasally from the center on the horizontal scan. In MPH, the OCT profile was a steepened contour with increased perifoveal retinal thickness and normal or slightly increased centrofoveal thickness. In LMH, the OCT profile was an irregular contour, with near-normal perifoveal thickness and thinner than normal centrofoveal thickness. Using these OCT criteria, the study indeed showed two clearly different groups that the authors termed MPH and LMH (1).

Witkin et al. (2) used qualitative image analysis of ultrahigh-resolution OCT sections in an attempt to define criteria for LMH diagnosis that do not necessitate measurement of retinal thickness. They presented four basic criteria for an OCT diagnosis of LMH: (i) an irregular foveal contour, (ii) a break in the inner fovea, (iii) a dehiscence of the inner foveal retina from the outer retina, and (iv) an absence of a full-thickness foveal defect with intact foveal photoreceptors. To avoid confusion between MPH and LMH, they proposed that the definition of MPH be expanded to include any macular lesion that has the appearance of a macular hole but lacks a full-thickness foveal defect. An LMH would then be a subcategory of MPH in which there is a lamellar defect caused by separation of the inner from the outer retinal layers (2).

It is clear that one of the major problems encountered in an OCT diagnosis of a foveal defect is the difficulty of determining with certainty whether there is loss of retinal tissue. Furthermore, if there is loss of foveal tissue, it is difficult to determine the anatomic location of this loss.

Fundus AF Imaging

In vivo imaging of fundus AF can be performed with commercially available adapted fundus cameras (Topcon USA, Paramus, NJ) or a confocal scanning laser ophthalmoscope (see Chapter 5) (14). The usefulness of this technique has already been demonstrated for the diagnosis of FTMH (see Chapter 14A), and its accuracy has been reported to be comparable to that of fluorescein angiography (16,17).

Fundus AF has challenged the current OCT concepts regarding the differentiation between MPH and LMH (19). In a study of patients with stage 2 macular holes based on OCT classification (9) and further classified as MPH and LMH according to the OCT profiles established by Haouchine et al. (1), we found that the foveal AF intensity did not differ between these two conditions (18). In both LMH and MPH, an increase in the foveal AF signal with respect to background was found (Figs. 14B.2 and 14B.3). However, in patients with epiretinal membrane and macular pucker (Fig. 14B.4) diagnosed by slit-lamp biomicroscopy, and in patients with impending macular holes (foveal detachment) (Fig. 14B.5), no focal increased AF at the fovea was detected. As noted above, fundus AF derives from lipofuscin-laden RPE (13) (see Chapter 3), which in the macula is attenuated by the luteal pigment. Most of this pigment in the fovea resides in the outer plexiform layer (15), interposed between the foveal photoreceptors and the stimulating light. Thus, even very thin foveal defects, such as those affecting only the outer plexiform layer and sparing the photoreceptors, as in LMH (2), may increase the foveal AF. Thus, the AF findings (i.e., increased AF

(text continues on page 264)

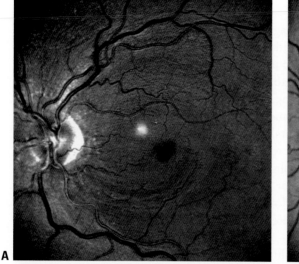

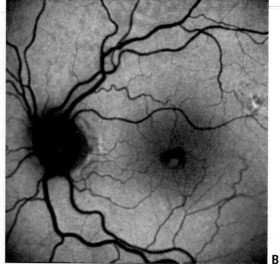

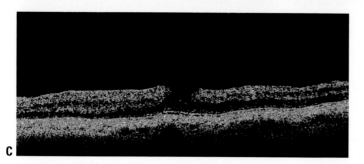

FIGURE 14B.2. **(A)** Red-free image, **(B)** AF image, and **(C)** vertical OCT scan. On the basis of OCT (centrofoveal thickness 149 μm, nasal perifoveal thickness 331 μm, temporal perifoveal thickness 282 μm) the diagnosis of MPH was established. However, fundus AF demonstrated an increased in the foveal AF signal, indicative of loss of foveal tissue and the presence of an LMH.

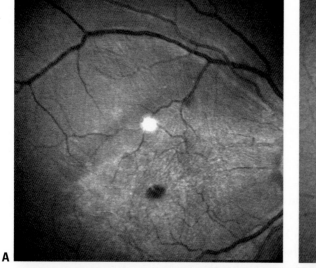

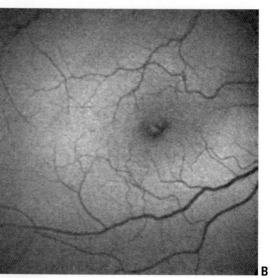

FIGURE 14B.3. **(A)** Red-free image, **(B)** AF image, and **(C)** vertical OCT scan. On the basis of OCT (centrofoveal thickness 93 μm, nasal perifoveal thickness 356 μm, temporal perifoveal thickness 390 μm) the diagnosis of LMH was made. This diagnosis was confirmed by fundus AF imaging demonstrating the presence of an increased AF signal at the fovea.

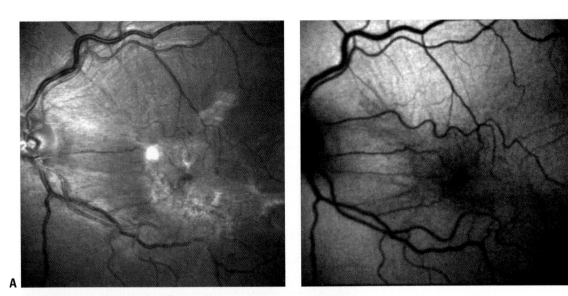

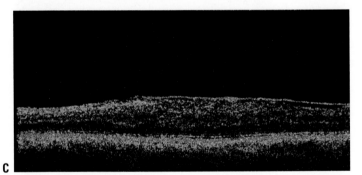

FIGURE 14B.4. **(A)** Red-free image, **(B)** AF image, and **(C)** horizontal OCT scan in a patient with macular pucker. No increased AF at the fovea is observed, indicating a lack of tissue loss at the fovea.

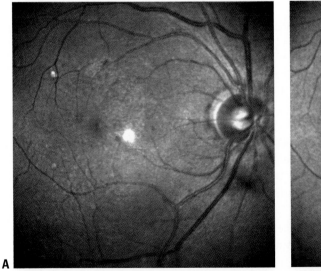
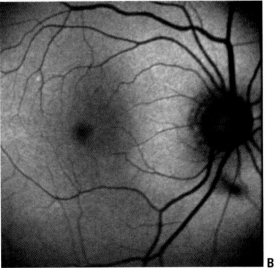

FIGURE 14B.5. **(A)** Red-free image, **(B)** AF image, and **(C)** vertical OCT scan of a patient with an impending macular hole (stage 1a). No increased foveal AF is present.

at the fovea) in patients with MPH and LMH defined by OCT suggest that in both conditions there is loss of foveal tissue (Figs. 14B.2 and 14B.3). There was also a lack of correlation between the amount of AF and the thickness of residual retinal tissue at the bases of either MPH or LMH. A likely explanation for this is that once the outer plexiform layer in the fovea is affected, the absence of masking pigment allows the AF originating from RPE cells to be easily detected, irrespective of the thickness of the overlying photoreceptor-cell layer. This is also supported by the lack of increased foveal AF recorded in patients with macular pucker and impending macular holes, in which there is no defect at the level of the outer plexiform layer or, therefore, on the luteal pigment (Figs. 14B.4 and 14B.5).

Fluorescein Angiography

Fluorescein angiography (FA) has been used in the past to diagnose FTMH (19). At the site of the macular hole, the fluorescence from the underlying choroid becomes clearly visible due to the lack of luteal pigment, which would normally attenuate the choroidal fluorescence. Therefore, foveal hyperfluorescent lesions are typically observed in stages 2, 3, and 4 FTMH (19); in stage 1 FTMH and in LMH, the hyperfluorescence may vary depending on the attenuation caused by the foveal luteal pigment; however, if present, it is usually mild.

Fundus AF imaging appears to be as accurate as FA in the diagnosis of FTMH (see Chapter 14A) (16,17). Likewise, AF imaging is sensitive enough to detect a small loss of luteal pigment in cases of LMH, and the lack of loss of luteal pigment in MPH (Fig. 14B.6) (18). Together with the fact that, unlike FA, AF is noninvasive, these findings favor the use of AF instead of FA in the evaluation of patients with FTMH, LMH, and MPH.

CLINICAL IMPLICATIONS OF AF FINDINGS

The lack of a significant difference in foveal AF between LMH and MPH, as diagnosed by means of OCT imaging, raises questions concerning the validity of this differentiation. Fundus AF may be a more valuable tool to evaluate the loss of inner retina in such cases by demonstrating the presence or absence of the luteal pigment, which is located predominantly at the level of the outer plexiform layer in the human fovea. An absence or decrease of macular pigment (i.e., a loss of outer plexiform tissue) would increase foveal AF. In such cases, a diagnosis of LMH should be established. Fundus AF imaging can thus be used clinically to establish a differential diagnosis between LMH and MPH, conditions that are usually difficult to tell apart even by expert ophthalmologists (20).

Fundus AF imaging may replace FA in the evaluation of FTMH, LMH, and MPH. Fundus AF imaging has many advantages over FA: it is noninvasive, rapid, and shows an accuracy comparable to that of FA (16). Fundus AF imaging cannot replace OCT examination in all cases. For example, OCT may still be needed when the diagnosis of FTMH is not clear on slit-lamp biomicroscopy. In such cases, OCT will demonstrate a full-thickness defect, whereas AF, as in LMH, will show an area of increased foveal AF at the site of the hole. The similarly increased foveal AF in LMH and FTMH implies that fundus AF imaging is not suitable to differentiate a lamellar from a full thickness macular hole. Therefore, OCT may be more appropriate than AF imaging to monitor the progressive thinning of a LMH. OCT, however, does not appear to be sensitive enough to differentiate between an LMH (where AF will

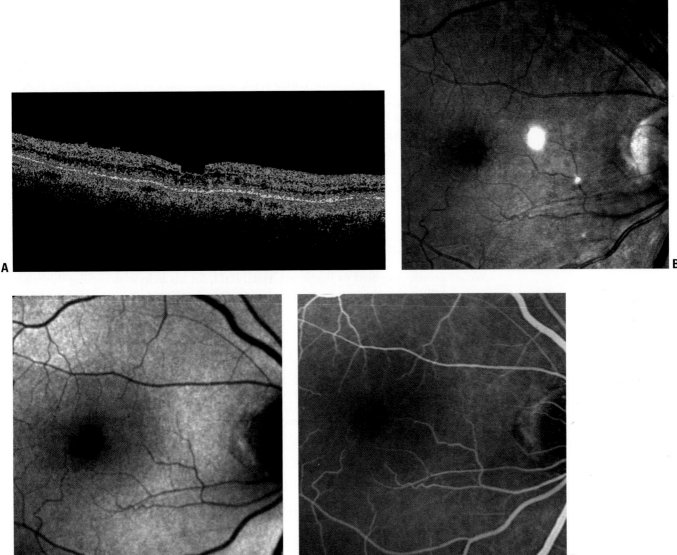

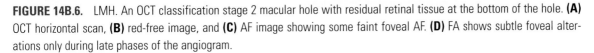

FIGURE 14B.6.   LMH. An OCT classification stage 2 macular hole with residual retinal tissue at the bottom of the hole. **(A)** OCT horizontal scan, **(B)** red-free image, and **(C)** AF image showing some faint foveal AF. **(D)** FA shows subtle foveal alterations only during late phases of the angiogram.

demonstrate increased foveal AF) and an MPH (where AF will show a normal pattern of foveal AF).

An accurate diagnosis of FTMH, LMH, and MPH is important to determine the proper surgical treatment of these lesions. Different options may be selected according to the OCT and fundus AF imaging findings. For instance, in the absence of foveal AF, the integrity of the foveal tissue is almost certainly confirmed. Therefore, it is likely that removal of the epiretinal membrane alone is all that is needed in such cases. However, if foveal AF is present, a loss of foveal tissue has very likely occurred and the decision to operate will depend on many factors, such as the residual visual acuity and progression of signs and symptoms. Some recent reports have suggested that early intervention in LMH should probably be avoided because of the often disappointing results (2).

SUMMARY

Fundus AF imaging is becoming increasingly important in the examination of many macular diseases, including macular holes. FTMHs may be properly diagnosed by means of slit-lamp biomicroscopy and OCT examination. In contrast, lesions characterized by the presence of residual retinal tissue at the bottom of the foveal defect (OCT classification stage 2 according to Azzolini et al. [9]) may be more difficult to classify because OCT cannot indicate with certainty the loss of retinal tissue. Both LMH and MPH may produce a similar degree of functional loss. In such cases, fundus AF is sensitive enough to differentiate an LMH (AF positive) from an MPH (AF negative), and thus should be performed routinely for the clinical diagnosis and follow-up of patients with these macular diseases.

ACKNOWLEDGMENTS

We are greatly indebted to Francois Delori, PhD, for his help in designing this study and providing the picture of macular pigment distribution in a macaque (Fig. 14B.1).

REFERENCES

1. Haouchine B, Massin P, Tadayoni R, et al. Diagnosis of macular pseudoholes and lamellar macular holes by optical coherence tomography. Am J Ophthalmol 2004;138:732–739.
2. Witkin AJ, Ko TH, Fujimoto JG, et al. Redefining lamellar holes and the vitreomacular interface: an ultrahigh-resolution optical coherence tomography study. Ophthalmology 2006;113:388–397.
3. Allen Jr AW, Gass JD. Contraction of a perifoveal epiretinal membrane simulating a macular hole. Am J Ophthalmol 1976;82:684–691.
4. Gass JD. Idiopathic senile macular hole. Its early stages and pathogenesis. Arch Ophthalmol 1988;106: 629–639.
5. Gass JD. Reappraisal of biomicroscopic classification of stages of development of a macular hole. Am J Ophthalmol 1995;119:752–759.
6. Hee MR, Puliafito CA, Wong C, et al. Optical coherence tomography of macular holes. Ophthalmology 1995;102:748–756.
7. Gaudric A, Haouchine B, Massin P, et al. Macular hole formation: new data provided by optical coherence tomography. Arch Ophthalmol 1999;117:744–751.
8. Tanner V, Chauhan DS, Jackson TL, et al. Optical coherence tomography of the vitreoretinal interface in macular hole formation. Br J Ophthalmol 2001;85:1092–1107.
9. Azzolini C, Patelli F, Brancato R. Correlation between optical coherence tomography data and biomicroscopic interpretation of idiopathic macular hole. Am J Ophthalmol 2001;132:348–355.
10. Haouchine B, Massin P, Gaudric A. Foveal pseudocyst as the first step in macular hole formation: a prospective study by optical coherence tomography. Ophthalmology 2001;108:15–22.
11. Watzke R, Allen L. Subjective slitbeam sign for macular disease. Am J Ophthalmol 1969;68:449–453.
12. Tsujikawa M, Ohji M, Fujikado T, et al. Differentiating full thickness macular holes from impending macular holes and macular pseudoholes. Br J Ophthalmol 1997;81:117–122.
13. Delori FC, Dorey CK, Staurenghi G, et al. In vivo fluorescence of the ocular fundus exhibits retinal pigment epithelial lipofuscin characteristics. Invest Ophthalmol Vis Sci 1995;36:718–729.
14. von Ruckmann A, Fitzke FW, Bird AC. Distribution of fundus autofluorescence with a scanning laser ophthalmoscope. Br J Ophthalmol 1995;79:407–412.
15. Snodderly DM, Auran JD, Delori FC. The macular pigment. II. Spatial distribution in primate retinas. Invest Ophthalmol Vis Sci 1984;25:674–685.
16. von Ruckmann A, Fitzke FW, Gregor ZJ. Fundus autofluorescence in patients with macular holes imaged with a laser scanning ophthalmoscope. Br J Ophthalmol 1998;82:346–351.
17. Ciardella AP, Lee GC, Langton K, et al. Autofluorescence as a novel approach to diagnosing macular holes. Am J Ophthalmol 2004;137:956–959.
18. Bottoni F, Carmassi L, Cigada M, et al. Diagnosis of macular pseudoholes and lamellar macular holes: is optical coherence tomography the gold standard? Br J Ophthalmol 2008;92:635–639.
19. Gass JD. Idiopathic senile macular hole. Its early stages and pathogenesis. Arch Ophthalmol 1988;106: 629–635.
20. Martinez J, Smiddy WE, Kim J, et al. Differentiating macular holes from macular pseudoholes. Am J Ophthalmol 1994;117:762–767.

CHAPTER 15

Daniel Lavinsky
Rubens Belfort Mattos Neto
Eduardo V. Navajas
Rubens Belfort Mattos Jr.

Fundus Autofluorescence of Intraocular Tumors: Choroidal Nevus and Melanoma

choroidal melanoma is the most frequent primary intraocular tumor and the second most frequent malignant melanoma of the body (1). Although it is a malignancy of the melanocytic cells of the choroid, it directly affects the retinal pigment epithelium (RPE). This secondary epitheliopathy appears as areas of atrophy, drusen, lipofuscin accumulation, and localized detachment of the RPE (2).

Large tumors are not difficult to diagnose as malignant, but the differential diagnosis and management of small choroidal melanomas remains controversial. Documented growth of a recently diagnosed small choroidal melanocytic lesion is considered a hallmark for the diagnosis of choroidal melanomas, and quantitative (tumor size) and qualitative factors, such as symptoms, drusen, subretinal fluid, RPE changes, juxtapapillary location, and orange pigmentation, may be predictive of tumor growth in patients with these melanocytic lesions (3).

Secondary epitheliopathy and particularly orange pigmentation overlying the lesion have been described as a major risk factors for progression to melanoma (2,4–6). Orange pigment, indicative of lipofuscin accumulation within the RPE, overlying small choroidal melanocytic lesions has been found to be significantly correlated with the risk of subsequent growth (3,7).

Recently, several groups have investigated the role of fundus autofluorescence (AF) in the diagnosis and prognosis of choroidal lesions (8–12). It is accepted that the AF signal in the fundus comes predominantly from lipofuscin in the RPE (see also Chapter 3). Thus, AF imaging may provide important information regarding patients with choroidal tumors.

BASIC PRINCIPLES

In 1976, Shields et al. (13) demonstrated that lipofuscin accumulates in RPE cells and macrophages of malignant choroidal tumors from incomplete degradation and digestion of photoreceptor outer segments. It is usually seen as orange pigment over the lesion; however, depending on whether the tumor is melanotic or amelanotic, the color may vary from orange to brown or red-brown, respectively.

Lipofuscin is a mixture of proteins, lipids, and small chromophores, and its accumulation in the RPE results from impaired or overwhelmed lysosomal digestive activity (see Chapters 1 and 2). Evidence demonstrates that lipid peroxidation-derived protein modifications are able to induce lysosomal dysfunction and lipofuscinogenesis in the RPE, and suggests that such lipid peroxidation-induced lysosomal dysfunction

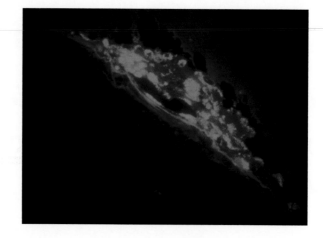

FIGURE 15.1. Autofluorescent deposits within the RPE and macrophages overlying the choroidal melanoma seen by fluorescence microscopy.

considerably contributes to cell damage and subsequent retinal degeneration (14). The exact mechanism by which choroidal melanoma induces lipofuscinogenesis remains to be elucidated.

In one histopathologic study (15), retina overlying choroidal melanoma showed areas of degeneration of outer retinal layers with a reduction in the number of nuclei of photoreceptors. Sheets of proliferated RPE cells and clusters of pigment-laden macrophages were present under the degenerated neurosensory retina, corresponding in position to the orange pigment observed in the macroscopic view of the tumor. On electron microscopy, most of the pigment granules appeared round to oval and demonstrated moderate homogeneous density with irregularly indented outlines, similar to typical lipofuscin granules normally observed throughout the retina to a lesser extent, and different from melanin granules.

Histochemical analysis indicates that orange pigment in macrophages and RPE cells of tumors stains positive for PAS, Sudan black B, and Long Ziehl-Nielsen (8); reduces silver salts with the Fontana-Masson method; bleaches partially with potassium permanganate; and is acid-fast and oil red O positive in paraffin sections. It also exhibits a golden-yellow AF when examined with ultraviolet light or a fluorescence microscope, suggesting that this pigment is in fact lipofuscin (Fig. 15.1) (15). Lohmann and colleagues (16) studied the endogenous fluorescence of ocular malignant melanomas and found that lipofuscin granules were cleaved off and broken into small remnants in the melanoma.

CLINICAL CHARACTERIZATION AND FUNDUS AUTOFLUORESCENCE FEATURES

Choroidal Nevus

A choroidal nevus can be classified clinically according to the Collaborative Ocular Melanoma Study (COMS). Benign lesions are usually less than 1 mm in height and 5 mm in basal diameter according to ultrasound measurements, and have no risk factors for growth, such as specific symptoms, orange pigmentation, subretinal fluid,

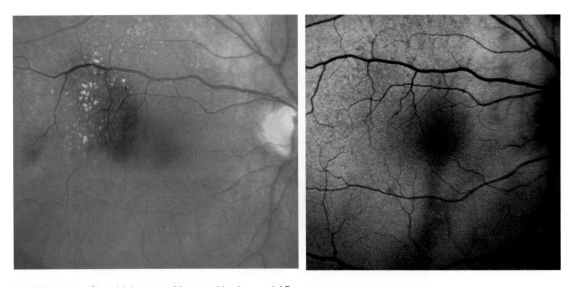

FIGURE 15.2.   Choroidal nevus with normal background AF.

juxtapapillary location, and "hot spots" on angiography. Nevi may be brown to gray in color and their appearance may vary from homogeneous, small, flat, and well delineated to more heterogeneous with secondary changes overlying the nevus, such as drusen and pigment mottling.

AF in choroidal nevus may show a normal pattern of background fundus AF, with no areas of increased or decreased AF signal, indicating a lack of RPE involvement (Fig. 15.2). Most nevi will demonstrate this pattern (8). In a minority of cases, nevi may also reveal areas with mild decreased or increased AF signal (11). The size of these lesions does not appear to influence the AF pattern, since large lesions may show normal background AF and small lesions with some RPE chronic degeneration may have a faint increased or decreased AF signal.

Drusen, often overlying nevus, when large or coalescent, may appear as areas of localized increased AF. However, the increased AF signal under these circumstances may not be a sign of lipofuscin accumulation in the RPE, such as occurs in choroidal melanoma; rather, it may result from the accumulation of different fluorophores inside these large drusen of drusenoid detachments, or relate to the presence of detached RPE cells within the latter.

Pirondini et al. (11) observed drusen in 56% of nevi, the majority of which demonstrated no changes in the distribution of AF or a traced increased AF signal. Less commonly, a reduced AF signal was also detected. Another clinical feature of nevus, although seen less commonly than drusen, is overlying RPE atrophy, which is easily identified as areas of low AF signal on AF images.

Choroidal Melanoma

Choroidal melanoma may appear as a pigmented lesion with orange pigment in a reticular or confluent pattern throughout its surface. Other features present in this lesion are subretinal fluid, superficial fibrosis with RPE metaplasia, and adjacent retinal detachment.

In the majority of cases, fundus AF correlates with the presence of orange pigmentation within choroidal melanoma. Gunduz et al. (9) found a complete

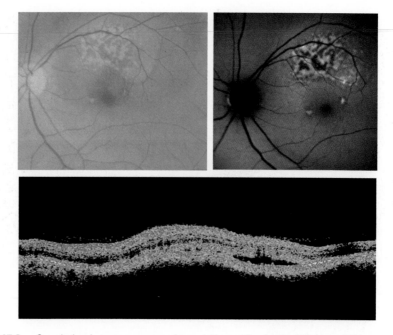

FIGURE 15.3.   Correlation between orange pigmentation and subretinal fluid on AF images and OCT (horizontal scan) in a choroidal melanoma.

correlation between an increased AF signal and orange pigment in 61.5% of tumors, a partial correlation in 23.1%, and no correlation in only 15.4%.

AF areas in small, medium, and large choroidal melanomas share common characteristics, such as a homogeneous increased AF signal and a confluent plaque-like configuration. An increased AF signal can be seen even before the appearance of orange pigment on ocular fundus photography (8).

Materin et al. (10) studied small choroidal melanoma and noted that all tumors that presented with orange pigment had increased AF signal, although of different intensities, and the majority of lesions showed mild increased AF (Fig. 15.3). Subretinal fluid associated with choroidal melanoma disclosed increased AF signal in 61% of the cases. Gunduz et al. (9) found that nearly 90% of the choroidal melanoma showed at least one focus of increased AF signal corresponding to the location of lipofuscin or hyperpigmentation over the lesion. In 75% of amelanotic choroidal melanomas, increased AF was observed in areas of hyperpigmentation (9). Shields et al. (12) demonstrated that the AF signal over small choroidal melanomas was indistinguishable from that of the background, but that areas of subretinal fluid and overlying orange pigment disclosed increased AF that seemed to be accentuated by the low AF signal present between each clump of orange pigment. A direct correlation between areas of increased AF and orange pigment was identified clinically (Fig. 15.4).

Medium and large choroidal melanomas also appear to have increased AF. In larger tumors, superficial fibrosis and subretinal fluid have been noted, and an increased AF signal has been observed throughout the surface of the lesion corresponding to areas of increased pigmentation and fibrous metaplasia of the RPE. However, in highly elevated tumors, artifacts related to the imaging technique may limit the interpretation of fundus AF images (8).

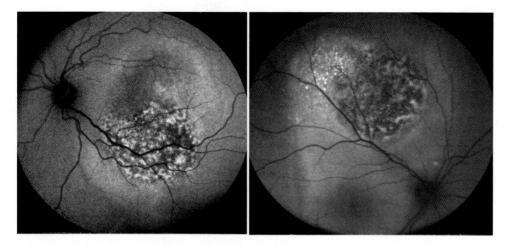

FIGURE 15.4.   Choroidal melanoma with increased AF areas over the lesion (photograph obtained using a 55 degree lens) corresponding to areas of orange pigment.

OTHER ANCILLARY TESTS

Fluorescein Angiography

Fluorescein angiography (FA) has been used extensively for the diagnosis and differentiation of choroidal tumors, although its accuracy in evaluating suspected choroidal melanomas is limited. There is no pathognomonic angiographic sign for a choroidal melanoma; however, certain features can be identified, such as blockage of the background fluorescence, punctuate hyperfluorescence due to changes in the pigment epithelium, an independent vascular network, and late staining as the dye leaks from the tumor vessels. In larger, dome-shaped melanomas, a characteristic "double circulation" pattern is evident in the early phase of the angiogram (17). Confocal FA may reveal vessels within the tumor, although these are only visualized in the very early arterial phase of the angiogram.

Bernard and Dhermy (18) performed a histological study in a choroidal melanoma with orange pigment and pinpoint foci of hyperfluorescence on FA. The former relates to areas of increased lipofuscin, whereas the latter relate to exudative, hyaline, and gluco-lipido-proteic "blebs" in connection with Bruch's membrane or in the subretinal space. The authors concluded that these findings are an expression of choriocapillaris and/or RPE dysfunction, and today we are able to identify these findings by AF. However, the complete correlation and value for diagnosis of FA and AF remain to be determined.

Indocyanine Green Angiography

It has been reported that certain histologically identified microcirculation patterns are an independent risk factor for the metastatic behavior of choroidal melanomas (19,20). These patterns can be classified as "parallel with cross-linking" or "networks," both of which indicate higher risk for metastatic disease, or as "silent" and "parallel without cross-linking," which suggest a better prognosis.

Confocal indocyanine green angiography (IGA) is capable of detecting microcirculation patterns and appears to be superior to FA with a conventional fundus camera (21). Today, with videoangiography we are able to image very early phases of the angiogram, which can facilitate the identification of these patterns.

Fluorescein and IGA are better suited for large tumors with more prominent vessel structure, and although AF might add data on the status of the overlying retina and RPE to the differential diagnosis, as the tumors get larger, the role of AF probably becomes more limited. However, for smaller lesions, AF could be helpful for the early diagnosis of choroidal melanoma in combination with other imaging techniques by demonstrating areas of increased AF signal related to the presence of orange pigment or subretinal fluid, which is rarely observed over benign choroidal nevus.

Optical Coherence Tomography

Optical coherence tomography (OCT) provides cross-sectional imaging of the retina with a resolution of 10–15 μm (STRATUS OCT™; Carl Zeiss Meditec) to more recent instruments such as spectral domain OCT, which reaches ~3-μm axial image resolutions. Several studies used this technique to evaluate choroidal melanocytic tumors, including choroidal nevi and small choroidal melanoma. OCT findings of choroidal nevi and melanomas are limited to the anterior portion of the mass, since the laser is scattered by the RPE, causing a weak reflectivity within the tumor. Therefore, OCT is not useful for studying the choroidal tumor itself. However, it may help identify changes in the RPE and neurosensory retina (22,23).

Shields and colleagues (22) studied retinal findings at the site of choroidal nevi by OCT, which included overlying retinal edema, subretinal fluid, retinal thinning, drusen, and RPE detachment. They also determined the thickness of the overlying retina and the status of the photoreceptors (i.e., whether there was a loss or attenuation of this layer). Findings specific to the lesion are more difficult to identify; however, in one study (8) we were able to show in the majority of nevi an increased thickness of the RPE/choriocapillaris layer with an attenuation of the reflectivity beneath that area. AF in these cases was useful for determining the functional status of the RPE, rather than the anatomical status, since most cases of choroidal nevus appear with normal background AF, suggesting a normal or at least relatively healthy RPE and neurosensory retina overlying the tumor. Therefore, the combination of OCT and AF for choroidal nevus is probably recommended for early detection of signs of malignancy, and is certainly better than clinical examination for detecting related retinal edema, subretinal fluid, retinal thinning, and overlying RPE damage (8).

OCT can also be very useful for early diagnosis of small choroidal melanomas because localized subretinal fluid is strongly associated with tumor growth (24,25). Espinoza and colleagues (26) identified an active OCT pattern of subretinal fluid with localized full-thickness retinal detachment overlying or adjacent to choroidal melanoma, which may indicate an active tumor that is more prone to grow. They compared these features with a more chronic pattern featuring retinal thinning or intraretinal cysts that could be confused with fluid and could suggest a lesion less likely to grow. Moreover, subretinal fluid demonstrates increased AF signal in cases of choroidal melanoma, and this feature may be associated with findings of OCT to better differentiate and diagnose melanocytic tumors (8,12).

DIFFERENTIAL DIAGNOSIS

AF may also be useful for the differentiation of choroidal and retinal lesions other than nevus and melanoma.

Congenital Hypertrophy of the Retinal Pigment Epithelium

Congenital hypertrophy of the RPE (CHRPE) is normally identified as a flat, pigmented lesion at the level of the RPE, and it can be usually differentiated from choroidal nevi and small melanoma by its clinical appearance. However, when the diagnosis is not straightforward, fundus AF may be beneficial because CHRPE appears, in the majority of cases, as lesions with low AF signal. This correlates to the histopathological finding of absence of lipofuscin in these lesions, probably due to extensive photoreceptor degeneration and a defect in the phagocytosis of photoreceptor outer segments (Fig. 15.5) (27). There is often a pigmented halo surrounding CHRPE, which generally appears with normal or slightly increased AF. Using fluorescence microscopy, Lloyd et al. (28) demonstrated an increase in the amount of lipofuscin in the surrounding RPE of CHRPE, which may explain the halo present clinically. Since choroidal nevus often does not interfere with the normal background AF, these features are helpful for the diagnosis and differentiation of CHRPE (Fig. 15.5).

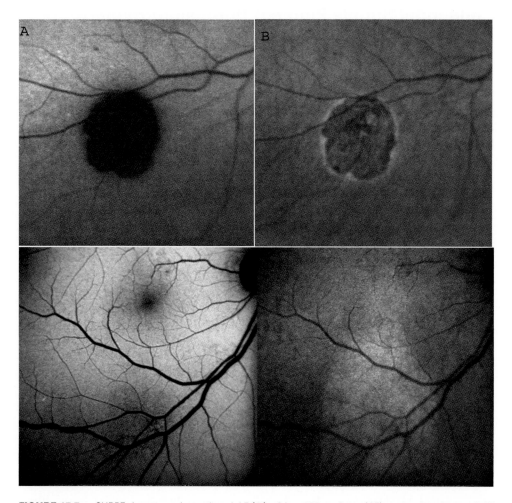

FIGURE 15.5.   CHRPE demonstrating reduced AF **(A)** with a 488 nm laser (AF), and reduced-normal AF **(B)** with a halo of increased AF with a 787 nm laser (NIA), in contrast to the choroidal nevus, which has normal AF **(C)** and increased AF with NIA **(D)**.

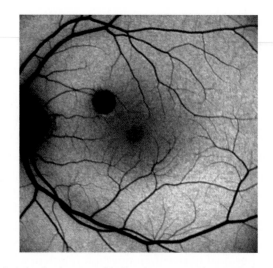

FIGURE 15.6. Congenital simple pigment epithelium hamartoma demonstrating reduced AF.

Congenital Simple Pigment Epithelium Hamartoma

Congenital simple pigment epithelium hamartoma is generally found in routine examinations in asymptomatic children and young adults. It is composed of hyperplastic RPE, with a variable vascular component. Shields and colleagues (29) described subtle feeder vessels in the clinical exam, although this finding was not confirmed angiographically. This lesion has a superficial, full-thickness retinal involvement and consequently will appear as a lesion with low AF signal due to blockage of normal background AF (Fig. 15.6) (30).

Retinal Astrocytic Hamartomas in Tuberous Sclerosis

Tuberous sclerosis is a hereditary disease characterized by multiple hamartomas in several organs, such as the central nervous system and the eye. Retinal astrocytic hamartomas may arise from the inner surface of the retina or from the optic nerve head. They can be a circular or oval solitary, flat, gray mass without calcification (type 1), or they may contain several lesions with multiple calcified nodular areas (type 2). A third type combines features of the other two and appears with a whitish-gray glistening central calcification and a peripheral irregular rim (type 3). AF may be useful for differentiating these types of lesions from each other, as well as from other retinal and choroidal tumors. Type 1 hamartomas can have either normal background AF or reduced AF signal due to blockage of normal background AF. Types 2 and 3 may have lesion-specific AF, but they may also have areas of reduced AF signal due to blockage of background AF (31).

Near-Infrared Autofluorescence

Near-infrared AF (NIA) uses a laser diode excitation at 787 nm and a detection filter with transmitted light at 800 nm (see also Chapter 6). The NIA signal appears to originate in the RPE and the choroid, and has been related to oxidized melanin or compounds associated with melanin (32).

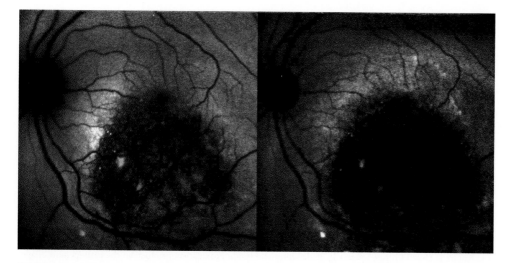

FIGURE 15.7. Choroidal hemangioma demonstrating reduced AF with both a 488 nm laser and NIA with a 787 nm laser.

Weinberger and colleagues (33) studied NIA images of several patients, including two cases with choroidal nevi that presented with increased NIA signal but lacked blue-light-excited AF, demonstrating the absence of lipofuscin accumulation in these lesions.

We studied choroidal melanocytic lesions using NIA, and both choroidal nevus and choroidal melanoma showed an increased signal that correlated with near-infrared reflectance and did not correlate with blue-light-excited AF (488 nm). Although this technique may not be useful for the differentiation of nevus and melanoma, it could be useful for the differentiation of retinal and choroidal lesions, such as CHRPE, choroidal hemangiomas, and other nonmelanocytic tumors. CHRPE and choroidal hemangiomas show decreased NIA, in contrast to the increased signal of nevus and melanoma (Figs. 15.5 and 15.7).

SUMMARY

Choroidal melanomas appear to have a pattern of confluent increased AF signal over the tumor, secondary to accumulation of lipofuscin. Most nevi do not have areas of increased AF, although secondary changes such as large drusen may appear occasionally as areas with mildly increased AF signal. It is possible that transforming lesions may be identified by detection of subclinical lipofuscin (orange pigment) by AF imaging or by a newly diagnosed area of increased AF. Therefore, serial AF images of choroidal nevus and melanoma are advisable in the follow-up of patients with choroidal melanocytic lesions. However, prospective studies with a larger number of patients are necessary to confirm these findings.

REFERENCES

1. Margo CE. The collaborative ocular melanoma study: an overview. Cancer Control 2004;11:304–309.
2. Damato BE, Foulds WS. Tumor-associated retinal pigment epitheliopathy. Eye 1990;4:382–387.
3. Singh AD, Mokashi AA, Bena JF, et al. Small choroidal melanocytic lesions: features predictive of growth. Ophthalmology 2006;113:1032–1039.
4. Augsburger JJ, Schroeder RP, Territo C, et al. Clinical parameters predictive of enlargement of melanocytic choroidal lesions. Br J Ophthalmol 1989;73:911–917.

5. Shields CL, Cater J, Shields JA, et al. Combination of clinical factors predictive of growth of small choroidal melanocytic tumors. Arch Ophthalmol 2000;118:360–364.
6. Smith LT, Irvine R. Diagnostic significance of orange pigment accumulation over choroidal tumors. Am J Ophthalmol 1973;76:212–216.
7. Shields CL, Cater JC, Shields JA, et al. Combination of clinical factors predictive of growth of small choroidal melanocytic tumors. Arch Ophthalmol 2000;118:360–364.
8. Lavinsky D, Belfort RN, Navajas E, et al. Fundus autofluorescence of choroidal nevus and melanoma. Br J Ophthalmol 2007;91:1299–1302.
9. Gunduz K, Pulido JS, Bakri SJ, et al. Fundus autofluorescence in choroidal melanocytic lesions. Retina 2007;27:681–687.
10. Materin MA, Pirondini C, Bianciotto C, et al. Autofluorescence features of small choroidal melanoma in 23 cases. In: Proceedings of the Meeting of ISOO, Siena, Italy, 2007.
11. Pirondini C, Bianciotto C, Demirci H, et al. Autofluorescence features of choroidal nevus in 63 cases. In: Proceedings of the Meeting of ISOO, Siena, Italy, 2007.
12. Shields CL, Bianciotto C, Pirondini C, et al. Autofluorescence of orange pigment overlying small choroidal melanoma. Retina 2007;27:1107–1111.
13. Shields JA, Rodrigues MM, Sarin LK, et al. Lipofuscin pigment over benign and malignant choroidal tumors. Trans Sect Ophthalmol Am Acad Ophthalmol Otolaryngol 1976;81:871–881.
14. Kopitz J, Holz FG, Kaemmerer E, et al. Lipids and lipid peroxidation products in the pathogenesis of age-related macular degeneration. Biochimie 2004;86:825–831.
15. Font RL, Zimmerman LE, Armaly MF. The nature of the orange pigment over a choroidal melanoma. Histochemical and electron microscopical observations. Arch Ophthalmol 1974;91:359–362.
16. Lohmann W, Wiegand W, Stolwijk TR, et al. Endogenous fluorescence of ocular malignant melanomas. Ophthalmologica 1995;209:7–10.
17. Atmaca LS, Batioğlu F, Atmaca P. Fluorescein and indocyanine green videoangiography of choroidal melanomas. Jpn J Ophthalmol 1999;43:25–30.
18. Bernard JA, Dhermy P. [Orange pigment and hyperfluorescent pin-point dots on the angiographic datas of malignant melanoma (author's transl)]. J Fr Ophtalmol 1978;1:529–534.
19. Rummelt V, Folberg R, Rummelt C, et al. Microcirculation architecture of melanocytic nevi and malignant melanomas of the ciliary body and choroid. Ophthalmology 1994;101:718–727.
20. Rummelt V, Folberg R, Woolson R, et al. Relation between the microcirculation architecture and the aggressive behavior of ciliary body melanomas. Ophthalmology 1995;102:844–851.
21. Mueller AJ, Bartsch DU, Schaller U, et al. Imaging the microcirculation of untreated and treated human choroidal melanomas. Int Ophthalmol 2001;23:385–393.
22. Shields CL, Mashayekhi A, Materin MA, et al. Optical coherence tomography of choroidal nevus in 120 patients. Retina 2005;25:243–252.
23. Muscat S, Parks S, Kemp E, et al. Secondary retinal changes associated with choroidal naevi and melanomas documented by optical coherence tomography. Br J Ophthalmol 2004;88:120–124.
24. Shields CL, Cater J, Shields JA, et al. Combination of clinical factors predictive of growth of small choroidal melanocytic tumours. Arch Ophthalmol 2000;118:360–364.
25. The Collaborative Ocular Melanoma Study Group. Factors predictive of growth and treatment of small choroidal melanoma. COMS Report No. 5. Arch Ophthalmol 1997;115:1537–1544.
26. Espinoza G, Rosenblatt B, Harbour JW. Optical coherence tomography in the evaluation of retinal changes associated with suspicious choroidal melanocytic tumors. Am J Ophthalmol 2004;137:90–95.
27. Shields CL, Materin MA, Walker C, et al. Photoreceptor loss overlying congenital hypertrophy of the retinal pigment epithelium by optical coherence tomography. Ophthalmology 2006;113:661–665.
28. Lloyd WC, Eagle RC, Shields JA, et al. Congenital hypertrophy of the retinal pigment epithelium. Electron microscopic and morphometric observations. Ophthalmology 1990;97:1052–1060.
29. Shields CL, Shields JA, Marr BP, et al. Congenital simple hamartoma of the retinal pigment epithelium. A study of five cases. Ophthalmology 2003;110:1005–1011.
30. Shukla D, Ambatkar S, Jethani J, et al. Optical coherence tomography in presumed congenital simple hamartoma of retinal pigment epithelium. Am J Ophthalmol 2005;139:945–947.
31. Stefan Mennel S, Meyer CH, Eggarter F, et al. Autofluorescence and angiographic findings of retinal astrocytic hamartomas in tuberous sclerosis. Ophthalmologica 2005;219:350–356.
32. Keilhauer CN, Delori FC. Near-infrared autofluorescence imaging of the fundus: visualization of ocular melanin. Invest Ophthalmol Vis Sci 2006;47:3556–3564.
33. Weinberger AW, Lappas A, Kirschkamp T, et al. Fundus near infrared fluorescence correlates with fundus infrared reflectance. Invest Ophthalmol Vis Sci 2006;47:3098–3108.

Autofluorescence (AF) *(continued)*
  lipofuscin formation in, 44–45
  lipofuscin inhibition in, 45–46
  mouse models of disease, 41–42, 42f
  normal mouse, 40–41, 40f, 41f
  cell-specific, 3
  crystalline lens absorption and, 28–29, 30f
  distribution of, 28, 34, 34f, 99–102, 100f, 101f
  excitation and emission spectrum of, 27, 28, 29f
  focally increased, 102–103
  in healthy eye, 99–104
  imaging of, 27, 38–40, 48–58
  increased, 72–74
  interpretation of, 28, 60, 70–76
  irregular, 74
  longer wavelengths in, 103
  mathematical model for, 102–103, 103f
  normal pattern, with vision loss, 70–72, 71f
  quantification of, 78–94
  reduced, 74
Autofluorescent storage material, 3. *See also* Lipofuscin
Autophagosome, 7
Autophagy
  cellular stress and, 9
  chaperone-mediated, 7
  definition of, 7
  forms of, 7
  and lipofuscin accumulation, 5, 7–8, 10f, 16
Autosomal dominant cone and cone-rod dystrophies, 153, 155t, 156–160
Autosomal dominant drusen, 115–116
Autosomal dominant pattern dystrophy, 184
Autosomal dominant retinitis pigmentosa, 141–142
Autosomal recessive cone and cone-rod dystrophies, 153, 155t, 161–163
Autosomal recessive pattern dystrophy, 184
Autosomal recessive retinitis pigmentosa, 141
AVMD. *See* Adult vitelliform macular dystrophy
AZOOR. *See* Acute zonal and occult outer retinopathy

B

Bardet-Biedl syndrome, 141
Basal laminar deposit (BLD), 108
Basal linear deposit, 108
Basement membrane deposit (BMD), 108
Best disease, 197–204
  age of onset, 197
  autofluorescence in, 143–144, 198f, 201–204, 203f
  clinical presentation of, 197, 199
  diagnostic techniques in, 200–202
  differential diagnosis of, 204
  electrophysiology of, 201, 204
  fibrotic stage of, 197, 198f, 203f
  fluorescein angiography of, 48, 200
  functional testing in, 201
  fundus examination in, 198f
  genetics of, 197–200
  histopathology of, 197–200
  imaging of, 200–204
  indocyanine-green angiography of, 200

optical coherence tomography of, 200, 201f, 203
  vs. pattern dystrophy, 193–194, 204
  previtelliform stage of, 197, 198f, 201, 201f
  pseudohypopyon stage of, 197, 198f, 202
  vitelliform stage of, 48, 197, 198f, 201–202, 203, 204
  vitelliruptive or "scrambled egg" stage of, 197, 198f, 202, 203
BEST1 mutation, 185, 197–204
Bestrophin, 197–200, 202
Biomicroscopy. *See* Slit-lamp biomicroscopy
Birdshot choroidopathy, 234, 236f, 238, 240
BLD. *See* Basal laminar deposit
Blood-retinal barrier (BRB), 232, 233f
Blue shift, 31–33
BMD(s). *See* Basement membrane deposit; Bruch's membrane deposits
Boxcar principle, 81
BRB. *See* Blood-retinal barrier
Bruch's membrane, lipofuscin in, 15f
Bruch's membrane deposits (BMDs), 31–32, 32f. *See also* Drusen
Bull's eye appearance
  in cone and cone-rod dystrophies, 154, 154f
  in fundus autofluorescence, 73–74, 74f
  in Stargardt disease, 206
Butterfly-shaped pattern dystrophy, 184, 187, 188f

C

Calcium, in lipofuscin, 4–5
Camera(s)
  conventional fundus, 48, 49f
  modified fundus, 48, 50–52
    vs. confocal scanning laser ophthalmoscopy, 52–58
    excitation and emission filters of, 51, 51f
    excitation and emission spectrum of, 52–53, 53f
    image acquisition in, 56
    image processing with, 56–58
    mode of excitation and detection in, 53–56, 55f
    noise with, 56–58
    sensitivity of, 56–58
Carbohydrates, in lipofuscin, 4
Cathepsins, and lipofuscin accumulation, 6–7
CCR2/CCL2 knockout mice, 41, 42f
Cell death, lipofuscin and, 9–11
Cellular stress
  and lipofuscin accumulation, 5, 8–9, 10f, 16
  and retinal degeneration, 19–21
Central areolar choroidal dystrophy, 213
Central areolar choroidal sclerosis, 222
Central macula, autofluorescence of, 52–53, 53f
Central nervous system, lipofuscin/ceroid in, 9–11
Central serous chorioretinopathy (CSC), 243–249
  acute, 243, 247–249
  autofluorescence in, 246–249, 246f–248f, 250f
  chronic-recurrent, 243, 246–249
  clinical presentation of, 243
  differential diagnosis of, 249

fluorescein angiography of, 245, 247f, 248–249, 248f
  follow-up of treatment in, 249, 250f
  idiopathic, *vs.* age-related maculopathy, 115
  imaging of, 244–249
  indocyanine-green retinopathy of, 244, 245, 248–249
  optical coherence tomography of, 245–249, 246f–248f, 250f
  pathology of, 244
  vs. pattern dystrophy, 193–194
  slit-lamp biomicroscopy of, 243, 244–245, 249
  treatment of, 243–244
CEP290 mutation, 175–176, 177
Ceroid material, 3–5, 6t
CFH knockout mice, 41–42, 42f
Chaperone-mediated autophagy (CMA), 7
Chloroform-soluble lipofuscin, 16, 17f, 21
Chloroquine, and lipofuscin accumulation, 6
Chloroquine retinopathy
  vs. age-related maculopathy, 116
  NIA imaging of, 66, 67f
CHM. *See* Choroideremia
CHM mutation, 225–226
Cholesterol, in lipofuscin, 4
Chorioretinopathy
  central serous, 115, 243–249
  serpiginous, 235, 236f, 239
Choroid
  autofluorescence of, 33–34, 267–268
  dark
    in cone-rod dystrophies, 154
    in pattern dystrophies, 190
    in Stargardt disease, 208, 211
  excitation and emission spectra of, 87, 88f
  fluorescence lifetime of, 89, 89t
Choroidal atrophy, areolar, 131
Choroidal dystrophy, central areolar, 213
Choroidal melanoma. *See* Melanoma, choroidal
Choroidal neovascularization (CNV), 119–127
  with atrophic AMD, 131
  autofluorescence of, 72, 72f, 122–127, 123f–126f, 239, 239f
  in Best disease, 200
  in central serous chorioretinopathy, 243
  classic, 120, 121, 123f, 125
  drusenoid detachment in, 111
  fluorescein angiography of, 120, 121, 123f, 127, 234, 239
  histopathology and pathogenesis of, 119–120
  indocyanine green angiography of, 121–122, 127
  inflammatory, 232, 234, 235, 239
  mixed, 125
  mouse model of, 41, 42f
  occult, 120, 121–122, 125, 126f
  optical coherence tomography of, 122, 123f, 126f, 127, 131, 235, 239
  in pattern dystrophy, 184, 186, 189, 190, 191
  slit-lamp biomicroscopy of, 120–121, 131
  therapeutic targets in, 23–24
  type 1, 120
  type 2, 120
Choroidal nevus. *See* Nevus, choroidal
Choroidal sclerosis, central areolar, 222
Choroidal silence, in Stargardt disease, 208